Nursing Law and Ethics

Fourth Edition

Edited by

John Tingle

Reader in Health Law, Head of International Development,
Nottingham Law School, Nottingham Trent University, Nottingham, UK

and

Alan Cribb

Director, Centre for Public Policy Research,
King's College London, London, UK

WILEY Blackwell

Registered office: John Wiley & Sons, Ltd, The Atrium, Southern Gate, Chichester, West Sussex, PO19
                       8SQ, UK

Editorial offices: 9600 Garsington Road, Oxford, OX4 2DQ, UK
                       The Atrium, Southern Gate, Chichester, West Sussex, PO19 8SQ, UK
                       111 River Street, Hoboken, NJ 07030-5774, USA

For details of our global editorial offices, for customer services and for information about how
to apply for permission to reuse the copyright material in this book please see our website at www.
wiley.com/wiley-blackwell

Library of Congress Cataloging-in-Publication Data

Nursing law and ethics / edited by John Tingle, Reader in Health Law, Head of International
Development, Nottingham Law School, Nottingham Trent University, Nottingham, UK and Alan Cribb,
Director, Centre for Public Policy Research, King's College London, London, UK. – Fourth Edition.
       pages cm
   Includes bibliographical references and index.
   ISBN 978-0-470-67137-5 (softback : alk. paper) – ISBN 978-1-118-49231-4 (mobi) – ISBN 978-1-118-
49232-1 – ISBN 978-1-118-49233-8   1. Nursing–Law and legislation–Great Britain.   2. Nursing ethics–
Great Britain.   I. Tingle, John.   II. Cribb, Alan.
   KD2968.N8N87 2013
   344.4104'14–dc23
                                                                                   2013007105

A catalogue record for this book is available from the British Library.

Wiley also publishes its books in a variety of electronic formats. Some content that appears in print may
not be available in electronic books.

Cover image: Peter Dazeley/Photographer's Choice/Getty Images
Cover design by Cyan Design

Set in 10/12 pt Palatino by Toppan Best-set Premedia Limited, Hong Kong
Printed in Singapore by Ho Printing Singapore Pte Ltd

1   2014

Nursing Law and Ethics

Contents

v

Notes on Contributors

Richard E. Ashcroft Professor of Bioethics, School of Law, Queen Mary, University of London, London

Robert Campbell Pro Vice Chancellor (Academic), University of Bolton, Greater Manchester

Alan Cribb Director, Centre for Public Policy Research, King's College London, London

Fiona Culley Independent Consultant, formerly Professional Adviser, Nursing and Midwifery Council, UK

Michael Dunn Lecturer in Health and Social Care Ethics, The Ethox Centre, Department of Public Health, University of Oxford, Oxford

Tracey Elliott Lecturer in Health Care Law, School of Law, University of Leicester, Leicester

Bobbie Farsides Professor of Clinical and Biomedical Ethics, Brighton and Sussex Medical School, University of Sussex, Brighton

Charles Foster Barrister, Outer Temple Chambers, London, and Fellow of Green Templeton College, University of Oxford, Oxford

Lucy Frith Senior Lecturer in Bioethics and Social Science, Department of Health Services Research, University of Liverpool, Liverpool

Natasha Hammond-Browning Lecturer in Law, Southampton Law School, University of Southampton, Southampton

Jonathan Herring Fellow in Law, Exeter College, University of Oxford, Oxford, and Professor in Law, Director of Undergraduate Studies, Faculty of Law, University of Oxford, Oxford

John Hodgson Reader in Legal Education, Nottingham Law School, Nottingham Trent University, Nottingham

Harry Lesser Honorary Research Fellow in Philosophy, Centre for Philosophy, University of Manchester, Manchester

Vanessa L. Mayatt Director, Mayatt Risk Consulting Ltd, Cheshire

Jean McHale Professor of Health Care Law, Director of the Centre for Health Law, Science and Policy, Birmingham Law School, University of Birmingham, Birmingham

Leon McRae Lecturer in Law, Birmingham Law School, University of Birmingham, Birmingham

Jo Samanta Principal Lecturer in Law, Leicester De Montfort Law School, De Montfort University, Leicester

David Seedhouse CEO of VIDe Ltd, and Visiting Professor, University of Cumbria

Anupama Thompson Head of the Regulatory Legal Team, Nursing and Midwifery Council, UK

John Tingle Reader in Health Law, Head of International Development, Nottingham Law School, Nottingham Trent University, Nottingham

Peter Walsh Chief Executive, Action against Medical Accidents (AvMA)

Preface to the Fourth Edition

Once again we are very pleased to have been given the chance to update and revise this book into a fourth edition. Health care legal and ethical issues continue to dominate social and political agendas and the courts, as they have done in the periods covered by all the previous editions of our book. Litigation in health care is now a fairly constant feature of the NHS health care environment. Not a week seems to pass without a case being sent to court. The popular media in recent times have abounded with stories of things going wrong in hospitals and elsewhere, where patients have been caused avoidable injury and sometimes death. Nurses feature along with doctors in litigation and claims; and nurses play a key role in making health care safe. Along with lots of other legal and ethical issues and topics covered in this book, we consider the ways the Government and the NHS have tried to grapple with the rising tide of health litigation, and the risk management and patient safety strategies that have been put into place to deal with this.

It is worth highlighting a couple of basic but important truths here:

Errors in health care are inevitable
We are dealing with human beings who sometimes make mistakes. None of us is infallible. Add to this complex medical technology, the busy nature of a health care setting, and you have the recipe for problems. The best we can try to do is to minimise the risk of errors and adverse events occurring, through the proper application of clinical risk management and patient safety strategies. What is more worrying, however, is that the same errors are often repeated and we don't always seem to learn from the errors of the past.

A lot of errors made are simple ones and involve failures of communication
When health care errors are looked at in totality, it seems that a lot could have been easily avoided if doctors, nurses and other health carers properly

communicated with each other and with patients. When surveys and error reports are analysed, many involve simple communication errors such as wrongly noting a patient's name or drug or missing out and failing to convey other key information. Again, this seems to be an area where, sadly, we do not appear to be learning sufficiently from past mistakes. It is easy to feel as an observer that record-keeping is seen as a chore by health carers, when it should be regarded as a key duty and skill.

On the other hand, the NHS has much to be proud about in this area. The NHS is arguably getting better at ensuring good-quality and safe health care. Our patient safety, health quality infrastructure is copied in many parts of the world and is very highly regarded. But it is important to keep the momentum of improvement, and there are considerable challenges to doing so. Since the last edition of this book, the NHS has been in an almost constant state of reform and, as we said in the previous edition's preface, this unstable platform brings about its own problems, as NHS organisations struggle to implement government health quality, risk and patient safety policies and at the same time manage root-and-branch change.

We repeat here the warning about health law changes that we made in previous editions. Health care law is always in a state of flux, and it is simply impossible, for practical reasons, to represent all the legal changes that took place before this book went to press. We have tried to regularly capture the changes to the law as this book's production has progressed, particularly up to September 2012.

For this fourth edition we have been able to retain many of the authors who contributed to earlier editions but a number have now retired. We wish them well in their retirement and extend our deepest gratitude for the contributions they have made. A number of new contributors have joined us for the fourth edition and to them we extend a warm welcome. We, once again, very much hope that this new edition of the book will prove to be of practical benefit – and theoretical interest – to the nursing community.

John Tingle and Alan Cribb
Nottingham and London
January 2013

Preface to the Third Edition

We are pleased to have been given the chance to update and revise this book into a third edition. Health care legal and ethical issues continue to dominate social and political agendas and the courts. Since the last edition a myriad of ethical and legal dilemmas have flowed through the media and the courts, and we have tried to reflect many of these in this new edition. Such dilemmas arise in the context of an NHS that appears to be in a constant state of reform and subject to a number of increasingly contentious and competing political agendas. This unstable platform brings about its own problems, as NHS organisations struggle to implement government health quality, risk and patient safety policies, and at the same time manage root-and-branch change. Nursing law and ethics, as an academic discipline, continues to develop and is now often seen to sit alongside these patient safety, quality and risk topics. The focus now, practically speaking, is the practical and holistic integration of these topics (the Government, for example, currently puts all this under the umbrella of 'Integrated Governance'). We suggest that nursing law and ethics, to be understood properly, should be seen in this broader context, which includes the wider policy context of the NHS. The nursing law and ethics student cannot ignore the work of NHS organisations such as the NPSA, NHSLA and Healthcare Commission and the related governance agendas. An understanding of these broader institutional and policy frameworks is essential for a fully informed discussion, and we hope this book helps to support such a discussion, as well as to properly represent the more focused and disciplinary demands of law and ethics.

The preface to the first edition set out the rationale for, and the structure of, the book. We hold true to this for the third edition as we did for the second. There have been changes, particularly to the law, and we have tried to capture these up to August 2006. That health care law is in a fairly constant state of flux is a self-evident truth, and it is simply impossible, for practical reasons, to represent all the legal changes that took place before the book went to press. We would note, however, that the NHS Redress Act 2006 was eventually passed into law. Positive changes were made to it as it progressed through Parliament, and it now has the potential to make a real difference to patients who have been harmed through lack of care in the NHS.

We, once again, very much hope that this new edition of the book will prove to be of practical benefit – and theoretical interest – to the nursing community.

Alan Cribb and John Tingle
London and Nottingham

Preface to the Second Edition

We are, of course, pleased that the first edition of this book was so well received; and we are delighted to have had the chance to update and revise it. There is comparatively little to add to the preface produced for the first edition; this set out the rationale for, and the structure of, the book, and these remain the same. But there are many changes to the content of the book. The last six years have seen an extraordinary amount of change in many aspects of health care law and ethics, in the regulation and management of health services, and in conceptions of health professional accountability. The contributors to this new edition have sought to reflect and illuminate these changes and also to provide clear overviews of their subject matter.

There is a new chapter in the first part of the book which summarises the changing policy context and legal environment of nursing; and in the second part there is a new 'pair' of chapters on clinical governance. We are grateful to all the authors who have updated their work and/or written material for the first time in this edition. We very much hope that this new edition will prove to be of practical benefit – and theoretical interest – to the nursing community.

Acknowledgements

We would like to thank Professor Jean McHale, Faculty of Law, University of Leicester and Mr Harry Lesser, Centre for Philosophy, University of Manchester, for acting as editorial advisers.

Alan Cribb and John Tingle

Preface to the First Edition

One of the key indicators of the maturation of nursing as a profession and as a discipline is the growing importance of nursing law and ethics. A profession which seeks not only to maintain, and improve on, high standards but also to hold e chof its individual members accountable for an increasing range of responsibilities is inevitably concerned with legal and ethical matters. It is not surprising that these matters have come to prominence in nurse education, and to enjoy a central place along with clinical and social sciences in the disciplinary bases of nursing. There is now a substantial body of literature devoted to nursing law and to nursing ethics.

This book is distinctive because it is about both law *and* ethics. We believe it is of practical benefit, and academic value, to consider these two subjects together. Put simply, we need to be able to discuss 'what the law requires' and 'what is right', and to decide, among other things, whether these two are always the same.

The book is divided into two parts. The first part is designed to be an overview of the whole subject and includes introductions to the legal, ethical and professional dimensions of nursing, as well as a special chapter on patient complaints. The second part looks at a selection of issues in greater depth. These chapters contain two parts or perspectives – one legal and one ethical. The legal perspectives take the lead – the authors were invited to introduce the law relating to the subject at hand. The ethics authors were invited to write a complementary (and typically shorter) piece in which they took up some of the issues but then went on to make any points they wished. Thus the terms of invitation for the ethics authors were different, and more flexible, than those for the lawyers. This difference in treatment of the two perspectives is quite deliberate.

The essential difference is this: it makes good sense to ask lawyers for an authoritative account of the law, but it is not sensible to ask authors for an authoritative account of what is good or right – which is the subject matter of ethics. An account of the law will not simply be factual; it will inevitably include some discussion of the complexity and uncertainties involved in identifying and interpreting the implications of the law. But it is in the nature of the law that lawyers should be able to give expert guidance about legal judgments. There are no equivalent authorities on ethical judgement. Instead some nurses with an interest in ethics and some philosophers with an interest in nursing ethics were invited to discuss some of the issues and/or cases raised in the first part of the chapter. Clearly, these responses are of different styles and are written from different standpoints. Each author is responsible for his or her piece and any of the views or opinions expressed within them. This difference between the two sets of perspectives is indicated (indeed, rather exaggerated) by giving the former the definite, and the latter an indefinite, article – 'The Legal Perspective' but 'An Ethical Perspective'!

These differences in presentation reflect deeper differences between the two subjects. In short, law and ethics are concerned with two contrasting kinds of 'finality' – in principle, ethics is final but, in practice, law is final. It is important to appreciate the need for both open-ended debate and for practical closure. When it comes to making judgements about what is right and wrong, acceptable or unacceptable, the law is not the end of the matter. Although it is reasonable to expect a considerable convergence of the legal and the ethical, it is perfectly possible to criticise laws or legal judgments as unethical (this is the central impetus behind legal reform). On the other hand, society cannot organise itself as if it were a never-ending philosophy seminar. There are many situations in which we need some authoritative system for decision-making, and mechanisms for closing debate and implementing decisions – this is the role of the law. Any such system will be less than perfect, but a society without such a system will be less perfect still.

Of course there are also areas in which there is little or no role for the law. The way in which nurses routinely talk to their patients raises ethical issues, and may also raise legal issues (e.g. informed consent, negligence), but unless some significant harm is involved, these ethical issues can fall outside the scope of the law. For example, it is a reasonable ideal for a nurse to aim to empathise with someone she is advising or counselling; she might even feel guilty for failing to meet this ideal, but she could hardly be held legally guilty. Laws which cannot be enforced, or which are unnecessary, could be harmful in a number of ways. They could detract from respect for the law and its legitimate role, and they could create an oppressive and inflexible climate in which no one benefitted. So even if we are clear that a certain practice is ethically unacceptable, it does not follow that it should be made illegal. However, the opposite can also be true. The overall consequences of legalising something which many people regard as ethically acceptable (e.g. voluntary euthanasia) may be judged, *by these same people*, to be unacceptable – as raising too many serious ethical and legal complications. Both lawyers and ethicists have to consider the proper boundaries of the law.

Even these few examples show that the relationship between the law and ethics is complicated. Professional values, such as those represented in the UKCC Code of Conduct, act as a half-way house between the two. They provide a means of enabling public discussion of public standards. They address the individual conscience but, where necessary, they are enforceable by disciplinary measures. We hope that this book will illustrate the importance of considering all of these matters together, and will help to provide nurses with insight into what is expected of them, and the skills to reflect on what they expect of themselves.

Alan Cribb and John Tingle

Part One: The Dimensions

1

The Legal Dimension: Legal System and Method

John Hodgson

Reader in Legal Education, Nottingham Law School, Nottingham Trent University, Nottingham

We live in a society dominated to an increasing – some would say excessive – extent by legal rules and processes. Many of these apply to all of us – for instance, the rules relating to use of the road as driver, passenger, cyclist or pedestrian, while others apply only to specific groups. In this chapter we will concentrate on the law as it affects the provision of health care. It is easier to do this than to look at the law relating to nurses or nursing, since for many purposes there is no legal distinction between different health care professionals and their contributions to the overall health care system. Before we do this, however, it is necessary to look briefly at the main features of the legal systems in which health care operates. There are four distinct legal systems within the United Kingdom. Northern Ireland has had a substantial measure of legislative and executive devolution since the 1920s, although this was often suspended due to civil unrest. A new devolution settlement for Northern Ireland and first-generation ones for Scotland and Wales were enacted in the 1990s.[1] The Welsh initially sought and obtained more restricted powers, but these have since been extended. The devolved legislatures are not sovereign, they exercise defined powers formally delegated by the Westminster Parliament, although any attempt to curtail or modify either the legislative or executive competence of the devolved provinces would be politically hazardous. The provision of health care through the National Health Service (NHS) was originally established throughout the United Kingdom by legislation of general application, but health is now a devolved matter, therefore in Scotland and Northern Ireland it is under the authority of the Scottish and Northern Irish Ministers, and legislative changes are made by the Scottish Parliament and Northern Ireland Assembly. In Wales the Welsh

Nursing Law and Ethics, Fourth Edition. Edited by John Tingle and Alan Cribb.
© 2014 by John Wiley & Sons, Ltd. Published 2014 by John Wiley & Sons, Ltd.

Assembly Ministers have had executive authority for over a decade, but the Welsh Assembly has only recently acquired legislative competence in relation to primary legislation. The Westminster Government and Parliament now have direct authority only over the NHS in England.

This chapter will concentrate on the English position. It is also possible to draw valuable illustrations and guidance from other countries outside the United Kingdom, particularly in relation to general legal principles, rather than the detail of legislative provisions, although these are influential rather than decisive.

1.1   The law and its interpretation

In this section we will look briefly at the various sources of law operating in England[2] and at some of the methods used by judges when they have to interpret and apply the law.[3]

1.1.1   Statute law

Most English law is in the form of statutes. These are made by the Crown in Parliament. Since 1689, by virtue of the Bill of Rights, the Crown in Parliament has been the supreme legislative body in England, and subsequently in the United Kingdom. A statute, or Act of Parliament, results from a bill or proposal for a statute. The bill may be proposed by the Government or by any individual MP or member of the House of Lords. It is debated and approved, with or without amendment, in both Houses.[4] Once approved in Parliament by both Houses, the bill receives formal Royal Assent. Statutes have been passed on almost every topic imaginable. Among those of direct relevance to the health care professions are the following:

- The series of statutes establishing the NHS and subsequently modifying its structure and organisation. The National Health Service Act 1946 carried through Nye Bevan's project to secure a national, public, health service. Today the principal Act is the National Health Service Act 1977, but this has been amended and supplemented many times – for example, by the National Health Service and Community Care Act 1990, which introduced NHS Trusts and the internal market; the Health Act 1999, which introduced Primary Care Trusts and the Commission for Health Improvement; the Health and Social Care Act 2001, which made numerous changes to community health provision; the Health and Social Care (Community Health and Standards) Act 2003, which among other things created Foundation Trusts; and the Health Act 2009, which among other things introduced the NHS Constitution. The Health and Social Care Act 2012, which among other things extends GP commissioning and restructures NHS management regulation, recently continued this process of amendment and development.

- The Acts regulating the health care professions, such as the Medical Act 1983 for doctors, and the Nurses, Midwives and Health Visitors Act 1997.[5]

Statutes generally provide the broad framework of rules. Thus section 1(1) of the National Health Service Act 1977, in its latest form after amendment, provides:

> It is the Secretary of State's duty to continue the promotion in England and Wales of a comprehensive health service designed to secure improvement – (a) in the physical and mental health of the people of those countries, and (b) in the prevention, diagnosis and treatment of illness, and for that purpose to provide or secure the effective provision of services in accordance with this Act.

This is called 'primary legislation' because it sets out the principal foundational rules. More detailed regulations are contained in statutory instruments, which are made by ministers (or in practice by their civil servants) under powers conferred by a relevant statute. This is referred to as 'secondary legislation' because it deals with matters of detail dependent on the general powers given by primary legislation. So, for instance, the provision of general medical services is governed by sections 28C to 34A of the National Health Service Act 1977, which provide for regulations on a variety of topics, including: the manner in which, and standards to which, services are to be provided; the persons who perform services; the persons to whom services are to be provided; and the adjudication of disputes.

In theory the Crown in Parliament can pass a statute on any subject whatever, and may also repeal any existing legislation. So in theory Parliament can accordingly legislate for the execution of people on some arbitrary ground, such as having red hair. This is subject to three very different qualifications, as follows:

(1) Parliament can only operate within the scope of what is politically and socially acceptable. This not only means that the Red-haired Persons (Compulsory Slaughter) Act will never see the light of day, but more importantly that legislation on such contentious issues as abortion or euthanasia is not undertaken lightly.
(2) By virtue of the European Communities Act 1972, Parliament has granted supremacy to the legislation of the European Union (EU) in those areas covered by the Treaty of European Union and the Treaty on the Functioning of the European Union. This can mean that existing parliamentary legislation is found to be incompatible with EU law, although the courts will always try to interpret the two pieces of legislation consistently with each other, and it can even mean that new legislation must be disregarded.[6] In practice EU law does not really have much specific bearing on medico-legal and ethical issues, although since it does deal with recognition of qualifications and many equal-pay and equal-opportunity issues in employment law, it may have an impact on the professional life of many nurses. EU free trade and competition rules apply to drugs and medicines as they do to any other products, and they feature in much of the case law. The EU also regulates the provision of services, and this includes private medical services

with a cross-border element, as well as public medical services to the extent that they are in competition with private provision.

(3) The Human Rights Act 1998 came into full effect on 2 October 2000. This Act is designed to give effect in English law to the rights conferred by the European Convention on Human Rights and Fundamental Freedoms (ECHR) ('Convention rights'). This has been in effect since 1954, and was originally binding on the United Kingdom internationally through the European Court of Human Rights and the Council of Europe, but not as part of our own legal system. So even if rules of English law, whether in statutes or otherwise, were inconsistent with the Convention, they prevailed, although the United Kingdom might then be held to be in default by the European Court of Human Rights. This has now changed as follows:

- Each new bill must be certified by the Minister responsible to comply with the Convention rights, or an explanation given as to why it is appropriate to legislate incompatibly.
- English law must be construed so far as possible to be compatible with the Convention rights. The courts have now made it clear that they will exercise this power robustly, as explained later.
- If an Act is found by the courts to be incompatible with Convention rights, the judges may make a declaration to that effect and it will be up to the Government to invite Parliament to make the necessary changes.
- The courts will have regard to decisions of the European Court of Human Rights when interpreting English law.
- All public bodies must act in accordance with the Convention. This includes the various component parts of the health service.

Judges must interpret all statutes to conform to Convention rights 'so far as it is possible to do so'. Although the full implications of this are still being worked through, the approach of the judges is to first consider what the social or other policy purpose of the legislation is, then whether there is a breach of Convention rights if the legislation is interpreted naturally. If there is, but this was clearly intended because of the overall structure of the Act, or the issues are complex and far-reaching, the judges will be reluctant to impose an alternative interpretation. Where they can work 'with the grain' of the legislation, especially where the incompatibility appears accidental and there is no need to address fundamental policy issues, the courts will 'read down' the actual words used and substitute a form of words that secures respect for Convention rights.[7] The Convention confers a number of rights on people. Some of them are substantive in nature, such as the right to life and the right to freedom of expression, while others are procedural, such as the guarantee of a fair trial. This applies to disciplinary proceedings and requires that there be an independent and impartial tribunal. This may be problematic for bodies such as the Nursing and Midwifery Council (NMC) which have been responsible for the investigation and adjudication of complaints and have had difficulty in developing systems which provide for the necessary degree of independence.

Some areas of medico-legal significance are likely to be affected by the Act. One example is the detention of mentally impaired people. This is permitted in principle under Article 5, where it is necessary for the protection of the patient or others and there is the safeguard of an appeal to an independent judicial body independent of the executive government.[8]

In 1998 in the case of *R* v. *Bournewood NHS Trust, ex parte L* the House of Lords approved under the doctrine of necessity the use of informal measures to keep 'compliant' patients who lacked the capacity to consent in hospital without using the powers under the Mental Health Act 1983. In *HL* v. *United Kingdom* (2004) the European Court of Human Rights ruled that this did not provide adequate safeguards.[9] In *R (Sessay)* v. *South London & Maudsley NHS Trust* (2011) any notion of the use of necessity when dealing with a non-compliant incapacitated patient was rejected; the Mental Health Act 1983 and the Mental Capacity Act 2005 together provide a complete statutory framework regulating compulsory detention, assessment and treatment. The acts both of the police and of the hospital, outside the statutory framework, breached the claimant's right to liberty under Article 5 of the Convention.

The right to life would appear to be of direct concern to the health care community, but in practice it focuses on negative aspects (preventing officially sanctioned killing), rather than positive ones (requiring states to provide resources and facilities to cure the sick).[10] In *D* v. *United Kingdom* (1997) it was held that, while deporting an HIV-positive prisoner to St Kitts, where treatment was not available, amounted to inhuman and degrading treatment, it was not necessary to consider whether the state was failing to ensure the right to life. Indeed recent decisions of the UK courts have held that deportation of HIV-positive patients will not even amount to inhuman or degrading treatment in the absence of extreme circumstances.[11] It is also clear as a result of one of the first cases under the Act that withdrawal of hydration and nutrition from a patient in persistent vegetative state (PVS) does not entail a breach of the right to life (*NHS Trust A* v. *Mrs M., NHS Trust B* v. *Mrs H.* (2001)).

Both the UK courts and the European Court of Human Rights have held that the refusal of the state to allow assisted suicide is neither an infringement of the right to life (this was a rather convoluted argument that the right to life included a right to terminate one's own life) nor a failure of proper respect for the privacy and autonomy of the patient. In this latter instance it was held that while there was a right to die, safeguards might be necessary against abuse and coercion, and the existing rules were not disproportionate for achieving this.[12] However, doubts persisted, and it was eventually determined that it was appropriate to require the Director of Public Prosecutions to promulgate a policy on prosecution in cases of assisted suicide.[13]

1.1.2   Common law

The rules of the common law pre-date statute. However, there are now so many statutes in so many areas of law that the common law rules are normally of secondary importance. These rules are legal principles laid down over the centuries by the judges in deciding the cases that came before them. In theory the judges were simply isolating the relevant principles from a body of law that already existed and which represented the common view of the English people as to what was right and lawful, but in practice the judges were really developing a coherent and technical set of rules based on their own understanding of legal principle. We will look at the techniques the judges currently use later. For the moment it is important to recognise that there are some areas where, despite the rise of statute, the common law remains of considerable importance.

The best example is tort, in particular negligence. This is important to nurses, as this branch of the law deals with whether a patient who has suffered harm while being treated will be able to recover compensation because the treatment he received was inadequate.

The judges also have the task of interpreting statutes and statutory instruments and giving effect to them. They have developed their own techniques and principles for this task, which are themselves part of the common law.

An important function of the judges today is controlling the activity of central and local government and other public bodies by means of judicial review. This is now the responsibility of the Administrative Court, which is part of the High Court. Judicial review is essentially a means of ensuring that decisions and policies are made lawfully and by the correct procedures. The judges themselves have developed the rules on which decisions can be challenged and what grounds of challenge are available.[14] In principle, the judges accept that they have not been given responsibility for making the decisions in question, and so do not consider the merits. In *R* v. *Central Birmingham Health Authority ex parte Walker* (1987) the court had to consider a failure to provide treatment to a particular patient, as a result of decisions not to allocate funds to this particular aspect of the health authority's operations. It was held that the authority was responsible for planning and delivering health care within a given budget and the resulting decisions on priorities. The court could not substitute its own, inexpert, judgment, particularly as it would only hear detailed arguments about the needs of this one patient and not about the whole range of demands. However, in *R (Coughlan)* v. *North & East Devon HA*[15] the court did address the question of what constituted health care and what constituted social care, as the financial arrangements for these were different. This was a question of statutory interpretation, not of relative priorities. The issue of health care resources is more fully discussed in Chapter 8.

1.1.3   European Union law

Throughout the post-World War II period, the states of western Europe have been engaged in a complex and long-term project of economic cooperation and integration. The first major stage in this was the Treaty of Rome, which established the European Economic Community in the 1950s. The United Kingdom joined this Community in 1974. The initial objective was the establishment of a common market, an area within which there was to be free movement of the various factors of production of goods and provision of services, namely goods, labour, management and professional skills and capital. Initially this meant the removal of obvious barriers, such as customs duties, immigration controls, exchange controls on money and other restrictions. Subsequently other objectives, such as environmental protection, have been added, and indeed the entity has been renamed the European Union, although the main impact of the Union is still on economic affairs.

Free movement of workers, guaranteed by Article 45 of the Treaty on the Functioning of the EU (TFEU), implied many additional social policies, as workers would not, in practice, move around the EU unless their social security entitlements were ensured and they were allowed to bring their families with them. Genuine freedom of movement also required a common approach to qualifications, with no discrimination on grounds of nationality, and also equal opportunity, at least between men and women. This has resulted in much legislation and many decisions of the European Court of Justice. Article 53 of the TFEU specifically gives power to regulate mutual recognition of diplomas and qualifications. Directives 77/452 and 80/154 made provision for general nurses and midwives, respectively, but there are now general frameworks for the recognition of degree-level and other vocational qualifications in Directive 2005/36, which deals in detail with many medical, nursing and allied qualifications.

The case of *Marshall* v. *Southampton and SW Hants AHA* (1986) established that UK law permitting differential retirement ages as between men and women in the health service was incompatible with EU law requiring equal treatment, and as a result the UK law had to be disregarded.

The member states of the EU have agreed, in effect, to transfer to the EU institutions their sovereign rights to make and apply laws in those areas for which the EU is to be responsible. As a result EU law prevails over national law in these areas where they are in conflict. However, there are a number of different mechanisms for securing this, and it is not simply a question of ignoring national legal provisions.

The European Council, which comprises an elected president, the heads of government of the member states and the president of the European Commission, is the principal policy-making body for the EU. It meets in regular summits which discuss current economic and international relations issues. The European Council should not be confused with the Council. This is a legislative and administrative body, comprising relevant departmental ministers from each member state. In most cases the legislation is made jointly by the Council and the Parliament, on a proposal from the European Commission. In many cases the Council can act by a majority, and thus legislate against the wishes of one or more member states. The majority is usually a 'qualified' or weighted majority designed to ensure that there is very substantial support for the measure. In practice great efforts are made to ensure a consensus of opinion. The Parliament does not initiate legislation but, as noted above, does have to approve and join in making most important legislation, so it has at least a blocking power and can suggest amendments. The Parliament must also approve the EU budget and the members of the Commission. It may also remove the whole Commission, and although it has never voted to do so, the likelihood of this occurring led to the resignation of the Commission in 1999 as a result of allegations of financial irregularities against one of its members.

The Commission is the administrative arm of the EU. It implements policies and proposes legislation, and can itself make detailed regulations, particularly in relation to the Common Agricultural Policy. It also makes decisions on alleged infringements of EU law – for example, in relation to competition law. It is responsible as 'guardian of the treaties' for ensuring that member states comply with their EU obligations.

The European Court of Justice, assisted by the General Court, has the sole responsibility, to the exclusion of the national courts of the member states, for interpreting EU law. It does so by means of rulings on points of law referred by national courts (Article 267 of the TFEU), deciding cases brought against the member states for alleged failure to comply with their obligations under EU law by the Commission (Articles 258 and 260) and by judicial review of the validity of acts of the institutions (decisions on particular cases or secondary legislation) on the application of other institutions, the member states and others directly affected (Article 263).

There are two forms of Act that amount to secondary legislation, namely, Regulations and Directives; both are governed by Article 288 of the TFEU. Regulations, which may be made by the Council, with or without the Parliament, or by the Commission, are directly effective rules of EU law that must be obeyed by all persons and companies within the EU and will be enforced by national courts. Directives, which are normally made by the Council and Parliament, are used where the EU wishes to ensure that national law in all member states achieves the same results, but it is not appropriate to do this by way of regulation. One example is in relation to company law, where the law of the states is very variable in its form and terminology, so regulations would be meaningless.

EU law applies not only to states but also to individuals. This was not clear from the beginning, but the Court of Justice ruled in *van Gend & Loos* (1962) that an individual could rely on a treaty provision which was clear and complete and capable of conferring direct rights (in this case a prohibition on new customs duties) to defeat a claim by a state based on its own incompatible legislation. In *Defrenne* v. *Sabena* (1976) it was held that a treaty provision meeting these requirements (in this case the right to equal pay for women) could be relied on against a person or company, notwithstanding incompatible national legislation.

The position with regard to directives is more complex. They normally provide for an implementation period; while this is running they have no legal effect (*Pubblico Ministero* v. *Ratti* (1979)), unless the state passes implementing legislation early, while the period is still running. In that case, the state is bound by the terms of the directive (*Pfeiffer* (2005)).

After the implementation date directives are binding on the state,[16] therefore the state is prevented from relying on its own incompatible law. In addition, the state can be obliged to act in accordance with them (*Marshall* v. *Southampton and SW Hants AHA* (1986)).

This binding effect applies to the courts, which must interpret national legislation 'as far as possible' in accordance with the directive, even in cases involving two private litigants with no state involvement (*Marleasing* (1992)). This applies particularly to rules relating to remedies, which must be effective (*von Colson*

(1986)). However, where the two cannot be reconciled, national law will prevail (*Wagner Miret* (1993)).

A directive cannot be relied on as such against a private individual or company (*Faccini-Dori* v. *Recreb* (1995)), although the court can be asked to interpret national law, as above.

Where an individual or company suffers loss as the result of the failure of the state to implement a directive properly or at all, as a last resort the state may be held liable in damages (*Francovich* (1993)) provided that the breach is sufficiently grave (*Brasserie du Pêcheur/Factortame* (No. 3) (1996)). In principle this liability extends to a court decision that fails to apply community law (*Köbler* (2004)). Note also that this remedy may be available where the state fails to comply with EU law in other ways, as was the case in *Factortame*.

English courts have been willing to apply very radical interpretative methods to English legislation introduced specifically to give effect to EU requirements, even 'reading them down' to the extent of reversing the apparent meaning of the English legislation. The reasoning behind this is that it was the primary intention of Parliament to comply with the EU requirement, and the words used were believed to achieve this, so any reinterpretation meets that underlying purpose, even if it is not the obvious interpretation of the particular passage (*Pickstone* v. *Freemans* (1989); *Litster* v. *Forth Dry Dock* (1990)). After considerable uncertainty it seems that the same will apply to other legislation not passed specifically to meet EC requirements (*R* v. *Secretary of State for Employment ex parte Equal Opportunities Commission* (1994); *Webb* v. *EMO Air Cargo* (No. 2) (1995)), although there has been some suggestion that the English courts are happier to see damages claims for non-implementation, rather than radical interpretation (*Kirklees MBC* v. *Wickes* (1993)).

1.2   The English legal system

The English legal system has developed over many centuries, and although there have been piecemeal reforms, many old procedures and systems remain in place. This applies particularly to titles. Why should the principal judge of the civil side of the Court of Appeal be called the Master of the Rolls? He has nothing to do with either baking or high-end motor cars. What actually happened was that an official responsible for keeping the official records, or rolls, of the Chancery was gradually given a judicial role and by the 19th century, when the Court of Appeal in its modern form was established, he had become a senior judge and was therefore the right person to be appointed to preside over the Court of Appeal.

Effectively there are two court systems in England. The criminal courts concentrate on crime, while the civil courts deal with everything else. There are some exceptions, where specialised tribunals have been set up. The most important of these are probably the Employment Tribunals[17] and the Employment Appeal Tribunal, which deal with most employment-related issues, including equal opportunities, although the various tribunals within the social security system deal with more cases. There are also separate tribunals for income tax and VAT.

1.2.1   Criminal justice system

All cases start with an appearance in the magistrates' court. Usually the case will have been investigated by the police and will be prosecuted by the Crown Prosecution Service, but other government departments and agencies, local authorities and bodies such as the RSPCA also prosecute cases. Private individuals may prosecute, but rarely do. There are a total of some 1,720,000 cases each year,[18] of which 60 per cent are purely summary offences (motoring offences such as speeding, careless driving and defective vehicles, and other minor offences of drunkenness, vandalism, etc.). These must be dealt with in the magistrates' court. The great majority of defendants plead guilty or do not contest the case. The remaining more serious offences fall into two groups. The most serious offences, such as murder, rape and robbery, are actually a small proportion of the total and can only be tried at the Crown court, 'on indictment' – the magistrates' court only deals with bail and legal aid. The others are the middle range of offences (e.g. most assaults, theft, fraud and burglary). These are said to be triable 'either way'. This means that if the defendant admits the charge when it is put to him in the magistrates' court, he is convicted there, although he may be committed to the Crown court for sentence if the magistrates' powers of sentence[19] are inadequate. If the defendant does not admit the offence, the magistrates must decide whether they have power to hear the case, having regard to its seriousness and complexity. If they decline to hear it, the case must go to the Crown court. If they agree to hear the case, the defendant may still elect trial at the Crown court.

Where a case is heard by the magistrates, the defendant may appeal against sentence (and, if he pleaded not guilty, conviction) to the Crown court. These appeals are heard by a judge sitting with magistrates. Although an appeal against conviction is a full rehearing, it will not be before a jury. Both prosecution and defence may appeal to the Queen's Bench Division of the High Court,[20] where they consider that the final decision is wrong on a point of law (as opposed to being a wrong decision on the facts). They may also apply to the same court for judicial review of any preliminary decision (e.g. on bail or legal aid).

The Crown court deals with about 130,000 cases a year, of which about 30,000 are contested trials. About 30 per cent of these result in acquittals. These trials are before a judge and jury, with the judge responsible for decisions on matters of law, evidence and procedure, and the jury responsible for matters of fact and the final verdict.

The defendant may appeal to the Court of Appeal (Criminal Division) on the ground that the verdict is unsafe. The Court considers whether the defendant was prejudiced by irregularities at the trial, such as rulings of the judge on law, or the admissibility of evidence, or errors in the judge's summing-up. In effect the Court is asking, 'Can we rely on the jury's verdict, or do we feel that they would have decided otherwise if the irregularity had not occurred?' The prosecution may not appeal against an acquittal, although they may ask the Court of Appeal to consider the point of law involved in an acquittal on a hypothetical basis by an Attorney General's reference. They may also challenge a ruling made by the trial judge which has the effect of terminating the proceedings in favour of the defendant. The defendant may, with leave, appeal against sentence, and the prosecution may appeal against an unduly lenient sentence. There is an appeal to the Supreme Court, formerly House of Lords, for both prosecutor and defendant from the Court of Appeal where the case raises a point of law of public importance.

Although nurses may commit crimes, there is usually no direct connection with their professional activities. The availability of controlled drugs in a hospital environment may lead nurses into temptation, and there may be cases of deliberate harm to patients, which will be prosecuted as assaults under the Offences Against the Person Act 1861, or in extreme cases as murder, as in the notorious case of Beverley Allitt, a children's nurse at Grantham Hospital, who in the 1990s murdered or seriously harmed a number of children in her care. Nurses have no general privileges in relation to the physical management of patients, but most actions undertaken reasonably and in good faith will be protected by the ordinary law of self-defence, actions taken to prevent crime (restraining one patient to prevent an attack on another) and necessity. Restraint is also specifically authorised in some circumstances under the Mental Health Act. Prosecutions usually result from actions that go well beyond normal practice, for which there is no apparent explanation, and that are clear abuses of the nurse's professional responsibilities. In extreme cases health professionals may find themselves facing criminal charges arising from decisions made and actions taken within normal professional parameters, such as the following:

- Manslaughter by gross negligence. Where one person owes another a duty of care (and a nurse owes this duty to a patient), there may be criminal liability where there is a clear and obvious breach of this duty that obviously exposes the victim to a specific risk of death, and the victim dies (*R* v. *Adomako* (1994)). In *R* v. *Misra and Srivastava* (2005) this principle was applied in a case where junior doctors failed to recognise that a post-operative patient was suffering from an iatrogenic infection. Arguments that the offence was incompatible with the ECHR were rejected, as were arguments that negligence, even gross negligence, was inappropriate as a basis for criminal liability.
- 'Mercy killing' or active euthanasia. Any action that results in the shortening of life, and that is undertaken with that intent, is murder. It is irrelevant that the victim is terminally ill and in acute distress or severely disabled, and whether or not the victim or the next of kin consents. Juries are notoriously unwilling to convict in mercy killing cases,[21] and reliance is often placed on 'double effect', which legitimises the use of strong pain control, even if life is incidentally shortened.

1.2.2 Civil justice system

The general civil court system was, in the late 1990s, significantly reformed by the introduction of new Civil Procedure Rules.[22] These create a new overriding objective of dealing with cases justly, having regard to ensuring that the parties are on an equal footing, expense and proportionality to the importance and complexity of the case. In practice this means that all cases are allocated either to the 'small claims track' for speedy and informal disposal of small-scale disputes, to the 'fast track' for routine cases requiring limited court time, or to a 'multi-track' which allows for more complex cases to be handled as they deserve. Procedural judges take charge of the timetable of the case and the parties have to comply with the standard timetable of the fast track, or the agreed timetable in the multi-track. In the process the distinction between the county court and the High Court has been blurred. Most cases will actually be tried in the county court, including many high-value claims, but High Court judges will continue to hear the most complex cases. A decision of a procedural judge may be appealed to a circuit judge, and an appeal from the decision at a trial may be made to the Court of Appeal. There are special arrangements for family law cases.

Much of the work of the High Court is now judicial review. This is, in effect, a review of the legality and propriety of decisions by government departments and other public bodies while exercising statutory powers. The main grounds of review are: illegality, where the decision is outside the powers given; procedural impropriety, such as a failure to give the applicant notice of the allegations against him; and irrationality, or reaching a decision that no reasonable body, carefully considering all relevant considerations, could have reached.

There is an appeal from the county court or High Court to the Court of Appeal, provided that the leave of either court is obtained. There is an appeal from the Court of Appeal to the Supreme Court, but as in criminal cases there must be an issue of public importance.

One aspect of civil law that impinges directly on the health care profession is negligence. This is dealt with in depth in Chapter 6. At this stage it is important to note that liability for negligence is essentially liability for failure to reach a proper standard of care in dealing with someone to whom a legal duty is owed. In many cases this duty is imposed by the law in general terms, but in others it arises from a prior contractual agreement.

Since the 18th century it has been established that a physician or surgeon (and by extension any health care professional who takes responsibility for a patient) owes a duty to that patient. This general duty covers all NHS patients. It does not extend to practitioners who are 'off duty' and may be required to intervene if, for example, they come upon an accident victim in the street. In private medicine there is a contract between the practitioner and the patient. Ordinarily, this contract will merely require the practitioner to use reasonable care and skill,[23] and this is the same standard as under the general law. However, in some circumstances the patient may have greater rights under the contract. For instance, the contract may specify a particular model of artificial hip, and failure to provide this is a breach. There would be liability to an NHS patient only if the device fitted was one that was not regarded as suitable by a responsible body of opinion. Normally a practitioner undertakes to use proper care and skill, but does not guarantee a cure. However, a contract may include a warranty of a cure, although this would be unusual (*Thake* v. *Maurice* (1986)).

Another important function is the inherent jurisdiction of the court to protect the interests of the incompetent. This is particularly relevant to 'end of life decisions' but also occurs in relation to consent to treatment. These cases often take the form of an application for a declaration. However, often the issues at stake are essentially questions of trespass to the person. Touching or restraining a person is normally wrong, but if it is in the best interests of an incompetent person it may be justified by necessity. Examples include the PVS cases of *Bland v. Airedale* (1993) and the 'informal detention' cases of *R v. Bournewood* (1998) and *Sessay* (2011) which we have already met. These issues are dealt with in depth in Chapter 7.

1.3   Legal method

Judges have two roles. First, they are responsible for ensuring that the facts of the particular case are ascertained. They do this directly in civil cases, and supervise the jury in criminal cases. This is an important task, and vital for the parties to the case. It is not, however, the more legally significant of the two roles. The crucial judicial role is in ascertaining the law, so that it can be applied to the facts of the case. The facts are usually quite specific, and affect only the parties,[24] but the legal principle is of general application. As indicated above, ascertaining the law may involve a review of existing common law rules or an interpretation of statute, EU law or the ECHR.

In English law, judges have the power to state the law. In this they differ from judges in most Continental European systems, who have no status to declare the law but merely a duty to interpret and apply the law that is to be found in the national legal codes. Of course these interpretations are entitled to respect and are usually followed for the sake of consistency and because they reflect a learned opinion on the meaning of the texts. However, if judges can state the law, it is necessary to have rules as to which statements are authoritative and must be followed (whether later judges agree with them or not).

1.3.1   Binding authority

The following statements of law, forming the basis of legal principle on which a case was decided, are binding on later judges:

- Decisions of the European Court of Justice bind all English courts.
- Subject to the above, decisions of the Supreme Court of the United Kingdom (which replaced the Judicial Committee of the House of Lords as the highest court in the United Kingdom in 2009) bind all other English courts. The Supreme Court itself may, if it is persuaded that there is good reason to do so (either because there is a strong case that the earlier decision was wrong, or because the earlier decision is no longer appropriate to modern social and economic conditions) depart from an earlier decision and restate the law.
- Decisions of the Court of Appeal bind the Court of Appeal and all lower courts.
- Decisions of the Divisional Court bind magistrates' courts.

Judges may consider any other material; this will, however, merely be persuasive. It can include *obiter dicta* or comments in a judgment that do not form part of the basis of the decision,[25] statements in dissenting judgments,[26] statements by more junior judges,[27] decisions in other jurisdictions and academic comments. Decisions of the European Court[28] of Human Rights come into this category.[29] An earlier statement of law will only be binding if the present case raises the same legal issue. It is possible to distinguish cases by explaining how, while similar, they do not raise the same legal issues. It is also possible to cheat by claiming to distinguish cases where the judge does not want to follow the earlier ruling, or vice versa, and it is often difficult to be sure whether judges are using this technique properly or not. Applying the law is an art, not a mechanical process.

In practice judges need to go beyond earlier statements of the law. New issues arise and social and economic conditions change. In the past judges were very coy about admitting that they did make new rules rather than reinterpreting old ones, but they now accept that they do. They are usually very conservative, preferring to go no further than strictly necessary. When in *Airedale NHS Trust v. Bland* (1993) the House of Lords was asked to rule on whether treatment could be withheld from a patient in an irreversible persistent vegetative state, they did so on the narrow basis that there was no justification for intrusive treatment as it did not serve the patient's best interests, and expressly stated that they could not consider general arguments based on the legality or desirability of general rules on euthanasia. That was a matter for Parliament.

1.3.2 Interpreting statutes (and EU Law)

The law has been laid down here by Parliament (or the EU institutions). The judges may or may not approve, but in principle they must apply the law as passed. Unfortunately not all law is clear. There may be inconsistencies or ambiguities, or there may be situations that Parliament did not foresee and therefore did not cover.

Over the years the judges have worked out an approach to interpretation which allows some flexibility but stays as close as possible to the words actually enacted by Parliament. The approach will depend to some extent on the type of legislation. Criminal and tax legislation is always interpreted against the state in cases of doubt, while legislation intended to meet an EU law requirement will be interpreted to achieve that purpose.

The priority is to give effect to the words of the statute if they have a plain and unambiguous meaning. This will be applied even if it is not what Parliament 'meant', as in the case of *Fisher* v. *Bell* (1961), where Parliament had clearly introduced legislation designed to prohibit trading in flick knives. However, it created an offence of 'offering' such a knife for sale, and when a shopkeeper was prosecuted because he had one on display in the window, the court ruled that since it had already been decided that it was the customer who made an offer for goods on display, he was not guilty of the offence. The words used were clear, and it was wrong to look back at what the underlying intention was as this was a criminal case and the statute had to be interpreted in favour of the defendant anyway. Where wording is ambiguous various approaches may be used, as follows:

- Preferring a sensible meaning to an absurd meaning. So the word 'marry' in the definition of the crime of bigamy was interpreted in *R* v. *Allen* (1872) as 'go through a form of marriage' rather than 'contract a [valid] marriage' which would have made the offence impossible to commit, as someone already married cannot validly marry again.
- Consideration of the underlying intention of the statute. In *Kruhlak* v. *Kruhlak* (1958) the expression 'single woman' in the context of affiliation proceedings was interpreted to mean any woman not living with her husband or supported by him; that is, it could include a divorcee or widow. The mischief was the need to ensure financial support for illegitimate children, whatever the marital status of the mother. Similarly in *Knowles* v. *Liverpool Council* (1993) a broad interpretation was given to the expression 'equipment' in the Employers' Liability (Defective Equipment) Act 1969, in order to give effect to the broad aims of the legislation in the light of the known mischief.
- Reference to any authoritative statement in Hansard by the sponsoring minister on the meaning of the particular provision (*Pepper* v. *Hart* (1993)).

The main danger in interpretation is that the greater the leeway the judges allow themselves, the more likely it is that they will be accused of interpreting to suit their own notions of what is right and proper. As most such cases either involve issues of political controversy or raise contentious ethical issues, and this will increasingly be the case under the Human Rights Act, there is increasing concentration on the judges, and questions are increasingly being asked about their qualifications to adjudicate on these controversial issues, as opposed to technical legal matters, where their expertise is acknowledged.

1.4   The legal context of nursing

Nurses are governed by three separate sets of legal rules,[30] quite apart from the law that establishes the framework of the NHS and the general law of the land. There are legal obligations to patients, normally arising in the context of allegations of negligence. There are professional obligations, imposed in the case of nurses by the Nursing and Midwifery Council (NMC), which is responsible for education, registration, professional standards and discipline. The essence of the professional standards established by the NMC in its Code of Practice is that each nurse must:

- Make the care of people your first concern, treating them as individuals and respecting their dignity.
- Work with others to protect and promote the health and wellbeing of those in your care, their families and carers, and the wider community.
- Provide a high standard of practice and care at all times.
- Be open and honest, act with integrity and uphold the reputation of your profession.[31]

Specific obligations in the Code of Practice require the nurse to respect the right of the patient to be involved in the planning of care, to work cooperatively with colleagues and to report anything that adversely affects the standard of care being provided.

The large majority of nurses work as employees in the NHS or the private health sector and thus have a legal employment relationship. Despite the reforms of the 1980s which were intended to create an internal market of independent NHS Trusts, each establishing its own terms and conditions of employment to replace the earlier national Whitley Council arrangements, in practice terms and conditions have remained relatively uniform. The employer is entitled to a professional standard of performance of the duties assigned, and the employee is entitled to be treated properly. Three aspects of employment law appear to be particularly relevant to the nursing profession, as examined below.

1.4.1 Equal opportunity

Equal opportunity, both between the sexes and in relation to ethnicity, has been a major issue for many years. The latter is a purely English matter, regulated by the Race Relations Acts, while the former is regulated by the Equal Pay Act and the Sex Discrimination Act, both supplemented by Community law. Direct discrimination is rare, and most difficulties concern disguised discrimination.

Disadvantageous treatment of part-time workers may amount to indirect discrimination because these part-time workers are predominantly female (*R* v. *Secretary of State for Employment ex parte Equal Opportunities Commission* (1995)). The salary scale for a particular group may be depressed because the profession or group is largely female, and this may constitute indirect discrimination (*Enderby* v. *Frenchay Health Authority* (1993)), although it is important that the two groups are actually comparable, and where one is objectively rated as more demanding, the case will fail.[32] The law will seek to deal with historical anomalies based on gender-specific recruitment, but cannot resolve complaints about the relative valuation of different jobs.

1.4.2 Psychological and stress-related industrial illness

Employers are increasingly being held liable for psychological and stress-related industrial illness where it arises from the way in which work is organised and allocated. In *Lancaster* v. *Birmingham City Council* (1999) the employer transferred an administrative employee to a new post in a significantly different area with a promise of training and support that did not materialise. The employer admitted liability for the resultant disabling stress. In *Walker* v. *Northumberland CC* (1995) the employee, a social work manager, became ill with work-related stress. On his return to work he received no support and his workload increased. The employer was held liable when he suffered a recurrence. In *Johnstone* v. *Bloomsbury Health Authority* (1990) the Court of Appeal held that a junior doctor had an arguable case that the conditions under which he was obliged to work constituted a reasonably foreseeable risk to his health. Since much of the work in some areas of the NHS, in particular A&E departments and ICUs, is inherently highly stressful, and other work can easily become so if poorly managed or short-staffed, this is clearly a significant area. The House of Lords has now confirmed that there may be liability in such cases provided that the employer is aware that there is a risk of such harm: *Barber* v. *Somerset CC* (2004).

1.4.3 'Whistle blowing'

'Whistle blowing' has been problematic. Nurses are under a professional duty to report circumstances that may adversely affect patient care. They may also be under a duty to the patient. Some employers, including NHS Trusts, place great weight on the management of information and resent adverse publicity, whether or not it is justified. Nurses who have publicised matters of concern have in the past attracted considerable attention and suffered serious consequences, like Graham Pink, a nurse at Stepping Hill Hospital, who became frustrated at what he considered to be managerial indifference to his complaints over staffing levels and in the early 1990s drew these to public notice, attracting disciplinary action from his employers as a result. Some protection is now given by the Public Interest Disclosure Act 1998. This protects an employee from dismissal or other retaliatory action if he discloses information relating to circumstances which disclose an apparent breach of legal duties or a threat to the health and safety of any person. The disclosure must be to the individual's employer, to the Secretary of State if the employee is in the public sector (including NHS Trusts, but not GP practices), to a prescribed regulator, which in the health context will generally be the Care Quality Commission, or to the press or public where the employer has not taken action on an earlier report to him and it is reasonable to do so.

Most of the time these three duties do not cut across each other. Most of the time employers and employees have a common interest in promoting the welfare of patients in an efficient and professional manner. There are problems, however. The employee may feel professionally obligated to report deficiencies in the employer's services to patients or may feel that other professionals are not respecting the patient's autonomy, or allowing the nurse to act as an effective patient advocate.[5]

The NMC states:

Make the care of people your first concern, treating them as individuals and respecting their dignity.

Treat people as individuals

1. You must treat people as individuals and respect their dignity. 2. You must not discriminate in any way against those in your care. 3. You must treat people kindly and considerately. 4. You must act as an advocate for those in your care, helping them to access relevant health and social care, information and support.[31]

In these circumstances the law is, at best, an imperfect instrument. Balancing the three duties is difficult, and a legal process that focuses on which of two cases has the better basis in law and in fact is not well adapted to weigh more complex issues.

1.5   Notes

1. Northern Ireland Act 1998, Scotland Act 1998, Government of Wales Acts 1998 and 2006.
2. Despite the changes to the constitutional position of Wales, much of this material still applies there.
3. We only have time for a brief consideration of these matters; for a more detailed treatment, see either Terence Ingman, *The English Legal Process*, 13th edn (Oxford, OUP 2011) or Michael Zander, *The Law-Making Process*, 6th edn (Cambridge, CUP 2004). The actual process of statutory interpretation is not significantly different in the other jurisdictions.
4. A bill may be voted down. This often happens to bills proposed by individuals (private members' bills) but rarely to government bills because the Government can usually guarantee that its MPs will support it. The Lords is less predictable, even after the recent reforms, but cannot block financial and tax bills, will not block bills that are part of the manifesto on which the Government was elected and can in any event only delay bills for one full year: Parliament Acts 1911 and 1949 and the Salisbury/Addison Convention.
5. There are over 1400 references to 'medical practitioner' in statutes, ranging from obvious ones such as the Mental Health Act to others such as the Deregulation and Contracting Out Act and the House of Commons (Disqualification) Act.
6. As occurred in the *Factortame (No. 2)* case [1991] 1 AC 603.
7. See *Ghaidan v. Godin-Mendoza* [2004] UKHL 3007.
8. The European Court of Human Rights (ECtHR) case of *X v. UK* (Case 7215/75, judgment 5.11.81) established that the original advisory role of the Mental Health Review Tribunal did not meet this requirement. As a result, the MHRT now makes the decision itself.
9. Measures to provide a review procedure for these patients have been introduced by the Mental Capacity Act 2005.
10. There may be a positive obligation on the police authorities where an individual is under specific threat: *Osman v. United Kingdom* (1998) ECtHR Reports 1998-VIII. In *LCB v. United Kingdom* (1998) ECtHR Reports 1998-III, the court considered 'that the first sentence of Article 2, section 1, enjoins the State not only to refrain from the intentional and unlawful taking of life, but also to take appropriate steps to safeguard the lives of those within its jurisdiction', but this was again in the context of non-health-related government action (exposure to radiation during nuclear tests).
11. *N v. Home Office* [2005] UKHL 31.
12. *Pretty v. DPP* [2001] UKHL 61; *Pretty v. UK* 2346/02.
13. *R (Purdy) v. DPP* [2009] UKHL 45.
14. These are, essentially, that the decision was illegal because it was made without power to act, was irrational or was in breach of procedural fairness.
15. [2001] QB 213.

16. Which includes state agencies such as the NHS.
17. Formerly Industrial Tribunals.
18. This excludes fixed penalties for motoring and parking offences. Source: *Criminal Justice Statistics in England and Wales* (2005–2011) http://www.justice.gov.uk/publications/statistics-and-data/criminal-justice/criminal-justice-statistics.htm.
19. Up to 6 months' (or in some cases 12 months') custody and usually fines of £5000 per offence.
20. Additionally, this may be done after the defendant has exercised his right of appeal to the Crown court.
21. *R v. Arthur, The Times* 5 November 1981, was a case where nutrition was withheld from a severely disabled neonate, who died. There was some evidence of acute ailments other than those initially identified, and which might have led to death. The doctor appeared to have decided, with the parents, that they did not want the child to survive, but was nevertheless acquitted by the jury. In *R v. Cox* [1993] 2 All ER 19 the jury were in tears as they convicted of attempted murder relating to an elderly terminally ill patient who had repeatedly asked for release from her intractable pain.
22. The so-called 'Woolf Reforms', following a report by Lord Woolf.
23. Section 13, Supply of Goods and Services Act 1982.
24. There are of course important cases where the facts affect many different people, such as industrial disease and drug defect claims, but these are in the minority.
25. The so-called 'neighbour principle' expounded by Lord Atkin in *Donoghue* v. *Stevenson* in 1932 has been extremely influential over the past 30 years in the development of liability for negligence.
26. A dissent by Lord Justice Denning in *Candler* v. *Crane Christmas* in 1949 ([1951] 2 KB 164) formed the basis of the decision of the House of Lords in *Hedley Byrne* v. *Heller* in 1964 ([1964] AC 465).
27. The so-called *Bolam* test for medical negligence was laid down by Mr Justice McNair, but has been endorsed by many senior judges in the Court of Appeal and House of Lords.
28. Also decisions of the European Commission on Human Rights and of the Council of Ministers of the Council of Europe, both of which formerly had a role in the application of the European convention.
29. Human Rights Act 1998, section 2.
30. Those working in mental health are also governed by the Mental Health Act, making four in all.
31. See http://www.nmc-uk.org/Publications-/Standards1/.
32. As in *Southampton & District HA* v. *Worsfold* (1999) LTL 15.9.99, where a female speech therapist's work was rated at 55 and a male clinical psychologist's at 56.5.

2 The Ethical Dimension: Nursing Practice, Nursing Philosophy and Nursing Ethics

Alan Cribb

Director, Centre for Public Policy Research, King's College London, London

What are the values that shape nursing practice? This is a much debated question. In fact most of the debate that takes place in nursing and in the academic nursing literature is about values. The only exception is debate about purely factual or technical matters. Value debates take place about the nature of professional–patient relationships, and about ideas like empowerment, partnership and advocacy. More specifically there are a host of particular debates about such issues as how midwives can best protect the interests of pregnant women, or how far the work of health visitors should be dictated by public health targets. Set alongside these are discussions about the professional standards of nursing, the framework of which is reviewed in Chapter 3. All these debates should be seen as continuous with nursing ethics, because they all involve making value judgements about the means or ends of nursing care; in short, they all ask: 'What is good nursing?' Anyone who has an interest in, and some grasp of, these issues is already 'inside' nursing ethics, although they may not have thought about their concerns in these terms.

This is not meant to imply that nursing ethics is easy – far from it: all of these issues are complex. In any case even if someone was very good at debating the nature of 'good nursing', this would not make them 'a good nurse'. If nursing ethics is to be of more than academic interest it should have something to say about how people might become good nurses. I will return to this question later, but notice that there is some apparent ambiguity in it. If we talk about a nurse being 'a good nurse' are we talking about her professional or technical skills or are we making an ethical judgement about her character, or perhaps both? It would certainly seem odd to call someone a good nurse if she could demonstrate

Nursing Law and Ethics, Fourth Edition. Edited by John Tingle and Alan Cribb.
© 2014 by John Wiley & Sons, Ltd. Published 2014 by John Wiley & Sons, Ltd.

many 'competences' but lacked any concern for or commitment to her clients or colleagues. In this respect it seems very different from calling someone a good mathematician – having a set of skills that is, on the face of it, compatible with being lazy, insensitive, and self-centred!

All nursing practice is necessarily informed, partly implicitly, by some nursing philosophy. Such a philosophy embodies answers to a range of questions that are faced by any nurse. These include questions about the aims of care, professional–client relationships, working in teams and with colleagues, and wider questions about institutional, local or national policies. Although nursing involves activities other than patient or client care, such as health care research and management, it seems reasonable to view care as central, and to see the other activities as supporting this central one. But 'care' is too broad a notion to be of much help in clarifying the aims of nursing; care is the focus, but what are the aims of care? One example of the debate about nursing philosophy and the aims of nursing is represented in what has been called the shift 'from sick nursing to health nursing'.[1] This shift – which is dramatic in some areas of practice and incremental in others – is from doing things to patients towards working with them; from an approach that is 'disease-based' and expert-centred to one that is 'health-based' and patient-centred. Such a shift follows from and reflects many developments, including changing patterns of ill health, emerging professional roles, an increase in consumerism, and emerging ideas about health promotion. But at its heart is what might be called an ethical shift, a shift in values which has two interrelated components. First, and rather crudely put, there is a move from treating people as passive towards treating them with respect as equals. This is not only because individuals have an important role to play in their own care, but also because individuals 'deserve' to be treated with respect, whether or not to do so is useful to professionals. Second, there is a move from equating the best interests of patients with being 'disease free' towards an acceptance that there is much more to well-being. Quality of life, peace of mind and self respect, for example, are legitimate concerns for a nurse, as well as disease management. These two components are closely related because one aspect of well-being, an aspect that many see as fundamental, is being able to make choices and have them treated with respect. These issues will be discussed more fully in the next section.

This example of a cultural shift shows the importance of what can be called 'habitual ethics':[2,3] the ethical judgements that individuals make as a matter of course; the values that are built into ways of working. Any shift in the philosophy or culture of nursing which entails that normal practice and expectations are changed, has enormous impact. Practice can be enhanced (or made worse) for literally thousands of people. Generally speaking much less rests upon the prolonged agonising about particular cases, however difficult they are. Of course these sorts of shifts in normal practice are difficult to implement: they involve reform of policies, institutions and so on. To reformers they might seem an overwhelming task, like trying to get the Earth to spin on a different axis, yet they are the bedrock for any practical ethic.

2.1   Promoting welfare and well-being

Let us say, to use a piece of shorthand, that nursing is about the promotion of well-being. This seems a useful phrase yet, at the same time, it throws up a lot of questions. Many of the key ethical issues faced by nurses and other health care workers can be identified and clarified by working through some of these questions.

Is this formulation of the nurse's role not too broad? There are many aspects of well-being; someone's well-being may be increased by a tour of the Mediterranean, by acquiring a new friend, or by learning Latin. None of these things, nor many others like them, seem to be the function of nursing. So perhaps it would be better to say that nursing is about the promotion of certain elements of well-being. One version of this, for example, is to equate nursing with the promotion of health. This is only an improvement if we can give a meaning to health that is less all-encompassing than well-being, and yet less narrow than the idea of absence of disease, which fails to capture all of the work of nurses. A number of authors have advocated a 'middle-order' conception of health, with the intention that such a conception would help clarify the central objectives and priorities of health workers.[4,5] Broadly speaking this conception identifies health with what others would call 'welfare': that is, someone is healthy to the extent that they have the resources to pursue and achieve well-being or fulfilment. In practical terms this would mean that nursing is about helping to ensure that individuals are in a position to travel, or to learn languages and so forth. This is not the place to review all of the discussions that have taken place on the theme. But it is possible to make a few comments on the central issues.

Although it is useful to try to clarify the aims of nursing, there is no reason to suppose that a single phrase or formula will capture everything that nurses aim at. It is reasonable to assert that the central or overall aim of nursing is to contribute to welfare, but this simple formula needs to be qualified, otherwise it is arguably both too broad and too narrow. First, the way in which welfare is promoted is, in the main, based around the management (including prevention) of suffering or risk rather than wider aspects of welfare promotion such as financial assistance or education, although there is a place for these within health care. That is to say that nurses rightly do not regard the promotion of all aspects of all people's welfare as within their remit. They respond to the suffering of individuals, or to the risks faced by certain populations. Second, once in a relationship with a client they need to have regard to all aspects of well-being that might be relevant to caring for that person. This is part of what is meant by holistic care, but it also follows from a concern with the promotion of welfare, for how can you know whether you are contributing to someone's welfare if you do not see what you do in the context of their whole life? Only by having regard to the whole can nurses ensure that their work is in the interests of their clients.

It is not possible to promote welfare, for example, without having regard to both the costs and the benefits of proposed interventions. Any intervention is likely to have some 'cost' or risk for the client which has to be weighed against the expected benefit; and there will be wider costs and benefits for others affected directly or indirectly. (We will return to this below.) Neither can welfare be promoted without having regard to the wishes or preferences of clients. This is because an important part of one's welfare consists in having one's wishes respected. So even if a nurse is clear about her aims, and has a clear view of what is in the interest of her client, she faces a number of potential problems of fundamental importance. What if the client disagrees about what is in his or her interest? What if the client agrees that in some respects the nurse's preferred intervention is in his or her interest but for some reason does not wish the intervention to take place? What if the client is not in a position to express an opinion? Under all of these sets of circumstances an appeal to 'promoting welfare' is not sufficient. A well-intentioned intervention is not necessarily in the best interest of clients, and even in those cases where it is, that is not sufficient to justify unwanted 'interference' in people's lives.

The possible tension between 'welfare' and 'wishes' is one of the key issues in health care ethics. Many of the contributions in this book discuss it in one form or another. How should nurses balance promoting the welfare and respecting the wishes of their clients? This is, for example, the background against which the importance of informed consent is discussed. This issue is so important in health care contexts because these typically involve, on the one hand, a patient who is in some distress and in a relatively powerless state and, on the other hand, a group of health professionals in relatively powerful positions who are charged with looking after the patient. This creates a constant temptation to 'take over' in one way or another for the sake of the patient, without proper regard for the patient's wishes. The ideal circumstances are those in which a client is able to discuss and understand the options facing him, and able to negotiate care and freely assent to any intervention. This assumes that the client is conscious, of sufficient maturity, mentally well and in an open and non-pressurised environment. When one or another of these conditions is not met, there is scope for ethical debate about how best to act. It is usually relevant to consider what the client would wish if they were able to express themselves freely. This might entail imaginatively 'putting ourselves in their shoes', or consulting their family and friends about their views. Sometimes health professionals or family members may be able to make an informed judgement based upon the wishes previously expressed by the client.

2.2   Respect for persons and respect for autonomy

Although it is certainly essential to take into account the views or wishes of clients, it should not be assumed that it is always right for these wishes to prevail. What is needed is an ethical account of why 'wishes' are of such importance, and when, if ever, they can be overridden. The intuitions that lie behind this judgement are so basic that it is difficult to produce an account. But the idea of 'respect for persons' helps to articulate it. In brief this is the idea that each of us has an intrinsic value which, if we are to recognise one another properly, cannot be ignored or 'traded off' for some other end. To treat someone only as an object, or only as a tool or resource, is to fail to treat them as a person. This way of expressing the value of persons is derived from part of Kant's moral philosophy, and for many people it expresses something close to the essence of ethics. One way in which respect can be exercised is by taking seriously the autonomous choices that people make and by not ignoring or overriding them. Hence the importance of consultation, partnership and informed consent.

However, respect for persons does not only involve respecting autonomous choices. Parents may recognise the choices of their teenage children as autonomous, and yet may choose to override some of their children's wishes without necessarily being guilty of treating them as 'objects'. Indeed they may be treating them with great respect and love, and they may be motivated purely by concern for their children's welfare. Acting in what one judges to be the best interests of someone else, in a way that overrides or limits the exercise of their autonomy, is called paternalism (or sometimes parentalism). As we have seen, paternalism is a constant temptation in health care, and if we are to respect autonomy there should be a presumption against it, but are there occasions on which it might be justified?

There are two reasons why nurses may, from time to time, be justified in acting paternalistically. First, autonomy is partly a matter of degree. How autonomous a choice is depends upon a number of factors, including the level of understanding and reasoning of the chooser. A choice made by a client may be judged autonomous at a minimum level, and as worthy of respect and serious consideration. Yet judged against a more demanding standard, the same choice may not be seen as sufficiently autonomous to decisively settle the matter. Second, it is often difficult to assess the degree of autonomy of a choice. Sometimes we cannot be clear what lies behind a decision or action, in particular how far it rests upon a misperception, a whim, a disturbed temperament, or external pressure. Under these conditions it might be justified to postpone a decision, or even override an apparently autonomous choice, in order to assess how far a choice is really autonomous. Both of these reasons are more likely to come into play if the risk to welfare is great (a suicide attempt is the paradigm case here).

Paternalism involves limiting a person's exercise of autonomy for his or her own sake, but there are, of course, other reasons to limit the exercise of autonomy. Respect for persons means taking into account the interests and wishes of all those affected. Normally this means that the client concerned has the overriding voice, but this is subject to important qualifications. A patient or client, even if we assume they are 'fully' autonomous, cannot merely demand an intervention whatever the cost to other people, or regardless of the views of health professionals. If we are to respect persons, then nurses cannot merely be used as objects or tools to meet the demands of other people – whether doctors or patients. This will happen unless they are involved in appropriate decision-making, and allowed to withdraw in a responsible fashion from involvement when they strongly object to what is decided. Also there is sometimes more than one client. A nurse may, for example, be supporting a bereaved family. Here respect for autonomy necessarily entails balancing the wishes of different individuals together, and having regard for the well-being of the family as a whole. Finally, a nurse acting as a budget holder or policy-maker has to consider the overall implications of decisions for the general population.

2.3   Utilitarianism and the public interest

This takes us on to a second cluster of problems concerning the promotion of welfare. How are nurses supposed to balance together the interests of different individuals, and how are they to consider both the needs of their immediate clients and a commitment to the general welfare or the public interest? A large number of practical dilemmas turn upon these two questions. Dramatic examples of the first kind include those cases where individuals donate organs to others, or cases in which the interests of pregnant women and fetuses can come into conflict. Dramatic examples of the second kind arise when clients are a potential danger to the health or safety of others. If someone has a highly infectious and serious condition, or is seriously mentally disturbed, under what circumstances should they be able to determine their own lifestyle in the community?

One way of thinking about these dilemmas is to see them as about considering the expected costs and benefits of alternative courses of action in order to see which course produces the best overall outcome. This way of thinking is often described as utilitarian, and there is a tradition of moral philosophy called utilitarianism in which it is defended as the basis of ethics. There are many debates about and within utilitarianism which cannot be summarised here. But it is possible to indicate both the plausibility and some of the difficulties of the central idea.

Its plausibility arises because it can seem odd to see ethics as simply about following rules or principles for their own sake. Surely what we are interested in is bringing about better, rather than worse, states of affairs. A nurse who is asked to adopt 'ethical standards' will expect to see how they are connected to protecting or promoting welfare, how they make the world 'a better place'. Yet a rule, principle or guideline that seems to work well most of the time may, on occasion, seem to do more harm than good. For example, it seems important to have rules to protect the confidentiality of clients, but it also seems that there are circumstances where the risks or costs of silence may be so grave that confidentiality could justifiably be broken. It appears that in this kind of example a more fundamental, and arguably utilitarian, ethic is being appealed to.

However, there are some problems with this way of thinking. There is no exact ethical accountancy by which the different sorts of costs and benefits can be optimised, and different individuals are likely to disagree about when a guideline is unhelpful and can be broken. At the extreme this could lead not only to a climate of uncertainty about policy, but to an individual nurse's idiosyncratic conception of what counts as a cost or benefit having undue influence.

More generally a concern about utilitarian thinking is that it can involve sacrificing some people's interests for the sake of others, and that this could amount to treating people merely as objects or resources. There is, on the face of it, a direct tension between certain applications of utilitarian thinking and the idea of respect for persons.

For example, consider resource allocation as an ethical issue that, on the face of things, lends itself to utilitarian thinking. A nurse manager might have to decide how to divide a budget between a number of patients and the professionals who work with them. It is plausible to suppose that she should use her experience, and research evidence, to determine which pattern of distribution would 'do the most good' (although note the complexity and uncertainty inherent in this), and opt for this pattern. This sounds fine in the abstract, but in the real world it would probably involve overriding the views and wishes of many of the patients and professionals involved. Certainly any decision that entailed not treating certain sick individuals at all because money 'wasted' on them might be better spent elsewhere would appear to treat the former with less than respect. For this reason many people react against utilitarian thinking, seeing it as amoral or even 'immoral'. Yet health professionals, including nurses, have some responsibility to the general welfare or the public interest, as well as to the individuals in front of them, and need to explore ways of balancing these responsibilities. This is merely one illustration of the way in which our basic approach to ethical thinking shapes the day-to-day practical decisions we might make.

2.4   Principles of health care ethics

One approach to health care ethics that has gained widespread currency is to set out fundamental principles, each of which needs to be taken into account when we make ethical judgements. This approach, and the so-called 'four principles', have been made famous by the work of Beauchamp and Childress[6] and Raanon Gillon.[7,8] The four principles are the following:

(1)   the principle of respect for autonomy
(2)   the principle of nonmaleficence
(3)   the principle of beneficence
(4)   the principle of justice.

In short, these principles mean that in deciding how to act health professionals ought to respect autonomy, avoid harming, where possible benefit, and consider (fairly) the interests of all those affected. This is not a formula for ethical decision-making, but rather a broad framework that can be used as a basis for organising ethical deliberation and discussion.

There is no substitute for reading about this approach in the source texts referred to above. These make quite clear the difficulties in interpreting and applying these principles, and the ways in which they tend to conflict with one another in practice. We have already seen that the idea of autonomy, and the ideas of costs and benefits, are open to different interpretations, and the idea of justice is, if anything, even more controversial. For example, some people would argue that a health care system in which health care is distributed by an open market, in which everyone has an opportunity to buy care, is perfectly just, whereas others would see this as profoundly unjust, arguing perhaps that health care ought to be distributed according to need.

This 'four principles' approach has come under criticism for being too superficial or too limited. Some of this criticism can be dismissed because it is based on misconceptions about what the proponents of this approach are advocating. They are not arguing that all ethical thinking can be reduced to a few key words, or that the four principles provide a quick and easy method for solving ethical dilemmas. Rather they are arguing that the principles provide a reminder of the key dimensions of ethical thinking, and that they can provide a common vocabulary and framework for individuals with different outlooks or philosophies. This approach is, in part, designed to avoid the paralysis of endless theoretical debate, and to be of practical help in real cases.

Leaving aside the question of its ultimate validity, the practice of applying the principles to cases provides important lessons for nursing ethics. It makes clear, for example, that although the principles supply 'rules of thumb', we cannot assess what we ought to do in a specific case without considering the particular circumstances of the case. Ethical judgement depends crucially on questions of fact as well as questions of principle, and it is worth noting in passing that a good deal of apparent ethical disagreement stems from disagreements about the facts. Also, because so much ethical thinking involves weighing together the conflicting demands of different principles, it is possible for a small difference between two similar cases to result in apparently contradictory conclusions. We have already seen, for instance, how a decision to act paternalistically can rest upon very fine judgements about a client's degree of autonomy. Hence not only abstract reasoning but also sensitivity and attention to detail are essential parts of ethical thinking.

2.5   Philosophical ethics: its value and limitations

Philosophy students study 'ethics' as an academic subject, albeit one that is normally seen to have an applied element. The questions typically considered in this context vary in their level of abstraction. The most abstract or general ones include, for example: What is the basis of ethics? Is it possible to have ethical knowledge? What are the meaning and the uses of the concept 'good'? Then there are middle-order questions that raise matters of practical substance but at a considerable level of generality, for example: What are the various conceptions of a fair society? Under what circumstances is it permissible to break promises? Finally, there are the most applied questions in which philosophers analyse the 'rights and wrongs' of specific policies or actions. In relation to health care these might include consideration of specific cases in which it is asked if nurse X was right to Y (e.g. breach confidentiality) in circumstances Z (where these could be spelled out in some detail). Nurses who are also philosophers, or nurses who are interested in philosophy – and there are increasing numbers of both – will be interested in all of these questions, but what is their relevance to nurses with other interests?

Philosophers who wanted to 'sell' their subject could offer the following argument: every nurse has to answer the applied or practical questions, and it is impossible to avoid answering them even if only by default (i.e. faced with circumstances Z, you either do or do not breach confidentiality; you cannot fail to 'answer' the question merely by not thinking about it). But, it could be argued, answers to the applied questions lower down the list depend upon having or assuming answers to the sort of questions higher up the list. Therefore, if you want to answer the practical questions responsibly, you must address the more philosophical questions. This is a very plausible argument. It takes the same form as all sales talk: 'You cannot do what you want to, or have to, without my product.' For this reason we should be suspicious of it; however, I would suggest that in essence it conveys a truth. The only way in which we can appraise specific circumstances is by standing back and comparing them with others. In so doing we will also find ourselves asking what kind of yardsticks, if any, we have. Are there some general standards we can apply, or do these vary from case to case, or from person to person?

Philosophical ethics is a discipline that is committed to this process of 'standing back' and systematic reflection and argument. There are a number of competing theoretical traditions that attempt to organise ethical reflection into systems of thought. At their most ambitious they attempt to produce a single theory (or a unified set of theories) to account for all our ethical judgements. Given such an overarching theory, we could identify any particular decision, action, policy or person to be right or wrong, or good or bad, in specified respects. Philosophers disagree about the extent to which it is possible or desirable to aim for such general accounts, and whether they should be satisfied with the 'untidyness' of competing or complementary accounts. They also disagree about the extent to which ethics lends itself to rational analysis, and the extent to which it is rooted in conventional codes and customs (note that these two things are not necessarily incompatible). However, anyone with an interest in applied ethics is interested in seeing how far systematic thinking can be of help in making or evaluating ethical decisions.

Hence one of the benefits of philosophical ethics is that it allows us to reflect in more depth about such things as utilitarianism, the idea of respect for persons, and the idea of principles of health care ethics. What are the different versions of utilitarianism? How far are utilitarian ways of thinking inevitable, how far are they useful? And so on. We can ask this sort of question in the hope that we might arrive at a definitive overview of the basis and nature of ethics, or merely in the hope that we will illuminate some of the complexity of the subject. Although there is a danger that health professionals may see these philosophical questions as irrelevant traps (and something like the 'four principles' approach may be preferred as a 'working model'), it is important for everyone to recognise that these basic questions are hotly disputed – that is, there is no definitive 'knowledge base' in nursing ethics.

For example, in the health care ethics literature there is frequent mention of the value of 'autonomy', and there are many references to 'informed consent'. It would not be unreasonable for someone coming to the subject for the first time to assume that, in relation to such basic building blocks, there was a clear consensus as to their meaning and role. Thus it might easily be supposed that each time an author uses such an expression he or she is making use of a shared technical vocabulary; that, for example, 'autonomy' always means precisely the same thing, that it is always valued for the same reason, and that its relative importance to other values is agreed. In reality there are both commonalities and differences in the way these terms are used, and this is not a product of poor 'coordination' but a function of the inherent contestability of ethics. (Incidentally some of these commonalities and differences are illustrated by the ethical perspectives in Part Two of this book, and some disagreements about the meaning and value of autonomy are discussed explicitly in the ethical discussions of consent.) There are a number of other things that the philosophical tradition can offer to nursing ethics. First, there is a considerable literature in which the terms and issues of ethics are clarified and debated. So much has been written over centuries, and over recent years, about well-being and justice and so on. Second, there are conventions for debate, based upon ideals such as disinterested and reasoned discussion, which can serve as useful models for people entering the subject. Third, there are many issues of health care ethics that have philosophical problems built into them. For example, questions about abortion and euthanasia do not turn only upon factual matters but also upon intrinsically philosophical matters to do with the nature and value of life. In these cases it is impossible to treat these issues seriously without some consideration of philosophical questions.

Finally, and paradoxically, one of the benefits of philosophical ethics is that it generates an awareness of its own limitations. Being philosophically skilled is not the same as being a good person. There may be some philosophers who believe that a full ethical theory would be sufficient to determine what should be done in every set of circumstances, but no one could think that this would be enough to make it happen. How would this perfect knowledge become embodied in practice? We all know that it is possible, sometimes all too easy, not to do what we regard as the right thing. For these reasons philosophers have to take an interest in character as well as in actions. What is it that makes people more or less likely to understand ethical demands, and to be inclined or disposed to meet them?

2.6   Being a good nurse

One tradition of philosophical ethics, which is concerned with 'the virtues', sees these questions about character as being at the heart of ethics. The tradition is usually associated with Aristotle's ethical writings but it is a thread that runs through all of ethics. The idea of 'virtues' may seem old-fashioned but it is a useful name for good qualities of character, in particular for admirable or desirable dispositions. To encourage children to do 'the right thing' we need not only to help them know what the right thing is but also to enable them to want to do it, preferably for it to become a habit or 'second nature'. The same goes for all of us. It would be no exaggeration to say that nurse education and development are about the cultivation of desirable dispositions as well as the transmission of clinical skills. Some of these dispositions relate to professional attitudes and behaviour – such as research awareness – but underpinning them all is a disposition to care for patients or clients, including the habit of paying attention and responding to needs. Unless a nurse has this quality she cannot be, except in very restricted circumstances, a good nurse. And this 'skill' of caring is intrinsic to ethics: it is not like other skills which may be used in good or bad ways. In fact caring is viewed by some as the pivotal concept of feminist ethics.[9] Caring does not necessarily mean a self-conscious emotional empathy or identification; there may be many instances where nurses are too tired or stressed to feel caring. The whole point of talking about a desirable disposition is to make clear that an attitude that is rooted in feelings will persist even when the requisite feelings are absent.

It would be an interesting, and perhaps useful, exercise to ask a group of experienced nurses to list the virtues necessary for nursing. At one time the Christian virtues of faith, hope and charity might have headed the list. Nowadays most people are likely to think of ideas such as honesty or integrity, whereas more 'old-fashioned' ideas such as patience or loyalty might be seen as more controversial. One thing is clear – as the conditions of nursing change, a different balance of virtues is called for. No doubt humility is a good quality but as the pressures of individual accountability increase, it needs to be tempered by courage and resolution. We all have some conception of what it is to be a good nurse. We can look at role models and try to identify which aspects of their character we admire. In this way we can set ourselves standards.

It is essential to note the difference between 'setting standards' for ourselves as individuals and the public kinds of standard-setting that have become increasingly important in health care – in the form of evidence-based guidelines, clinical governance, performance management and so on. Certainly the good nurse must take the latter into account and will, by and large, be happy to work towards publicly defined standards. But a nurse who has not only a sense of his or her personal accountability as a professional but also a strong sense of ethical integrity, and embodies nursing virtues such as courage, will want to 'aim above' public standards and – where necessary – critique, challenge or expose them. A number of the ethics authors in Part Two of this book point to ways in which ethics can be personally more demanding than the requirements of the law or of professional norms.

Hence, in the end, a serious engagement with ethics highlights some of the tensions between nursing as an ethical role and nursing as a professional or legal or institutional role – between the individual nurse and the nurse as part of the system. It is plausible to suggest that in the years since the first edition of this book was published there has been a substantial increase in these kinds of tensions, and hence a heightening of importance for nursing ethics. On the one hand more and more emphasis is given to personal accountability in an ever-growing range of health care agendas and settings. On the other hand there is a development and consolidation of both national and institutional policies, frameworks and guidelines. In many respects nurses are expected to 'do everything' – including being both personally responsible and jumping through other people's hoops!

This suggests that as well as cultivating courage nurses increasingly need to cultivate a form of constructive scepticism. They need, for example, to engage constructively with the systems of clinical governance that are put in place within their institution. Many things depend upon institutional systems and standards being in place. However, if nurses see aspects of these systems as misguided or ineffective – or if they find that they seem to be expressed only in apparently meaningless and self-referential jargon – they ought to explore means of saying so. In the health service the emperor is often quite naked and real standards sometimes depend upon people pointing this out!

So developing one's own personal standards is essential, but it is not a sufficient basis for establishing good nursing. Individual nurses cannot be expected to pull themselves up by their own boot straps. Only the exceptional few could achieve high ethical standards in an unethical environment. It is essential that the cultures and institutions of nursing foster the virtues of nursing. This is why it is important to continue the shift towards a philosophy of nursing founded upon ethical commitments. This is why it is important to have professional values and standards articulated in public documents and policies. This is why it is important for nurses to be able to debate the underlying principles and the particulars of ethics.

2.7   References

1. J. Macleod Clark, From sick nursing to health nursing: evolution or revolution?, in *Research in Health Promotion and Nursing* (eds J. Wilson-Barnett & J. Macleod Clark), (Basingstoke, Macmillan, 1993).
2. M. Oakeshott, The Tower of Babel, in *Rationalism in Politics* (London, Methuen, 1962).
3. R.S. Peters, Reason and habit: the paradox of moral education, in *Moral Development and Moral Education* (London, Allen and Unwin, 1981).
4. D. Seedhouse, *Health: The Foundations for Achievement* (Chichester, John Wiley and Sons, 2001).
5. L. Nordenfelt, *On the Nature of Health* (Dordrecht, Kluwer Academic Publishers, 1995).
6. T.L. Beauchamp & J.F. Childress, *Principles of Biomedical Ethics* (New York, Oxford University Press, 2008).
7. R. Gillon, *Philosophical Medical Ethics* (Chichester, John Wiley and Sons, 1986).
8. R. Gillon, *Principles of Health Care Ethics* (Chichester, John Wiley and Sons, 1994).
9. C. Gilligan, *a Different Voice* (Cambridge, MA, Harvard University Press, 1990).

3 The Regulatory Perspective: Professional Regulation of Nurses and Midwives

Fiona Culley[1] and Anupama Thompson[2]

[1]Independent Consultant, formerly Professional Adviser, Nursing and Midwifery Council, UK
[2]Head of the Regulatory Legal Team, Nursing and Midwifery Council, UK

3.1 Introduction

The current system of nursing and midwifery regulation, and that of doctors and all other health and social care professionals in the UK, is state-sanctioned professional regulation. This means that although the nine health and social care regulatory bodies work with the support of the four UK Governments to implement rules, and are accountable to Parliament through the Privy Council, they maintain a degree of independence in exercising their regulatory role. Their purpose is to bring important safeguards to users of health and social care services, and to help bring about safe and effective care.[1]

Overseeing the work of the statutory bodies that regulate health and social care in the UK is an independent body that is also accountable to Parliament, known as the Professional Standards Authority for Health and Social Care (PSA), previously known as the Council for Healthcare Regulatory Excellence (CHRE). Its role is to promote the health, safety and well-being of users of health and social care services, and promote a consistent and co-ordinated approach amongst the regulators.[2]

In addition to the statutory regulatory bodies, regulation of health and social care professionals in the UK is shared with Parliament, employers, registered practitioners, other health and social care workers, the people in their care, education providers, systems regulators, the public and those who raise concerns or make allegations about impaired fitness to practise. Between them, they legislate, implement, monitor, review and report on standards of professional conduct, performance and ethics.

Nursing Law and Ethics, Fourth Edition. Edited by John Tingle and Alan Cribb.
© 2014 by John Wiley & Sons, Ltd. Published 2014 by John Wiley & Sons, Ltd.

This chapter sets out to explore the professional regulation of nurses and midwives within its legislative context, principally focusing on the role of the Nursing and Midwifery Council (NMC), which has the legal authority through the Nursing and Midwifery Order 2001 (the Order)[3] to act as the regulator of nurses and midwives in the UK. It will consider the regulatory functions carried out by the NMC[4] through registration, standards for education, training, conduct, performance and ethics, and the processes that manage allegations of impaired fitness to practise.

This discussion is by no means exhaustive, and does not seek to replace the rules, standards, guidance and advice published by the NMC (www.nmc-uk .org), or the information provided in the *Nursing and Midwifery Council: Annual Fitness to Practise Report,* which has, by law, to 'indicate the efficiency and effectiveness of the arrangements it has put in place to protect the public from persons whose fitness to practise is impaired'.[5] Further understanding of the regulatory processes may be gained by observing any of the regulators' fitness to practise proceedings held in public on a regular basis across the UK. Further details are available from each of the regulators themselves.

An overview of the existing system of professional regulation now follows. It must be stressed that this reflects the position at the time of writing, and this, by its very nature, will alter. Regulatory function is constantly evolving as new legislation is implemented. For example, updated *Midwives Rules and Standards* were introduced in January 2013;[6] and the E ducation, Registration and Registration Appeals Rules were amended in 2012.[7] The NMC has a statutory duty to consult with representatives of registrants, employers, users of the services of registrants, commissioners and education providers, when establishing standards or providing guidance.[8] Further information is available on the NMC website at www.nmc-uk.org.

3.2   Overview of nursing and midwifery regulation

3.2.1   Background

Despite its long history, the statutory self-regulation of the professions has been described as a shadowy subject that is not well understood.[9]

The Medical Act 1858 established registration of qualified medical practitioners, and paved the way for other occupational groups, including nurses and midwives, to demand similar standing. Self-regulation is regarded by some as a privilege, and has, periodically, been criticised for promoting the self-interest of the profession, rather than protection of the public. For example, after the *Kennedy Report* into events at Bristol Royal Infirmary,[10] concerns were raised about the General Medical Council's (GMC) regulatory processes, an opinion repeated in the Shipman Inquiry.[11] More recently, the CHRE (now the PSA) set out eight elements of right-touch regulation, defined as 'the minimum regulatory force to achieve the desired result'.[12] These elements have transpired from the principles of good regulation identified by the Better Regulation Task Force[13] and recognise that regulation is not always the best answer to problem-solving, and is dependent on sharing good practice.[14] Such a model is being encouraged in an attempt to seek a balance between over-regulation, which may be seen as interference, and under-regulation, which may fail to sufficiently protect the public. Responsibility to ensure patient safety through early reporting is highlighted in *The Code: Standards of conduct, performance and ethics for nurses and midwives*[15] (the Code) and NMC guidance on raising and escalating concerns.[16]

Although about half of the recommendations in the *Fifth Report from the Shipman Inquiry*[17] related to the GMC, there are implications for all health and social care regulators and their fitness to practise procedures. In 2005 the Department of Health (DH)[18] announced a review by the Chief Medical Officer[19] into revalidation and regulation of doctors, and a separate review of the regulation of dentists, pharmacists, nurses, midwives, opticians, osteopaths, chiropractors and the 13 professions regulated by the Health Professions Council at that time.[20] The reviews led to further consultation, following which, in February 2007, the Government published its White Paper *Trust, Assurance and Safety: The Regulation of Health Professionals in the 21 Century*,[21] outlining further proposals for change. All of the health and social care regulators are working towards new systems of revalidation to enable them to provide further assurance that their registrants are fit to practise for as long as they are on their register. These developments have been driven by a number of factors, not least of which are the recommendations to '*reinforce the status and competence of registered nurses as well as provide additional protection to the public*' highlighted by the Francis Inquiry[22] into the events at Mid-Staffordshire NHS Foundation Trust. The NMC is committed to delivering and implementing an effective system for revalidation for nurses and midwives. However, it is not anticipated that this will be completely in place before the end of 2015.[23]

3.3   Registration of nurses and midwives

All nurses and midwives wishing to practise within the UK work within a jurisdiction, which means that it would be illegal to practise without effective registration. There are currently around 670,000 nurses and midwives registered with the NMC,[24] meaning that it holds the largest single register of health care professionals in the world. Nurses and midwives are also the largest occupational group employed by the UK health service.

Registration of midwives dates back to the Midwives Act 1902, with nurse registration following in 1919 when the Nurses Act established the General Nursing Councils for England and Wales, and for Scotland.

A single professional register for nurses, midwives and health visitors was introduced in 1983 by the Nurses, Midwives and Health Visitors Act 1979.[25]

In 1983, 11 parts to the register were established; these were later extended to 15 parts to identify the extra entry routes introduced by Project 2000, which saw a new system of nurse education whereby nurses studied to diploma or degree level within a higher education institution. Those 15 parts distinguished between first- and second-level nurses, with first level normally attained after a three-year preparation programme, and second level involving a shorter (two year) and more practical programme concluding with the qualification of the enrolled nurse. They also included midwives, and health visitors, and further separated the specialities of mental health and learning disabilities, adult and children's nursing. On 1 April 2002 the Order[26] established the NMC as the regulatory body for nurses and midwives in the UK, replacing its predecessor body, the United Kingdom Central Council for Nurses, Midwives and Health Visitors (UKCC). Since then a number of changes have taken place, including changes to the Council itself, to the NMC register, and to fitness to practise processes.

Since 2004 the rules relating to the NMC register[27] state that the register has to be accessible to the public at all times, and must include a part or parts for specialists in community and public health. Since 1 August 2004 the register has therefore been divided into three parts:

- nursing
- midwifery
- specialist community public health nursing.

The nursing part of the register is subdivided for first-level and second-level nurses and for adult, children's, mental health, learning disabilities and fever nurses. The midwifery part is open to all those with a midwifery qualification. The specialist community public health nursing part of the register includes health visitors that were previously registered on part 11 of the register, school nurses, occupational health nurses and family health nurses (in Scotland).

Registration processes are explained in Part IV of the Order, and allow names to be entered onto one or more parts of the register on completion of approved courses of education and training, and on receipt of a declaration of good health and good character. As part of the post–registration education and practice standards there are specific requirements for renewal of registration and returning to practice, when registration has lapsed after a break in practice of three years or more.[28]

The 2012 amendment to the Education, Registration and Registration Appeals Rules introduced for the first time provision for a nurse or midwife to apply to be removed from the register, even where they are subject to fitness to practise proceedings.[29]

3.3.1   Recordable qualifications

The NMC also has a number of recordable qualifications, meaning qualifications gained after initial registration, which are identified by a mark against the registrant's entry on the register. However, not all post-registration qualifications are recordable. The NMC only records qualifications for which it sets standards. These currently include programmes for prescribing medicines,[30] teaching nursing and midwifery,[31] and for specialist practice.[32] Where the programme leads to a recorded qualification, recording is to some extent optional, with the exception that for prescribers it only remains optional if they do not intend to use their prescriber qualification. Once it is recorded, the qualification remains on the register for as long as the nurse's or midwife's registration is active. There are currently no powers to have sanctions imposed against a recordable qualification, in isolation from registration, or to have a recordable qualification removed at the request of the registrant. Although all nurses and midwives are expected to demonstrate their continuing professional development in relation to their scope of practice, there are, as yet, no specific revalidation requirements for any recordable qualification.

3.4   Standards for education, conduct, performance and ethics

The Order requires the NMC to establish the standards for education, conduct, performance and ethics expected of nurses and midwives and prospective nurses and midwives.[33] This means that the NMC has to set out what is required of nurses and midwives up to, and at the point of registration, and beyond. It is chiefly concerned with satisfying the regulator, and others, that those on the professional register are not only appropriately qualified, but are also of good character, and physically and mentally fit to practise.

It does this by setting standards and guidance for education, conduct, performance and ethics, first through the Code,[34] which provides an overarching set of principles and a benchmark against which a nurse or midwife's fitness to practise will be measured. Since it was first published by the UKCC in 1983,[35] the Code has been reviewed around every four years. Whatever changes lie ahead, the Code's purpose remains constant. It emphasises individual accountability, highlighting that nurses and midwives are required to accept responsibility according to their particular knowledge, skills and competence, and have a duty to uphold the reputation of the profession, through their personal as well as professional conduct.

The Code draws attention to the values shared amongst all the UK health and social care regulatory bodies. There are implicit links with the four ethical principles upheld by Beauchamp and Childress,[36] which encompass ideals commonly used as a basis to help decide the acceptability of practice in health and social care: autonomy, non-maleficence (preventing harm), beneficence (doing good) and justice.

In 2010 the NMC produced guidance on professional conduct for student nurses and midwives[37] for the first time. The aim of this is to allow them to prepare towards working with a code once registered, as well as providing the public, approved education institutions, nurses and midwives and others with information about the conduct they may expect from student nurses and midwives.

The code is supported by a range of other standards, guidance and advice, which currently include separate rules and standards for midwives,[38] standards for pre-registration nursing education[39] and midwifery education,[40] medicines management,[41] prescribing,[42] record-keeping,[43] and good health and good character.[44]

3.5   The Council and its committees

The NMC is made up of distinct directorates, each dealing with different aspects of the NMC's functions. These directorates are overseen by a board known as 'the Council'. The Council makes the decisions that set the strategic agenda for the NMC and is the NMC's ultimate decision-making body. It decides on the direction of the organisation and sets the standards by which registered nurses and midwives must work. It is also the accountable body for the work and organisation of the NMC.[45]

The Council is made up of lay and nurse or midwife members appointed by the Privy Council, including one member from each of the four UK countries. As well as attending Council meetings, Council members sit on a number of Council Committees. These Committees explore in greater depth the issues affecting the organisation and feedback to Council as a whole.

The NMC also has three practice committees, as follows:

- the Investigating Committee
- the Conduct and Competence Committee
- the Health Committee.

Panels of these committees consider allegations of impairment of fitness to practise. Panels are made up of a mixture of lay and nurse or midwife members who are not Council members. As a matter of policy in substantive hearings at least one panel member will be registered on the same part of the register as the nurse or midwife against whom the allegation is made.

3.6   Fitness to practise

The purpose of fitness to practise proceedings is to protect the public and maintain confidence in the professions and the regulation of the professions. It is not to punish an individual nurse or midwife for wrongdoing. This can be a common misconception on the part of both the public and nurses and midwives themselves.

Fitness to practise is governed by Part V of the Order. When it was enacted, it brought into being for the first time the concept of impairment of fitness to practise and defined the following five categories of impairment:

- misconduct
- lack of competence
- a conviction or caution in the UK (or a conviction elsewhere for an offence which would constitute a criminal offence if committed in England or Wales)
- the nurse or midwife's physical or mental health
- a determination by another regulatory or licensing body that the nurse or midwife's fitness to practise is impaired.[46]

The question of impairment, although not defined in the Order or the rules, has been defined by the NMC as: 'a person's suitability to remain on the register without restrictions'.[47]

3.6.1   Misconduct

Defining professional misconduct can be testing, as it is a dynamic concept which not only is shaped by ethical and legal principles but also reflects social attitudes.

For example, in 1934 one nurse was reported to have been removed from the register for 'staying in a hotel with a married man (who was not her husband)', and a second, a matron, for 'having a child (out of wedlock) with a man employed on her staff'.[48] Nowadays, issues such as downloading illegal material from the internet have brought different challenges to the panels that consider fitness to practise.

Again, misconduct is not defined in the Order or the rules. Over the years there have been a number of definitions given. In the Nurses, Midwives and Health Visitors Act 1997 misconduct was defined as 'conduct unworthy of a nurse, midwife or health visitor'. In 2003 the NMC agreed a new definition of misconduct as 'conduct which falls short of that which can reasonably be expected of a nurse or midwife'.[49]

However, the courts have been reluctant to give too exhaustive a definition, Lord Clyde[50] stating in *Roylance* v. *General Medical Council* 2000:

> Misconduct is a word of general effect, involving some act or omission, which falls short of what would be proper in the circumstances.

Examples of some contemporary issues commonly arising from misconduct cases referred to the NMC are detailed in the *Nursing and Midwifery Council: Annual Fitness to Practise Report 2011–2012*[51] and shown in Box 3.1. There is no reliance on precedent with misconduct; however, decisions of the regulators, as well as the courts, can shape guidance and help determine and update standards. For example, in response to referrals in recent years relating to confidential information being placed on the internet, NMC advice was issued on the use of social networking sites.[52]

3.6.2   Lack of competence

Lack of competence means a lack of knowledge, skill or judgement of such a nature that the nurse or midwife is unfit to practise safely and effectively in any field in which he or she claims to be qualified or seeks to practise.[53] The NMC lack of competence procedures are designed to deal with intractable incompetence, after all other avenues have been exhausted at a local level.

Box 3.1   Details of types of allegations contained in new referrals.

- Neglect of patients
- Prescribing/drug administration
- Record-keeping
- Physical/verbal abuse of patients or clients
- Dishonesty (including theft of drugs)
- Failure to maintain professional boundaries
- Misconduct arising from social networking

Source: *Nursing and Midwifery Council: Annual Fitness to Practise Report 2011–2012.*[51]

3.6.3   Convictions or cautions

As well as a nurse or midwife's duty to inform the NMC of any conviction or caution they receive,[54] the police have a responsibility to inform the NMC when a registered practitioner is convicted of a crime.[55] It is not the NMC's role to retry the evidence, but rather to determine whether the conviction was proved and whether the nurse or midwife before them is the same person who was convicted. This is usually done by the submission of a certificate of conviction from the convicting court. The conviction does not need to relate to the practice of the nurse or midwife. Although not all criminal convictions will necessarily give rise to a finding of impairment of fitness to practise, more serious convictions may result in suspension or removal from the register.

3.6.4   Physical or mental health

Consideration of allegations surrounding unfitness to practise for reasons of physical or mental health is another important aspect of public protection. Allegations relating to the health of a nurse or midwife may come from the employer or occasionally from the nurse or midwife themselves, or a concerned relative or colleague. Complaints may relate to alcohol or drug abuse, or mental or physical illness. In 2011–12 over 3 per cent of referrals to the NMC related to the physical or mental health of the nurse or midwife concerned.[56] In almost all cases involving an allegation of physical or mental health, a medical examiner will be asked to examine and prepare a report on the nurse or midwife. The issue which has to be grasped is whether the health condition is one that currently impairs fitness to practise.

3.6.5   A determination by another regulatory or licensing body

If a nurse or midwife's fitness to practise is found to be impaired by another regulatory or licensing body (for example, Bord Altranais agus Cnáimhseachais na hÉireann/Nursing and Midwifery Board of Ireland (NMBI). The NMC can use this finding to evidence the nurse's or midwife's impaired fitness to practise in the UK. This provision can also be used where a nurse or midwife is registered with another regulator within the UK (for example, the Health and Care Professions Council), which has made a finding of impairment of fitness to practise. Usually there will be no investigation into the facts leading up to the other body's finding, simply evidence of the finding itself.

3.6.6   Referrals of allegations of fitness to practise

The NMC receives fitness to practise referrals about nurses and midwives in a number of ways, including from the following:

- members of the public (including patients and patients' relatives)
- employers
- the police or other public bodies
- local supervisory authorities
- proactive referral by the NMC itself (Article 26 of the Order).

In 2011–12 a total of 4407 new referrals were received by the NMC, 42 per cent of which were from employers and 19 per cent from members of the public.[57] In order for the NMC to progress the referral, the person making the allegation must be able to identify the nurse or midwife concerned, give an account of the incident complained of and provide any relevant documents that might support the allegation.

When an allegation is first received, it is assessed by the NMC's screening team, which ensures that the referral identifies a nurse or midwife who is on the register. Many cases do not progress beyond the screening stage. This could be because the allegation does not relate to that nurse or midwife's current fitness to practise or because the issue can be more suitably resolved by the employer at local level. If the case is to proceed, the screening team refers the case on for investigation. This investigation can simply be obtaining an up-to-date reference from the nurse or midwife's current employer or a more detailed investigation by the NMC's case investigation officers or solicitors engaged by the NMC for this purpose. When the investigation is complete, the case is referred to the Investigating Committee.

3.6.7   The Investigating Committee

The function of the Investigating Committee is to decide whether there is a case for the nurse or midwife to answer in respect of the allegation made against him or her.[58] In order to make this decision, a panel of the Investigating Committee meets in private to consider all the information gathered during the investigation together with any information submitted by the nurse or midwife concerned. It can ask for further information to be obtained before it makes this decision – for example, by directing further investigation or by inviting the nurse or midwife to undergo a medical examination. Once it has all the information it requires, the Investigating Committee can:

(a)   decide there is no case to answer and close the case (keeping a record for three years so that it can be re-opened if another allegation is made against the same nurse or midwife)

(b)   decide there is a case to answer and, in respect of an allegation of impaired fitness to practise by reason of physical or mental health, refer the case to the Health Committee

(c)   decide there is a case to answer, and in respect of an allegation of any other type of impaired fitness to practise, refer the case to the Conduct and Competence Committee.

3.6.8   The Health Committee

In order to determine whether a nurse or midwife's fitness to practise is impaired by reason of physical or mental health, a panel of the Health Committee usually holds a private hearing, although the Health Committee can also determine the allegation at a private meeting in the same way that the Conduct and Competence Committee does (see section 3.6.9). In most cases evidence is called from a medical examiner, who will have examined the nurse or midwife and who can give an opinion as to the nurse or midwife's health and fitness to practise. The nurse or midwife has the right to be present, represented and call evidence. If the panel concludes that the nurse or midwife's fitness to practise is impaired by reason of physical or mental health, it can impose a sanction (see section 3.6.10).

3.6.9   The Conduct and Competence Committee

When a case is referred by the Investigating Committee to the Conduct and Competence Committee, the Conduct and Competence Committee can decide to refer the case to a public hearing or to a private meeting. If a nurse or midwife requests that his or her case be considered at a public hearing, the case will automatically be referred for a hearing. In other cases the Conduct and Competence Committee must decide how the case should be determined. Common indicators for a meeting are where there are admissions by the nurse or midwife, where the allegations are straightforward and where there is no public interest in the case being dealt with at a public hearing. If a meeting is directed, the case is determined in private on the papers with no live evidence being called. The majority of cases are referred for a hearing.

Hearings of the Conduct and Competence Committee are usually heard in public. The rules do allow for hearings to be held in private.[59] This is usually on application by one of the parties, and common reasons for allowing the case to be heard in private include it being in the interests of a patient or witness or where evidence will be adduced about the nurse or midwife's health. The panel is assisted by a legal assessor, who advises on the law, but takes no part in the decision-making process. The NMC case is presented by a lawyer and the nurse or midwife has the right to be present and represented (usually by a lawyer or union representative, but sometimes by a friend or relative). Evidence is called from witnesses, either via live testimony or by the reading of their witness statement. Documentary evidence (for example, patient records, organisational policies, training and development records, duty rotas) may also be introduced. The nurse or midwife has the right to cross-examine witnesses called by the NMC, call evidence and give evidence on oath.

The panel is required to consider the allegations in three stages, as follows:

(a) Has the NMC proved the facts of the allegation on the balance of probabilities?[60]

(b) Is the nurse or midwife's fitness to practise impaired in light of the facts found proved?

(c) If so, what, if any, sanction should the panel impose?

At stages (b) and (c) particularly, the panel must balance the interests of the nurse or midwife against the duty to act to protect the public and maintain confidence in the profession. At each stage the panel must give written reasons for its decision. These reasons are sent to the nurse or midwife and published on the NMC website.

3.6.10 Sanction

Article 29 of the Order gives the Health Committee and the Conduct and Competence Committee the power to impose a sanction if either decides that it is not appropriate to take no further action. The sanctions available are the following:

- a caution order for one to five years
- a conditions of practice order for up to three years
- a suspension order for up to one year
- a striking-off order.

In health and lack of competence cases a striking-off order can only be imposed if the nurse or midwife concerned has already been suspended or subject to conditions of practice continuously for the preceding two years.[61]

In order to assist the panel in deciding what the most appropriate sanction to impose is, the NMC has issued indicative sanctions guidance to panels.[62] This sets out factors that should be taken into account and the general approach to be taken by the panel in reaching a decision on sanction.

When a suspension or conditions of practice order has been imposed, before the expiry of the order, a panel of the relevant committee must be convened to review the order. At this review the panel can extend the period of the order or impose any of the sanctions that would have been available at the original hearing.

3.6.11 Interim orders

At any stage after an allegation has been referred to the NMC, a practice committee can refer a nurse or midwife for consideration of the imposition of an interim order,[63] while the allegation is investigated and awaiting a final outcome. A panel of the relevant committee will consider the issue at a hearing. The nurse or midwife has a right to attend, to be represented and to call and give evidence. A panel can only impose an interim suspension or interim conditions of practice order if:

- it is necessary to protect the public or
- it is otherwise in the public interest or
- it is in the nurse or midwife's own interest.

The panel must give reasons for its decision, which are sent to the nurse or midwife and published on the NMC website.

An interim order can be made for up to 18 months. It must be reviewed by a practice committee after six months and every three months thereafter. If, at the end of the 18 months, the proceedings are not concluded, the NMC can apply to the High Court to extend the order for up to 12 months. There is no limit to the number of times that an application to extend can be made.

3.7   Appeals

The NMC makes a huge number of decisions in different contexts, many of which can be subject to challenge. The mechanism of challenge, however, differs according to the decision being appealed.

3.7.1   Registration appeals

Where an individual applies under Article 9 of the Order for admission to the Register or under Article 10 for renewal of registration, and such an application is refused by the Registrar, the individual has the right to appeal that decision under Article 37.

A registration appeal is heard by an appeal panel appointed by the Council, the chair of which must be a Council member. The individual has a right to attend, to be represented and to call and give evidence. If the appeal panel upholds the Registrar's decision not to admit the practitioner to the Register, the nurse or midwife can appeal to the County Court or, in Scotland, a Sheriff.

3.7.2   Statutory appeals to the High Court

A nurse or midwife who has been subject to fitness to practise proceedings can, under Article 38 of the Order, appeal any order (other than an interim order) made by the Health Committee or Conduct and Competence Committee to the High Court in England or Wales, the High Court of Northern Ireland or, in Scotland, the Court of Session. Typically, the appeal is against the decisions taken at a final hearing.

The nurse or midwife must lodge the appeal within 28 days of being notified of the decision in writing but does not need to demonstrate the merits of the appeal in order for it to be lodged. In England the substantive appeal is heard by a single judge sitting in the Administrative Court. In 2011–12 a total of 11 such appeals were concluded.[64]

3.7.3   Appeals against interim orders

Article 31(12) of the Order gives a nurse or midwife made subject to an interim order the right to appeal the decision by a practice committee to impose or continue the order. This appeal lies to the High Court in England and Wales, the High Court of Northern Ireland or, in Scotland, the Court of Session. Again, such appeals can result in decisions by the appellate courts that directly affect the way such cases are conducted before the practice committees.[65]

3.7.4 Judicial review

The NMC, being a public body, is an organisation capable of being judicially reviewed. The decision being reviewed must be a public law decision.[66] The significant point about judicial review is that it gives parties other than the nurse or midwife the opportunity to challenge decisions of the NMC. For example, it could be used where a person who has referred a nurse or midwife to the NMC wants to challenge a decision by the Investigating Committee that there is no case for the nurse or midwife to answer.

Unlike a nurse or midwife bringing a statutory appeal, a claimant applying for judicial review must first obtain the permission of the High Court by showing that there is an arguable case for judicial review.

3.7.5 Appeals by the Professional Standards Authority

All final decisions of the Health Committee and the Conduct and Competence Committee are reported to the PSA. The PSA regularly provides the NMC with 'learning points' on final decisions of the practice committees. These are used by the NMC to help to improve fitness to practise processes.

If the PSA considers any adjudication outcome to be 'unduly lenient'. it can appeal to the High Court (or the equivalent) under section 29 of the National Health Service Reform and Healthcare Professions Act 2002.

The decisions in these cases sit together with the cases being brought by way of statutory appeal to form a body of case law that is continually developing the law and practice relating to professional regulation.

3.8 Midwifery

Statutory supervision of midwives has operated within the United Kingdom since the beginning of the 20th century, when the majority of midwives practised independently or through charities. Since then, the role and function of supervisors of midwives have been shaped and defined by changes in social policy, professional development and practice. Now statutory supervision through the Local Supervisory Authorities (LSAs) sits alongside fitness to practise procedures within the Order.

Article 42 requires the establishment of rules to regulate the practice of midwives. This is done through the Midwives Rules and Standards 2012 ('the Midwives Rules'), which came into force on 1 January 2013.

LSAs are the organisations that hold statutory responsibilities for supporting and monitoring the quality of midwifery practice at local level. Each LSA in Scotland corresponds to each Health Board, in Wales to the Health Inspectorate, and in Northern Ireland, to the Public Health Agency. From 1 April 2013 England only has one LSA – the NHS commissioning body. Article 43(1)(b) requires the LSA to report to the NMC if it appears that the fitness to practise of a midwife within its geographical area is impaired. Echoing the NMC's function, the LSA's primary purpose is to safeguard and protect the public. Under rule 13 of the Midwives Rules, LSAs are required to complete and submit an annual report to the NMC. The annual report is an opportunity for the LSA to inform both the NMC and the public of its activities, and highlight any key issues.

Each LSA appoints a number of practising midwives as Local Supervisory Authority Midwifery Officers (LSAMOs). The LSAMOs are responsible for carrying out the LSA's responsibilities in terms of supervision of midwives.[67] Rule 8 requires the LSA to appoint what the NMC considers to be an adequate number of supervisors of midwives. (the current ratio is one supervisor of midwives to 15 midwives). Each practising midwife must have a named supervisor of midwives with whom he or she must meet at least once a year to review his or her practice and identify any training needs. A practising midwife must also have 24-hour access to a supervisor of midwives.[68] Supervisors of midwives are experienced practising midwives who have undergone additional training for the role.

Each LSA must publish its procedure for reporting and investigating any adverse incidents relating to midwifery practice or allegations of impaired fitness to practise against practising midwives within its area.[69] At the end of any investigation the investigating officer (usually a supervisor of midwives) recommends to the LSA what, if any, action should be taken. The LSA also has the power to suspend a midwife from practice pending referral to the NMC.[70]

Although the LSA system only applies to midwives, it is a model which reflects current political thinking with regards to professional regulation, namely as a move away from centralised regulation towards local oversight and responsibility. Whether this will eventually permeate through to other branches of the profession remains to be seen.

3.9   Conclusion

This chapter serves as a reminder of the individual and collective responsibility to regulate nurses and midwives, a minority of whom present an unacceptable risk to people in their care, the public or to the reputation of the profession. It also underlines the requirement upon nurses and midwives to work within their regulatory standards and the legal and ethical framework that informs them. It reiterates that all nurses and midwives and their employers need to understand the responsibility that registration brings, applying the standards to their own particular context, regardless of occupational setting.

A characteristic of any debate about health and social care regulation is that there can be no firm predictions about its future. All that can be said for certain is that the current system is likely to alter in response to public and professional opinion and lobbying. Whatever changes lie ahead, the importance of the regulatory requirements relating to nurses' and midwives' fitness to practise and accountability remains. Without them, public trust and confidence in the register and what it represents, will be compromised.

3.10   References and notes

1. *Enabling Excellence: Autonomy and Accountability for Healthcare Workers, Social Workers and Social Care Workers (Cmnd. 8008)* (London, The Stationery Office, 2011).
2. Health and Social Care Act 2012 c.7 part 7.
3. The Nursing and Midwifery Order 2001 (SI 2001/253).
4. See note 3.
5. The Nursing and Midwifery Order 2001 (SI 2001/253) Part X.
6. NMC (Midwives) Rules 2012 (SI 2012/2035).
7. Amended by the Education, Registration and Registration Appeals (Amendment) Rules 2012 SI 2012/2754.
8. The Nursing and Midwifery Order 2001 (SI 2001/253) Article 3 (14)
9. Davies C, Beach A, *Interpreting Professional Self Regulation: A History of the United Kingdom Central Council for Nursing, Midwifery and Health visiting* (London and New York, Routledge, 2000).
10. Bristol Royal Infirmary Inquiry (Kennedy Report), *Learning from Bristol: The report of the Public Inquiry into Children's Heart Surgery 1994-1995*, (Cmnd. 5207) July 2001, http://www.bristol-inquiry.org.uk.
11. The Shipman Inquiry, Fifth Report, 2004 *Safeguarding Patients: Lessons from the Past – Proposals for the Future*, www.the-shipman-inquiry.org.uk
12. *Council for Healthcare Regulatory Excellence, Right-touch regulation*, (London, CHRE, 2004).
13. *Better Regulation Task Force, Alternatives to Self Regulation* (London, The Cabinet Office, 2000).
14. See note 1.
15. Nursing and Midwifery Council, *The code: Standards of conduct, performance and ethics for nurses and midwives* (London, NMC, 2010).
16. Nursing and Midwifery Council, *Raising and escalating concerns: Guidance for nurses and midwives* (London, NMC, 2010).
17. See note 11.
18. Department of Health, *Government Widens Review into Healthcare Regulation*. Press release 2005/0121.
19. Department of Health, *Good doctors, safer patients: Proposals to strengthen the system to assure and improve the performance of doctors and to protect the safety of patients* (London, The Stationery Office, 2006).
20. Department of Health, *The regulation of the non-medical healthcare professions* (London, The Stationery Office, 2007).
21. Department of Health, *Trust, Assurance and Safety – The Regulation of Health Professionals in the 21st Century (Cmnd. 7013)* (London, The Stationery Office, 2007).
22. Report of the Mid-Staffordshire NHS Foundation Trust Public Inquiry chaired by Robert Francis QC February 2013: Presented to Parliament pursuant to Section 26 of the Inquiries Act 2005.
23. www.nmc-uk.org/Registration/Revalidation, November 2012, accessed 23 May 2013.

24. www.nmc-uk.org accessed 23 May 2013.
25. The Nurses, Midwives and Health Visitors Act 1979.
26. See note 3.
27. Nurses and Midwives (Parts of and Entries in the Register) Order of Council 2004, SI 2004:1765
28. Nursing and Midwifery Council, *The Prep handbook* (London, NMC, 2008 and refreshed in 2011).
29. See the Education Registration and Registration Appeals Rules Rule 14(2A) and (2B) and www.nmc-uk.org for restrictions on this process.
30. Nursing and Midwifery Council, *Standards of proficiency for nurse and midwife prescribers* (London, NMC, 2006).
31. Nursing and Midwifery Council, *Standards to support learning and assessment in practice* (London, NMC, 2008).
32. Nursing and Midwifery Council, *Standards for specialist education and practice* (London, NMC, 2001).
33. See note 3.
34. See note 15.
35. United Kingdom Central Council for Nurses, *Midwives and Health Visitors, Code of Professional Conduct for Nurses, Midwives and Health Visitors* (London, UKCC, 1983).
36. Beauchamp T L, Childress J.F, *Principles of Biomedical Ethics*, 5th edition (New York, Oxford University Press, 2001).
37. Nursing and Midwifery Council, *Guidance on professional conduct for nursing and midwifery students* (London, NMC, 2010).
38. Nursing and Midwifery Council, *Midwives rules and standards* (London, NMC, 2012).
39. Nursing and Midwifery Council, *Standards for pre-registration nursing education* (London, NMC, 2010).
40. Nursing and Midwifery Council, *Standards for pre-registration midwifery education* (London, NMC, 2009).
41. Nursing and Midwifery Council, *Standards for medicines management*, London, NMC, 2008.
42. See note 31.
43. Nursing and Midwifery Council, *Record keeping: Guidance for nurses and midwives* (London, NMC, 2009).
44. Nursing and Midwifery Council, *Good health and good character: Guidance for approved education institutions* (London, NMC, 2010).
45. www.nmc-uk.org.
46. Article 22(1)(a)(vi)-(vii) The Order creates two further categories of impairment – a barring by the Independent Barring Board in England or Wales or Northern Ireland or inclusion in the children's list or adults' list in Scotland. These provisions are yet to be brought into force.
47. See note 5.
48. Bendall E, Raybould E, *A History of the General Nursing Council* (London, H K Lewis, 1969).
49. Nursing and Midwifery Council, *Fitness to Practise Consultation Background Information* (London, NMC, 2003).
50. Roylance v. *General Medical Council* (No 2) [2000] 1 AC.
51. Nursing and Midwifery Council, *Nursing and Midwifery Council: Annual Fitness to Practise Report 2011–2012* (London, NMC, 2012).
52. Nursing and Midwifery Council, *Advice on social networking sites* (London, NMC, July 2011).
53. www.nmc-uk.org.

54. See note 7.
55. Home Office Circular 6/2006, *The Notifiable Occupations Scheme*.
56. See note 5.
57. See note 51.
58. The Nursing and Midwifery Order 2001 (SI 2001/253) Article 26.
59. Rule 19 Nursing and Midwifery (Fitness to Practise) Rules 2004.
60. Changed from the criminal standard of proof in November 2008 by virtue of section 112 of the Health and Social Care Act 2008
61. Although this power has been questioned see *Okeke* v. *NMC* [2013] EWHC 714 (Admin).
62. Nursing and Midwifery Council, *Indicative sanctions guidance to panels* (London, NMC, 2012).
63. The Nursing and Midwifery Order 2001 (SI 2001/253) Article 31.
64. See note 51.
65. See, for example, *Perry* v. *NMC* [2013] EWCA Civ 145.
66. For example, R (B) v. *The Nursing and Midwifery Council* [2012] EWHC 1264 (Admin).
67. NMC (Midwives) Rules 2012 (SI 2012/2035) Rule 7.
68. NMC (Midwives) Rules 2012 (SI 2012/2035) Rule 9.
69. NMC (Midwives) Rules 2012 (SI 2012/2035) Rule 10.
70. NMC (Midwives) Rules 2012 (SI 2012/2035) Rule 14.

4 The Complaints Dimension: Patient and Family Complaints in Health Care

Peter Walsh

Chief Executive, Action against Medical Accidents (AvMA)

This chapter will explore how complaints, reporting concerns about nurses and other health professionals, or litigation can be used by patients (or their family/advocate) to raise concerns and generate a suitable response from health care providers. This has been the subject of continual review and policy change over recent decades, and even the period since the last publication of this book has seen radical changes. For example, a whole Act of Parliament on the subject of providing suitable redress to patients harmed in NHS care – the NHS Redress Act – was passed in England in 2006 but, ironically, was never implemented in England, although it led to the Welsh Assembly for the first time using its new powers to enact the provisions in the Act in its own way for Wales. The NHS Complaints Procedure in England was reviewed and changed yet again with a new set of regulations coming into force in April 2009. The NHS Constitution for England was published in 2010, and the Patient Rights (Scotland) Act was passed in 2011. Arguably the biggest scandal to affect the NHS in its history, at least since the Bristol Royal Infirmary scandal, came to light in 2009 with a damning report by the Healthcare Commission into events at the Mid-Staffordshire NHS Foundation Trust. This led to public inquiry chaired by Robert Francis QC, which finally reported in February 2013 with 290 recommendations, with profound implications for the regulation of the NHS and patient safety. There continued to be upheaval in the administration of the NHS in England with the Coalition Government formed after the General Election in 2009 embarking with radical and controversial reforms contained in the hotly debated Health and Social Care Act 2012.

Nursing Law and Ethics, Fourth Edition. Edited by John Tingle and Alan Cribb.
© 2014 by John Wiley & Sons, Ltd. Published 2014 by John Wiley & Sons, Ltd.

As a result of devolution of power for health policy and the running of the NHS, the NHS in Wales, Northern Ireland and Scotland became increasing different to that in England. For practical reasons, this chapter will not attempt to cover the detail of arrangements for complaints in all parts of the United Kingdom and instead will concentrate mainly on England, with reference to developments in Scotland and Wales. Due to the nature of health care-related complaints it is necessary to deal with the interface with other processes which are the subject of more detailed consideration in other chapters of this book. In particular, the interface between complaints and litigation; complaints and health professional regulation; complaints and clinical governance and patient safety. As the vast majority of health care in the United Kindom is still provided as part of the NHS, we will concentrate mainly on the NHS but will also examine in less detail the corresponding arrangements in private health care.

4.1   The purpose of complaints and complaints procedures

There are certain common features to the making of a complaint and procedures for dealing with them that are common to any setting, be it in health care or any other service industry. A complaint is generally defined as an expression of dissatisfaction. Where there is a formal policy for dealing with complaints, there is an expectation that this expression of dissatisfaction necessitates some analysis and a response. It is not unusual for there to be either an informal or formal expectation that in certain circumstances a response might go beyond acknowledging and apologising for the cause of the dissatisfaction to providing explanations of what has or will be done to prevent the same thing occurring and even to providing some form of redress to the complainant. This might be by way of either putting right the cause of their dissatisfaction, or providing a material token of regret for the circumstances causing the dissatisfaction, or even some form compensation for time, inconvenience or costs incurred. Often where there is a formal policy, it is usual for there to be some mechanism for a complainant who is not happy with a response to his or her complaint to challenge the response and have it reviewed.

Generally speaking, the purpose of a complaints procedure will be to try to resolve the complaint to the complainant's satisfaction. Invariably, this will not always be possible, but at least the process can provide a degree of power to the consumer and a degree of transparency. In private industry complaints have for some time been seen not only as an opportunity to regain the loyalty (and business) of a customer, but also as a vital source of intelligence about how products and services can be made more attractive to customers and potential customers. British Airways, for example, claims to prize customer complaints for this reason as do many other successful businesses. In the NHS too, the emphasis of the policy intention at least has for some time changed from simply needing, as a public service, to be seen to be accountable and be responsive to patients' rights, to using complaints as a genuine learning opportunity. The degree to which this aim has been realised is very debatable as is discussed below, but in theory at least patient complaints should be able to provide vital intelligence to inform

NHS bodies' own work on clinical governance and patient safety. Patient complaints can also be used by regulators to help monitor quality and safety in health care organisations and to alert regulators as to when an intervention of some kind is needed. These issues became the subject of intense scrutiny in the public inquiry into the Mid-Staffordshire NHS Foundation Trust. The standard of health care and in particular the nursing standards at this trust had been shown to have dropped to quite appalling levels. Estimates based on standardised mortality statistics suggested that many more patients were dying at this hospital than should be expected, and eventually sparked an investigation by the national regulator, as it was then, the Healthcare Commission (subsequently replaced by the Care Quality Commission). However, patients or their relatives had for years been making complaints and raising concerns to the hospital trust and to anyone they could without anyone apparently recognising that these complaints indicated a fundamental breakdown in standards. Complaints were seen as things which needed to be processed. Responses were often at best formulaic and at worst overly defensive and even disingenuous. The emphasis was on meeting target times for issuing a response rather than grappling with the problem which caused the complaint. There was little connection with internal systems of clinical governance designed to monitor quality and safety. Even when complainants went beyond the hospital trust itself, those responsible for external monitoring and regulation did not take heed and referred the complainants back to the process for dealing with NHS complaints in a formulaic way, if indeed they responded at all.

Most of what happened at Mid-Staffordshire happened before the latest version of the NHS complaints procedure came into being in April 2009. Time will tell whether the new procedure will be more likely to deliver the kind of outcomes that the Government intended and help avoid future scandals like that at Mid-Staffordshire.

4.2   The 2009 NHS complaints procedure

Prior to the 2009 the NHS complaints procedure in England had consisted of three stages, as follows:

(1) **Local resolution.** A complaint needed to be raised with the organisation to which the complaint related. (In the case of GPs, dentists and other primary care professionals this means the practice.)

(2) **Independent review.** If a complainant was not happy with the response to a complaint, they could seek an independent review of the complaint from the Healthcare Commission. The Healthcare Commission could either take on the complaint for full investigation, refer it back for local resolution if this had not yet been attempted or exhausted, or take no further action if it considered that the complaint had been fully investigated and responded to.

(3) **The Parliamentary and Health Service Ombudsman.** A complaint could be referred to the Ombudsman if a complainant was dissatisfied with the

Healthcare Commission's review or if the Healthcare Commission declined to investigate.

The Department of Health's *Making Experiences Count*[1] set out a revised two stage system, as follows:

(1) **Local resolution.** As before but with more flexibility over target dates for response to allow more appropriate investigation and responses. Complaints about primary care professionals can be directed to the relevant primary care trust if preferred.

(2) **The Parliamentary and Health Service Ombudsman.** If dissatisfied, the complainant can refer to the Ombudsman who will screen the complaint and *may* conduct an investigation if the complaint meets their criteria.

The Healthcare Commission (which was to be replaced by the Care Quality Commission) had been overwhelmed with the number of independent reviews which it had to conduct and had had mixed reviews of its own performance. A backlog of independent reviews had led to long delays, and some complainants had expressed dissatisfaction with the response they eventually got from the Healthcare Commission. Yet, ironically, by the time its abolition was announced and a new complaints procedure was being put together, the Healthcare Commission had begun to whittle down the backlog and had become quite assertive in its findings against NHS bodies and cracking down on poor complaints handling.

The loss of the second 'independent review' stage was the biggest and most controversial change to the NHS complaints procedure. The theory was that removing a stage in the process would make the system more user friendly and less bureaucratic. The assumption was that independent reviews would be less necessary because complaints would be handled much better locally under the new procedure, and that when complainants were left dissatisfied, the Parliamentary and Health Service Ombudsman would be able to review the complaint and either intervene to ensure appropriate local resolution, deem that the complaint had been properly responded to and no further action was needed, or conduct a full investigation of its own. Critics of the change argued that the threshold used by the Ombudsman to decide when it would conduct a full investigation was higher than had been used by the Healthcare Commission, and that the Ombudsman had much more limited capacity to conduct investigations. This would mean that there would be less access to independent review of complaints and dissatisfied complainants would be left with nowhere further to go. Another criticism was that removal of dealing with complaints from the responsibilities of the national regulator (now the CQC) would mean that the CQC would not benefit from the insight this could give to patient's real experience, early warning signals about problems with quality in NHS trusts and how they were dealing with complaints. The Department of Health and the Ombudsman argued that the Ombudsman could cope and that it would also feedback issues both to individual trusts and the CQC. When the House of Commons Health Select Committee conducted a review of how the new complaints system was working in 2011, it became clear that whilst approximately 6000 independent reviews were being conducted by the Healthcare Commission each year, only around 300 investigations were being conducted by the Ombudsman. While the Ombudsman also screens each complaint that comes to her and may take some action without conducting a full investigation, there still seems to be a very substantial reduction in the ability of people to take their complaints about the NHS further, unless there has been a dramatic improvement overnight in the way that complaints are investigated and responded to and people no longer wanted to take their complaint further. This seems extremely unlikely and is not borne out by the experience of agencies which advise complainants such as Independent Complaints Advocacy Services, Action against Medical Accidents (AvMA), and the Patients Association. The Health Select Committee report is referred to in more detail later in this chapter.

Making Experiences Count was aptly named in that the stated intention of the new complaints procedure was to make the system more responsive to issues raised in complaints. NHS bodies were to be given more flexibility in how they investigated and responded to complaints, with the emphasis being on establishing with the complainant what outcomes they hoped for and investigating and responding appropriately, rather than being bound by tight deadlines for responding to complaints. Many commentators had argued that the pressure to meet deadlines for responding had led to a 'tick box' approach with investigations and responses being rushed. The new procedure allows response times to be extended, in consultation with the complainant, so as to do the complaint justice. This change has been welcomed by patients and NHS complaints staff alike, as has the emphasis given to trying to feed back lessons from complaints so as to make improvements to patient safety and quality of services. This 'closing the loop' between investigating and responding to complaints and actual learning of lessons and service improvements has long been the elusive holy grail of NHS complaints procedure. Whilst the intention and the exhortation to make this a reality is clear, there remains little evidence that it is happening consistently on the ground.

4.3   Complaints and litigation

Another significant but poorly publicised change to the complaints procedure in 2009 was the removal of the ban that had existed on investigating a complaint if legal action (usually a claim for clinical negligence) had been commenced or was specifically intended. It had been stipulated in the regulations underpinning the complaints procedure prior to 2009 that in those circumstances a complaint would be put on hold. AvMA and others had argued for years that this was unfair and at odds with the stated intention of the NHS to be open and transparent. Many felt that this sent the message that the NHS would hold back information which could help people make a successful claim. What other reason could there be for refusing to investigate and respond fully to a complaint? It also suggested a degree of disapproval or even intimidation of those who dared to challenge the NHS legally. If they did so, suddenly they would be denied some of the rights enjoyed by any other user of the NHS. The Department of Health accepted these arguments and accordingly the NHS Complaints Regulations (2009) were silent on this matter. However, because this change was not well publicised and because the Department of Health decided not to issue central guidance on implementation of the complaints procedure, unlike the approach with previous versions, the change was missed by many in the NHS.

AvMA continued to come across cases where the NHS was refusing to investigate a complaint on the basis that a claim was being made or there was a stated intention to make a claim, and continues to come across examples of this happening at the time of writing, in spite of the Department of Health having, at AvMA's suggestion, issued a letter to NHS bodies pointing out the change to the regulations. A snapshot survey of 20 NHS trust websites in 2011 (over two years after the change in the rules) revealed several examples of trusts' websites explicitly stating that a complaint would be put on hold if legal action was intended or commenced.

In one case where an NHS trust was flatly refusing to investigate a complaint because the complainant had stated an intention to make a claim for clinical negligence, the complainant decided to ask the Ombudsman to intervene or conduct their own investigation. The Ombudsman initially refused to investigate or intervene with the trust, so AvMA decided to step in and make representations to the Ombudsman to review the decision on the basis that the NHS trust was not acting in accordance with the NHS complaints procedure and was causing an injustice to the complainant. However, following a review, the Ombudsman upheld her original decision. She concluded that the NHS trust was within its rights to put the complaint on hold because, notwithstanding what the policy intention of the Department of Health was, its letter to NHS bodies on this subject was ambiguous. Whilst it stated that the 'default' position was that a complaint investigation should be conducted in the normal way even if legal action is in train, there is a provision for complaints being put on hold if progressing the complaint 'might prejudice subsequent legal or judicial action'. The complaint should be put on hold only if this is so, with the complainant being advised of this and given an explanation. Interestingly, in the case in question the only explanation that the complainant was given was that in the opinion of the NHS trust investigating the complaint might prejudice the clinical negligence claim. They offered no explanation of why this might be the case. The inference of this all is that an NHS trust can simply refuse to investigate a complaint quoting the 'prejudice' argument without justifying it. It implies that allowing the complainant to be more conversant with the facts of what happened with the benefit of a complaints investigation is considered prejudicial (i.e. it might help the complainant make a successful clinical negligence claim). This is completely at odds with Department of Health policy and with the spirit of openness expected of the NHS. It is an issue which at the time of writing, AvMA is taking up with the Department of Health.

There has for a long time been discussion about whether complaints should ever be connected to the notion of awarding compensation. In 2006 the NHS Redress Act was passed which provided for an NHS Redress Scheme whereby patients could be compensated without the need to take legal action, if the NHS deemed that there had been a liability in tort (clinical negligence). This was not what some people call a 'no-fault compensation' scheme, which successive governments have toyed with the idea of, but an in-house NHS administrative scheme which would have enabled issues forming the basis of a complaint to be considered for 'redress' (both remedial treatment and/or financial compensation) where appropriate. The scheme was not perfect but there was little doubt that it would benefit many people with relatively small claims which would be difficult to pursue through the courts. The scheme was also intended to promote more openness and to ensure lessons for patient safety were learnt and implemented as a result of the cases dealt with. A report explaining how this would happen was to be part of the redress package. Strangely, after devoting huge amounts of parliamentary time to debating the legislation and it having obtained royal assent, the Government decided to put the whole project on the back burner. The official position was that there would be a review of the new complaints procedure after a period of time to see if the initiative was still needed. However, the Government was fully aware that the complaints procedure was being revised, when it embarked on the legislation. This has led to some conjecture that the real reason for mothballing the project was that the Treasury were worried that it would lead to more claims and therefore more expenditure.

The Welsh Assembly Government, however, did decide to use the powers it had been given to develop its own scheme, called *Putting things Right – their* version of the NHS Redress Scheme – which was launched in April 2011. The scheme explicitly brings the consideration of compensation together with the investigation of complaints under the overall banner of responding to 'concerns'. Meanwhile in Scotland the Scottish Government has decided to go ahead with a full blown 'no-fault' compensation scheme based on the Swedish model. Details are yet to be announced. It is only a matter of time before alternatives to litigation, including the interface between complaints and litigation, will be considered again in England.

In spite of the fact that it is widely recognised that far fewer people make a clinical-negligence claim than might be expected, given the estimated rate of medical accidents, there continues to be a popular perception of there being a 'compensation culture', which is resulting in spurious claims and harming the NHS. However, the Department of Health estimates that around 10 per cent of hospital admissions result in a medical accident ('patient safety incident'). This would mean at least 1 million incidents in English hospitals alone. Yet, in 2010–2011 the NHS Litigation Authority received only 8655 claims. This figure itself is inflated because the Litigation Authority started recording claims in a different way that year (recording every 'letter before claim' sent to a trust, as opposed to the previous system, which only recorded claims which had progressed that point). Still, this is a tiny proportion of the number of claims we might expect and seems to fly in the face of theories of there being a 'compensation culture', at least when it comes to clinical cases. There is a considerable body of research evidence now which shows that on the whole people are reluctant to take legal action in respect of clinical negligence. For example, a MORI poll for the Department of Health report *Making Amends*[2] found that the most important things for people who had experienced a medical accident were as set out below.

Of those affected by medical injury:

- 34 per cent wanted an apology/explanation
- 23 per cent requested an enquiry into the causes
- 17 per cent asked for support in coping with the result
- 11 per cent expected financial compensation
- 6 per cent wanted disciplinary action.

In the experience of AvMA, a charity which advises some 3500 people a year who have been affected by a medical accident, less than 10 per cent express a desire to take legal action and many express embarrassment about even considering legal action. There appears to be a degree of stigma attached to seeking compensation. When people do take legal action, the charity says it is usually for one of two reasons or a combination of both:

(1)   because the NHS has not dealt with the matter openly and honestly, and legal action is a means of getting to the truth and holding the NHS to account, and/or
(2)   currently, taking legal action is the only way of obtaining compensation to help cope with life following what is often a catastrophic injury due to negligence. For example, paying for specialist care of a brain-damaged child for the rest of their life.

The importance of honesty or 'candour' when things go wrong and its potential to reduce claims and legal costs were strong themes of *Making Amends* in which there was for the first time a formal recommendation for a statutory 'duty of candour'. This issue is dealt with in more detail later in the chapter.

Nonetheless, it is true to say that the cost of settling clinical negligence claims has grown and in the year 2010–2011 had reached £863million.[3] Of this £257 million (30 per cent) is legal costs, as opposed to the actual damages paid to injured patients or their families. It is not surprising therefore that policymakers have looked at ways of reducing this burden. The Coalition Government published its Legal Aid, Sentencing and Punishment of Offenders Bill in 2011. This followed reports by Lord Young (*Common Sense, Common Safety*[4]), which amounted to an attack on the so-called 'compensation culture', and by Lord Justice Jackson (*Review of Civil Litigation Costs*[5]). Although there were fierce debates in Parliament, spurred by high-profile campaigns to retain legal aid in particular, the Bill became an Act in 2012. It represents a dramatic change to the legal system for civil litigation, including clinical negligence claims. The legislation takes up many of the reforms suggested by Lord Justice Jackson but chooses to ignore other recommendations of his. For example, Jackson was adamant that legal aid should be retained for clinical negligence in particular, although he did recommend a radical shake-up of how conditional fee agreements ('no-win no-fee' agreements) will work. The Government, however, decided to take clinical negligence out of scope for legal aid. Although a concession was won during the passage of the Act to keep certain clinical negligence cases involving birth-related brain damage to children in scope for legal aid, most commentators seem to agree that the package of reforms as a whole will make it much more difficult for the average person to pursue a clinical negligence claim. This is in spite of the Government's argument that the new system reduces legal costs but retains access to justice for claimants, albeit through a different route. Many argue that solicitors will not be able to afford to represent people with the more complex claims and those which do not, on initial screening, stand a very good chance of success. This is because of the high costs of investigating cases and the fact that under the new system solicitors will not be able to make as much money through success fees for the cases they win to compensate them for the cases which they lose or abandon following further investigation. Few would argue with the proposition that legal costs including success fees for conditional fee agreements have become disproportionate, and something needed to be done to address this. However, the Government's proposals have been described as unworkable and inevitably leading to a loss of access to justice to deserving claimants. The decision to take clinical negligence out of scope for legal aid is the hardest to understand. It is far more cost-effective for the NHS to settle a clinical negligence case brought under legal aid than a conditional fee agreement. That is one reason why the NHS Litigation Authority itself had called for the retention of legal aid for clinical-negligence cases. An independent report by King's College London[6] even estimated that taking clinical negligence out of scope for legal aid would cost the Government overall three times what it proposed to save by the measure. This is because whilst the Ministry of Justice would save a modest amount by not having to pay for legal aid, the NHS would be hit with an extra bill for insurance premiums in successful cases, whereas this would not arise if the cases continued to be legally aided. The Government itself conceded that taking clinical negligence out of scope for legal aid is at best 'cost-neutral'. All this has given rise to speculation about a more sinister possibility – that in spite of the stated policy intention the real motivation for this change is to prevent some of the cases progressing at all. As well as the access to justice and cost implications of this policy, another unintended consequence might be that the NHS is deprived of lessons to help it improve safety. It is often only after a claim which is initially staunchly defended succeeds, that there is insight into the fact there have been serious errors and how these might be avoided in the future.

4.4   House of Commons Health Select Committee inquiry into complaints and litigation, 2011

The first real independent scrutiny of how the new system was working came with the Health Select Committee inquiry into complaints and litigation in 2011. Its report[7] came as something of a wake-up call to the Department of Health and the NHS. Most notably it echoed many of the concerns expressed by patients' organisations about the removal of the independent review stage of the NHS complaints procedure and the capacity of the Ombudsman to fill that void. Under the heading 'The NHS Complaints System is not working' the Committee's press release covering publication of the report highlighted the following conclusions/recommendations:

- The legal and operational framework of the Health Service Ombudsman should be widened so that she can independently review any complaint which is referred to her following rejection by a service provider.
- The NHS still has no national protocol for the classification and reporting of complaints, and reporting by foundation trusts remains voluntary.
- The Government's recent consultation on information strategy in the context of the Health & Social Care Bill did not mention procedures for handling complaints.
- It remains unclear how patients' complaints about services delivered by primary care will be handled following passage of the Health & Social Care Bill.
- NHS culture is too often defensive and the service remains to be persuaded to adopt a more open culture.

The report criticised the ongoing culture of defensiveness with regard to complaints and was supportive of initiatives to promote and deliver openness, including the Government's proposed contractual 'duty of candour', which is discussed below. However, it was ambiguous about whether or not a statutory enforceable duty was required. On the one hand it seemed to imply that it was not, but on the other it did make a specific recommendation that a duty of candour with patients should form part of the licensing requirements with the CQC (which would be statutory). On litigation the Committee did not favour a 'no fault compensation' scheme, but did support plans to develop a fast-track scheme for lower-value claims. The Committee also warned of the effect that the removal of legal aid would have on access to justice in clinical-negligence cases.

How much clout the Health Committee actually has may be questionable. The Government subsequently fiercely resisted the recommendation to build a duty of candour into the CQC's registration requirements (but then reluctantly agreed to – see section 4.5) and pressed ahead with the removal of legal aid for clinical negligence.

4.5   A 'duty of candour' in health care ('Robbie's law')

Over 20 years ago a ten-year-old boy called Robbie Powell died in South Wales following failure of various doctors to diagnose and treat the Addison's disease from which he was suffering. Although liability for clinical negligence was established in this case, its most significant aspect in terms of health policy was the alleged cover-up that ensued following Robbie's death, including attempted forgery of medical records. The campaign to prevent cover-ups in health care by establishing a statutory 'duty of candour' has since been taken up by campaigners for patient safety and justice in health care, most notably the charity Action against Medical Accidents (AvMA), who called its campaign 'Robbie's law' in honour of his family and him. The case has been the subject of various investigations and procedures, including a case brought to the European Court of Human Rights, which established that doctors are under no legal obligation to tell the truth about a medical accident, even where it has caused serious harm or death of a child. Over the years various people have tried to address this alarming situation. As a result of the family's tireless campaigning the General Medical Council (GMC) amended its *Good Medical Practice* code to signal that covering-up of medical accidents causing harm is unacceptable, at least in theory. Other regulators of health professionals, including the Nursing and Midwifery Council, introduced similar provisions in their codes. However, when Robbie's case was eventually considered for investigation by the GMC in 2003, in spite of evidence of the alleged forgery and attempt to pervert the course of justice available from the police and crown prosecution service, they refused even to investigate. They invoked their so called 'five-year rule', which states that allegations about doctors will not normally be investigated if over five years old. The GMC had the power to use its discretion to waive the rule, but refused to do so in Robbie's case, in spite of requests to do so by the family, AvMA and even the NHS Health Board where some of the doctors still worked. The unique circumstances of the case and its significance failed to convince the GMC that it was sufficiently in the public interest to make an exception, even though the GMC was aware of the allegations well before five years had elapsed and only subsequently brought in the five year rule, having always said they would investigate once other procedures had been completed. The GMC even refused to review its decision when challenged by way of a judicial review brought by AvMA. The clear and chilling implication is that if doctors succeed in covering up their actions for more than five years, they can be reasonably confident that they will be in the clear as far as the GMC is concerned.

The case shattered public confidence in health professional regulators championing openness and transparency, but even if they could be relied upon to enforce their own codes rigorously, the codes only apply to individual health professionals. They do nothing to promote openness about medical accidents by organisations or managers who are not health professionals. Even by the start of the new millennium it remained the case that a health care organisation was in breach of no statutory rule if it chose to cover up medical accidents. Experts in patient safety, such as the ex-chief medical officer Sir Liam Donaldson, have decried the so-called culture of denial in the health service. This led him to formally recommend a statutory duty of candour which would apply to health care organisations and managers in his report *Making Amends* in 2003. The recommendation was never taken up by the Labour Government then in power and no explanation was forthcoming as to why. However, the ongoing campaign did result in a vaguely worded commitment to 'require' hospitals to be open when things go wrong and cause harm, which appeared in the Liberal Democrat manifesto for the General Election in 2010. The formation of the Coalition Government led to the same commitment in coalition government policy reflected in the NHS White Paper *Equity and Excellence: Liberating the NHS*.[8] Optimism grew that this was the dawn of Robbie's law – a statutory and enforceable duty to be open with patients or their families when harm was inadvertently caused. However, the Government, or at least Conservative ministers in it, voiced a strong ideological resistance to legislating over such matters, and in 2011 launched a consultation on their own version of a duty of candour. The consultation document made clear that there would be no consideration of other options such as a statutory, enforceable duty in the registration regulations of the Care Quality Commission (CQC), which registers and regulates all health care organisations in England. This was the option favoured by campaigners. Instead, what was proposed was a 'contractual' duty – a standard clause in commissioners' contracts with NHS trusts. The duty would not apply to primary care providers such as GPs and dentists and would only cover incidents which had already been reported to the CQC. (The CQC regulations require incidents causing harm to be reported to it, but place no obligation on health care organisations to be open with patients or their families about them.)

Campaigners were not impressed with the Government's proposals and took their argument to the House of Lords which were debating what is now the Health and Social Care Act 2012. An amendment was put forward which would have created a statutory duty on health care organisations to take all reasonable steps to ensure openness with patients about these incidents by making this a requirement for registration with the CQC. The CQC would be able to refuse or remove registration or take other measures over organisations who failed to comply, since the registration regulations have statutory force. In spite of considerable support, the amendment lost in a vote in February 2012 by 36 votes, following a three-line whip from the Government. Only one Liberal Democrat voted for the amendment, even though it was signed by a Liberal Democrat peer and senior Liberal Democrats spoke publicly in favour of it. It had, after all, stemmed from an original Liberal Democrat policy.

On the face of it, the lost vote in the Lords might suggest that campaigners for patient safety and patient's rights might have to be satisfied with at least having pressured the Government into committing to doing something about this issue, whatever the doubts about the adequacy of the contractual duty of candour. However, the issue is sure to return in the not-too-distant future. The Mid-Staffordshire NHS Foundation Trust public inquiry heard shocking evidence of cover-ups and the fact that people could not be held to account for them. Both the chair and counsel to the inquiry signalled that the final inquiry might have something to say on the matter, and the counsel to the inquiry clearly had reservations about the adequacy of the proposed contractual duty of candour. When the report from the public inquiry finally emerged in February 2013, much to the Government's embarrassment it did contain an explicit recommendation for a statutory duty of candour along the lines of what AvMA and other campaigners had been calling for. At the time of writing details were still awaited about how this would work in practice, but the Government has said that it will implement the recommendation even though it had fiercely resisted this previously. It has indicated it is less inclined to follow a related recommendation for there to be a corresponding legal duty on individuals with criminal sanctions for non-compliance. The long called-for creation of a statutory duty of candour on all health care organisations has nonetheless been described as potentially the biggest advance in patient safety and patient's rights since the creation of the NHS.

4.6   Independent support and advice for complainants

From 1974 the main source of independent advice and support for people wanting to make a complaint about the NHS came from Community Health Councils (CHCs). These were local statutory NHS watchdog organisations drawing on volunteers from the local community and facilitated by paid staff. They were also known as the 'patients' friend' in the NHS. Controversially, they were abolished in England in 2003, although they remain in Wales where the Welsh Assembly had allowed a public consultation on the matter and the overwhelming response was in favour of keeping them. England was left with the new Patient Advice and Liaison Service (PALS – a kind of internal customer services) which, being part of the NHS trusts themselves, is not independent. As a concession to the opponents of CHC abolition in England, the Government did establish an Independent Advice and Liaison Service (ICAS). However, whilst the original promise was for this service to be based at and run by staff of the new 'patients forums' being created in the place of CHCs, the service ended up being put out to tender by the Department of Health. Initially four and now three existing charities hold the contracts to provide the ICAS service in different parts of the country. At the beginning there were many teething problems with new staff and organisations unfamiliar with providing this kind of service, and considerable inconsistency between the different organisations with contracts to provide ICAS. To a large extent these difficulties were ironed out over the ensuing years, but doubts still exist about the model that has been adopted. For example, the Mid-Staffordshire NHS Foundation Trust Public Inquiry heard evidence about how the provider of ICAS in that area was not connected with any of the other patient and public involvement bodies and did not identify concerns from complaints it helped with and take the issues up with the trust. Witnesses pointed out that this may have not been the case, had the CHC model or an updated version of it been retained. CHCs combined the complaints support role (carried out by paid staff) with the strategic monitoring role of its members (volunteers). Information was passed seamlessly from complaints staff to the members to allow issues being identified to be taken up.

This lack of a joined-up system of patient and public involvement, with the complaints support service being part and parcel of it, has led to repeated calls for a return to a model nearer that of the original CHC – a local 'one stop shop' for the public concerning the local NHS. There were hopes that that might be achieved by the creation of yet another new system of patient and public involvement, which is one of the changes brought in by the Health and Social Care Act. This creates local 'Healthwatch' organisations. However, whilst the legislation allows for the possibility that complaints support would be provided by Healthwatch if they decide to and are in a position to tender for this, this is dependent on whether the local authorities, which will hold the budgets for both Healthwatch and the complaints support, decide to go down that line. As it stands, it seems likely that the new system will result in even more inconsistency and fragmentation than has been experienced so far since the abolition of CHCs.

4.7   Health professional regulation / fitness to practise procedures

One of the options available to patients, families or members of the public with serious concerns about individual health professionals is to raise their concerns via the relevant regulator's 'fitness to practise' procedures for the given profession. In the case of nurses, this is the Nursing and Midwifery Council (NMC). Lay people are often confused about the purpose of fitness to practise procedures and the terminology used with regard to them. For example, these procedures cannot be used to have a general complaint or dissatisfaction with a health professional investigated. They are there to help protect patients and uphold professional standards by investigating concerns about a health professional's 'fitness to practise'. Yet the word 'complaint' is often used in connection with raising these concerns. A member of the public raising a fitness to practise concern is initially treated as a complainant, but if the regulator takes a case on for investigation, they then become merely a 'witness'. They have no special role in the procedures themselves, which are driven by the regulator and its lawyers. They can find themselves on the witness stand having their integrity called into question by a defence lawyer acting for the health professional. Most 'complaints' do not get as far as an investigation anyway. The vast majority are screened out as being inappropriate (i.e. not calling into question fitness to practise) or are simply referred on to an employer. If an employer does not have evidence of similar concerns, no further action normally results.

In terms of nursing, the NMC has been the subject of very severe criticism in recent years regarding how it meets its responsibilities for fitness to practise of nurses. In 2008 following criticism by MPs, a highly critical report was published by its overseer, the Commission for Healthcare Regulatory Excellence (CHRE).[9] This led to a new chief executive and chair being appointed. Yet in 2012 problems with the governance and fitness to practise procedures of the NMC persisted and the Government asked the CHRE to conduct another review. The NMC is now committed to a challenging programme of improvement as a result, under a new chairman and chief executive.

The NMC must also be seen in the context of the world of health professional regulation generally. In 2007 the then Labour Government published its White Paper *Trust Assurance and Safety: The regulation of health professionals in the 21st century*.[10] This represented the Government's long- awaited plan for modernising health professional regulation, following a series of high-profile scandals and inquiries, including Harold Shipman, Ayling, Neale and Kerr/Haslam. There then ensued over a year of intensive work by various multi-stakeholder groups set up by the Department of Health to make recommendations about the detailed way forward within the context of the White Paper. Not all the work was specifically relevant to hearing and acting on the concerns of patients and members of the public about health professionals but much of it was. From the perspective of patients and the public, two of the most important recommendations came through the working group reporting on 'Tackling Concerns Locally', as follows:[11]

(1) The recommendation to develop a funded specialist advice service for people considering raising a concern with regulators. The report of the working group recognised that this was a significant gap which needed filling. Whilst millions of pounds are spent on 'independent complaints advocacy services' dealing with NHS complaints across the board, including general dissatisfaction, waiting times, rudeness as well as complaints about clinical issues, that service is restricted to NHS complaints and is not geared up to help with fitness to practise cases. At present there is no funded service available to do this, but specialist charities such as AvMA do what they can using their own limited resources.

(2) Recommendations to open up information about concerns which have been raised about health professionals and in particular to make information-sharing between different employers, commissioners and regulators mandatory. This was in response to concerns that problems with health professionals are not routinely shared. For example, if a GP were found to be liable in a whole series of clinical-negligence cases it is possible that the primary care trust which is responsible for clinical governance and patient safety monitoring of GPs and the GMC would know nothing about it. There is no requirement to report this. The same applies to nurses and other health professionals. Also, employers are not required to pass on concerns about nurses or doctors to their regulator or to other employers.

At the time of writing neither of these recommendations had been acted upon, nor is there a published plan for doing so.

4.8   The NHS Constitution

The NHS Constitution for England[12] was published in 2010 following a period of consultation. It sets out the principles which govern the running of the NHS, the 'rights' which patients have and also reminds them (and NHS staff) of responsibilities. It also makes a number of commitments or 'pledges'. With respect to patients' complaints and redress, the Constitution says the following:

'**You have the right** to have any complaint you make about NHS services dealt with efficiently and to have it properly investigated.

You have the right to know the outcome of any investigation into your complaint.

You have the right to take your complaint to the independent Health Service Ombudsman, if you are not satisfied with the way your complaint has been dealt with by the NHS.

You have the right to make a claim for judicial review if you think you have been directly affected by an unlawful act or decision of an NHS body.

You have the right to compensation where you have been harmed by negligent treatment.

The NHS also commits:

- to ensure you are treated with courtesy and you receive appropriate support throughout the handling of a complaint; and the fact that you have complained will not adversely affect your future treatment (pledge);
- when mistakes happen, to acknowledge them, apologise, explain what went wrong and put things right quickly and effectively (pledge); and
- to ensure that the organisation learns lessons from complaints and claims and uses these to improve NHS services (pledge).'

It is important to note that the NHS Constitution did not introduce any new rights. Rather, it is a pulling together of various existing rights coupled with a number of aspirational pledges. Even the existing rights might be described as questionable. The claim that patients injured by negligent treatment have a right to receive compensation, for example, might be better phrased 'You have the right to seek compensation through the courts if you have been injured as a result of negligent treatment'. One might question the usefulness of restating what is any citizen's right – to engage in civil litigation – in the NHS Constitution. Few would argue, however, with the spirit of the pledges above, and restating clearly what existing rights are and what the NHS aspires to do has been widely welcomed. However, the Government resisted any moves to make it easy for anyone to challenge the Government or NHS bodies as to whether these rights or pledges are being honoured in practice. The accountability of NHS bodies to abide by the NHS Constitution is restricted to a statutory requirement 'to have regard to the NHS Constitution'. In theory this gives the Department of Health, commissioners and regulators of NHS services the ability to take NHS bodies to task over how well they meet this requirement. In 2011, in response to a Freedom of Information Act request by AvMA, the Department of Health admitted that it did not know of one example of where any NHS body had been taken to task over its responsibility to have regard to the NHS Constitution.

4.9   Conclusion

There have been considerable changes to the different systems for dealing with patient and family complaints and concerns over recent years and a growing awareness of the need to do more to change what remains all too often a defensive culture in healthcare. The policy intentions of the new NHS Complaints procedure – particularly to finally 'close the loop' so that lessons are learnt and improvements made – have been universally welcomed, but it remains to be seen whether the outcomes will be realised. There continue to be huge challenges for patients or their families in participating in processes such as health professional regulators' fitness to practise procedures, and litigation. Do not be surprised to see further changes to these areas over coming years, including reconsideration of some modified version of an NHS Redress small claims scheme. The NHS Constitution in its current form is at best a useful statement of values, aspirations and existing rights. It has the potential to be a much more potent initiative if ways were made to make it binding and to give patients (and regulators/commissioners) a means of holding NHS bodies to account for failing to comply with it. The most exciting prospect for cultural change in how healthcare providers react to adverse events is the statutory Duty of Candour which has finally been agreed to. Only time will tell how robustly this is framed and enforced and whether it delivers the more open and fair culture that most stake-holders crave for.

4.10   References

1. Making Experiences Count, Department of Health, 2008.
2. Making Amends, Department of Health, 2003.
3. Annual Report 2010–2011, NHS Litigation Authority, 2012.
4. Common Sense, Common Safety, Lord Young of Graffham, Cabinet Office, 2010.
5. Review of Civil Litigation Costs, Jackson, Rt Hon Lord Justice; The Stationery Office, 2009.
6. G. Cookson, *Unintended Consequences* (London, Kings College London, 2012).
7. 'Sixth Report: Complaints & Litigation', Health Committee, House of Commons, June 2011.
8. *Equity and Excellence: Liberating the NHS* (London, The Stationery Office, 2010).
9. Performance Review of the Nursing & Midwifery Council, Council for Health Regulatory Excellence (CHRE), June 2008.
10. Trust Assurance and Safety: the regulation of health professionals in the 21st century' The Stationery Office, 2007.
11. Tackling Concerns Locally – report of the working group, Department of Health, 2009.
12. NHS Constitution for England, Department of Health, 2010.

5 The Policy Dimension: Moving Beyond the Rhetoric Towards a Safer NHS

John Tingle

Reader in Health Law, Head of International Development, Nottingham Law School, Nottingham Trent University, Nottingham

As the previous chapters have indicated, the legal and health policy contexts of nursing have changed significantly since the third edition of this book appeared in 2007. My chapter in the third edition included discussion of the NHS Plan, the concept of 'patient empowerment', the NHS Redress Bill, and the National Patient Safety Agency (NPSA). Writing in 2013, six years on, the new NHS Redress Scheme which the NHS Redress Act 2006 heralded and which maintained the potential to provide a significant alternative to the courts for patients seeking compensation for injuries caused by clinical negligence is still not in force yet. One wonders whether it ever will be? The 2006 Act cannot be implemented until the Department of Health draws up draft regulations, which then need to be laid before Parliament. None has yet been drawn up.

The NPSA, the new kid on the block for the third edition, has now been abolished as part of the Department of Health review of arm's length bodies.[1] These are explained by the Department of Health as follows:

> A network of organisations has been created at national level, but at 'arm's length' from the Department of Health, to regulate the system, improve standards of care, protect public welfare, support local services and provide specialist advice. The work these organisations undertake ranges from back office administrative functions to complex ethical or clinical-related work.
>
> Arm's-length bodies are Government-funded organisations which work closely with local services and other arm's-length bodies. The Department has three main types of arm's-length bodies: Executive Agencies; Executive Non-Departmental Public Bodies; and Special Health Authorities.[1]

Nursing Law and Ethics, Fourth Edition. Edited by John Tingle and Alan Cribb.
© 2014 by John Wiley & Sons, Ltd. Published 2014 by John Wiley & Sons, Ltd.

The review took place as part of the Government's drive to reduce costs, to reduce the number of quangos and to maintain a coherent policy framework to support increased autonomy and clear accountability at every level in the NHS.[1]

The NPSA, through its research and publications, made a significant contribution to the development of a patient-safety culture in the NHS. It acted as a readily identifiable 'patient safety champion' and its demise leaves a vacuum in this area which is yet to be filled.

The term 'compensation culture' is still being bandied about by various groups, and the Government still seems worried that the perception, rightly or wrongly held, of a 'compensation culture' may be inhibiting public services such as the NHS and schools from doing their jobs properly.[2] Stories have appeared in the media of schools banning conker matches or insisting that pupils wear goggles while playing conkers. Some schools ban the common style of pencil sharpeners because they have razor blades in them. The former chief executive of the National Health Service Litigation Authority (NHSLA) has given an unequivocal 'no' to the question of whether or not a compensation culture exists in the NHS.[3] However, the issue remains a hotly debated one.

The Government responded to the compensation culture debate by passing the Compensation Act 2006 on 25 July 2006. This Act does a number of things, including giving a stronger public focus to the issue of suing for negligence. Judges are reminded that when they assess the standard of care to be exercised in a case, perfectly innocent activities like school trips and conker matches may suffer as a result. Putting the standard at too high a level may have the effect of cancelling out very socially useful activities.

In a clinical context, Good Samaritan health professionals may be put off rendering assistance. For example, a renal dialysis nurse with no first-aid training may have done her reasonable best at a road traffic accident, but the patient feels that she should have done more and sues. Section 1 of the 2006 Act provides that, when considering a claim in negligence or breach of statutory duty, a court may, in determining whether the defendant should have taken particular steps to meet a standard of care (whether by taking precautions or otherwise), have regard to whether a requirement to take those steps might prevent an activity that is desirable from taking place (either at all, to a particular extent, or in a particular way), or might discourage persons from undertaking functions in connection with the activity. Section 2 provides that an apology, an offer of treatment or other redress shall not of itself amount to an admission of negligence or breach of statutory duty. This provision is intended to reflect the existing law, as Section 1 does. No new law is created, but the provision gently reminds the courts of what the law is, and it reassures the public and our institutions. We do not want to lose socially useful activities because of an unfounded fear of litigation, or through a risk-obsessed culture. Thinking they might be sued for something naturally puts people off doing things, but proving negligence in reality is a very hard thing to do. Sadly, the media and some claims companies present a false picture of this reality. The Compensation Act 2006 will hopefully work to redress the balance, and there is some evidence already in cases that it is so doing.

A related issue is whether the NHS has gone too far down the road of patient empowerment and has created, in the minds of patients, unrealistic expectations of what can be achieved. Is it time to try to introduce patients to the notion that the NHS cannot always guarantee a perfect outcome? In Michael Powers' terms,[4] to introduce them to 'the politics of uncertainty'?

5.1 Substantive developments since last edition

5.1.1 Clinical negligence litigation cost containment: abolition of the NPSA

The most notable substantive developments since the last edition in the clinical negligence litigation and patient safety field must be in the area of clinical negligence litigation costs management and the abolition of the NPSA.

5.1.2 Clinical negligence: cost containment

The NHSLA has long been concerned by high claimant clinical negligence solicitors costs. In the 2011–12 report and accounts it states:

> The proportion of the total legal costs accounted for by claimants' lawyers rose to almost 80%, in these cases, which remains a matter of real concern. The use of Conditional Fee Agreements in clinical negligence actions almost always results in legal costs which are much higher relative to the value of the damages paid. This is especially the case for lower value claims.[5]

The Legal Aid, Sentencing and Punishment of Offenders Act 2012 contains important provisions on litigation funding and costs which will impact on clinical negligence litigation. Other changes will be made through the Civil Procedure Rules.

There will be major changes to legal aid funding for clinical negligence cases, which will result in its general withdrawal for these types of claims and which will only be available in a number of very restricted incidences.

The Act takes forward recommendations made by Lord Justice Jackson in his review of civil litigation costs.[6] The report states on clinical negligence litigation:

> There are two objectives which have to be borne in mind in relation to this area of litigation. First, patients who have been injured as a result of clinical negligence must have access to justice, so that they can receive proper compensation. Secondly, this huge area of public expenditure must be kept under proper control, so that the resources of the health service are not being squandered unnecessarily on litigation costs . . . The general reforms proposed in Part 2 of this report will assist in achieving those objectives.[6]

The Jackson review proposals included the following:

- Case management directions for clinical negligence cases should be harmonised across England and Wales.

- Costs management for clinical negligence cases should be piloted.
- Regulations should be drawn up in order to implement the NHS Redress Act 2006.[6]

5.1.3   Demise of the NPSA

On Friday 1 June 2012 the key functions and expertise for patient safety developed by the NPSA transferred to the NHS Commissioning Board Special Health Authority (the Board Authority). The NPSA was abolished as part of the Government's, arm's length bodies review.[1] The Agency did maintain an impressive armoury of tools to help trusts develop and maintain an effective patient safety culture, including the National Reporting and Learning System(NRLS). The NRLS is still with us with operational management from April 2012 being with Imperial College Healthcare Trust (ICHT). ICHT will manage the team responsible for the existing NRLS function for a temporary period of two years. Current staffing levels supporting the NRLS have transferred to ICHT. The arrangements are covered in The National Patient Safety Agency (Amendment) Directions 2012, and The Imperial College National Health Service Trust Directions 2012 (updated 10 September 2012).

The publications of the NPSA can still be accessed through the NHS Commissioning Board. The work of the NPSA proved to be very significant in developing a sound infrastructure for reflective and safe clinical practice and was heralded in the last edition. The NPSA established the NRLS.

As was stated in the third edition the NRLS is the world's first comprehensive patient safety adverse-incident reporting system. The NPSA had been the subject of some criticism for its delay in introducing the NRLS and in its feedback to trusts. NHS trusts generally perceived that the NPSA had failed to maximise learning because it had not provided feedback quickly and regularly. There was also a question mark over the value for money being achieved by the NPSA.[7]

5.1.4   Health and Social Care Act 2012

Improving the quality of NHS care is a key tenet of the new Health and Social Care Act 2012. The Act contains a duty on the Secretary of State of improving the quality of services. The Secretary of State for Health has a duty to keep the performance of the health service under review and to report annually to Parliament on his findings. His annual report must include details of what has been done to improve the quality of services and to reduce health inequalities.

5.1.5   Managing health litigation in the NHS

5.1.5.1   The National Health Service Litigation Authority

The National Health Service Litigation Authority (NHSLA) continues to positively contribute to improving patient safety by the Clinical Negligence Scheme for Trusts (CNST) and its other schemes. The NHSLA is a Special Health Authority and part of the NHS. It has a number of functions, which include indemnifying English NHS bodies against claims for clinical negligence, NHS litigation management, and raising the standards of risk management in the NHS. Marsh Risk Consulting recently did a review of the functions of the NHLSA as part of the arm's length review.[8] The report highlighted the positive role of the NHSLA and the effective contribution it had made since its establishment in 1995 but also found that there were some areas where the NHSLA did not achieve optimum performance. There are a number of practices that are commonly applied by commercial organisations that, it suggests, would lead to better performance in these areas. The Department of Health responded to the report,[9] broadly accepting the conclusions and recommendations it made and actions will be taken to make appropriate changes.

5.1.5.2   Towards the development of an NHS patient safety culture

The NHS can now be seen to be developing, albeit slowly, an ingrained patient safety culture. It has been a long time coming and there is a long way to go, but positive steps have been made. The NHS would now seem to be a much safer place than it was when the third edition of this book was published. The difficulty remains, however, that there is at present no scientifically based outcome measurement to prove this. Also the chief clarion and champion of patient safety in England, the NPSA, has gone. Only time will tell whether the NHS Commissioning Board adequately fills the vacuum left by the NPSA.

5.1.5.3   Filling the vacuum left by the abolition of the NPSA

This mantle, however, can be seen to be partially filled by the World Health Organization (WHO) Patient Safety Unit, who have produced lots of interesting material and where now the former Chief Medical Officer for England, Sir Liam Donaldson, resides as the WHO Patient Safety Ambassador. WHO have produced patient safety curriculum guides and other very useful publications.[10]

Another clarion of patient safety and quality that is helping to fill the vacuum left by the demise of the NPSA is the Health Foundation, an independent charity working to continually improve the quality of health care in the United Kingdom. They commission research in the area and have produced a number of excellent publications in the patient safety and health quality area.[11]

5.2   NHS Litigation levels: still a problem

NHS clinical negligence litigation is still as much a problem in 2013 as it was when the third edition was published in 2007 and before. In 2004/2005, the NHSLA[12] paid out £503 million for all clinical negligence schemes (2003/2004: £422 million). However, there was a drop in the actual number of claims made, from 6251 in 2003/2004 to 5609 in 2004/2005. Currently clinical negligence claims continue to rise. The NHSLA *Report and Accounts 2011–12* state:

New Claims Received

The number of new claims received in the year rose by 6%, a significant increase but a substantially lower one than in 2010-11 and lower than each of the previous three years.

. . . clinical and non-clinical claims grew at a similar rate (5.6% and 6.3% respectively) after the sudden sharp rise of over 30% in clinical claims in the year before. Part of the growth in claims volumes in recent years is attributable to the earlier reporting of claims and incidents by Trusts, enabling us to close many claims more quickly and to hold down the legal costs as a consequence.[5]

On NHS outstanding liability for clinical negligence claims, the NHSLA states:

As at 31 March 2012, the NHSLA estimates that it has potential liabilities of £18.9 billion, of which £18.6 billion relate to clinical negligence claims (the remainder being liabilities under PES and LTPS). This figure represents the estimated value of all known claims, together with an actuarial estimate of those incurred but not yet reported (IBNR), which may settle or be withdrawn over future years.[13]

Clinical negligence claims are certainly a major NHS budgetary concern, and the claims and the costs associated with them continue to rise, as can be seen from the discussions in the NHSLA *Report and Annual Accounts 2011–12*.[5] The time duration of claims is not as long as it was in previous years and matters have speeded up considerably. The main clinical and non-clinical schemes are both now averaging a total claim duration of less than 16 months.[5] Litigation in the NHS can still be seen to be a big and expensive problem as, it was in the last and previous editions of this book, and the sentiments expressed by the former Chief Medical Officer in *Making Amends* still hold true today:

Legal proceedings for medical injury frequently progress in an atmosphere of confrontation, acrimony, misunderstanding and bitterness. The emphasis is on revealing as little as possible about what went wrong, defending clinical decisions that were taken and only reluctantly releasing information. In the past, cases have taken too long to settle. In smaller value claims the legal costs have been disproportionate to the damages awarded. In larger value claims there can be lengthy and expensive disputes about the component parts of any lump sum payment and the anticipated life span of the victim.[14]

The Bristol Royal Infirmary Inquiry Report expressed similar sentiments:

The system is now out of alignment with other policy initiatives on quality and safety: in fact it serves to undermine those policies and inhibits improvements in the safety of the care received by patients. Ultimately, we take the view that it will not be possible to achieve an environment of full, open reporting within the NHS when, outside it, there exists a litigation system the incentives of which press in the opposite direction. We believe that the way forward lies in the abolition of clinical negligence litigation, taking clinical error out of the courts and the tort system.[15]

The clinical negligence tort-based system, however, has not been abolished and remains largely intact. When all the arguments are considered and balanced, it is hard to see why it should be abolished in regard to clinical errors. The courts provide a very useful mechanism of accountability in health care. Doctors and nurses are called to account for their actions or omissions, and reported court cases provide a rich source of education. The tort system also can be seen to act as a deterrence mechanism for poor conduct. To avoid going to court health carers need to practise safely. The tort system exists perfectly well for other professional disputes, and the arguments used to support its abolition in respect of clinical negligence cases just do not measure up. The Woolf reforms discussed in the Department of Health's *Making Amends*[14] and in the second edition of this book have worked to improve the situation in regard to clinical negligence litigation, and the NHS Redress Scheme discussed below has the potential to offer a really good alternative.

5.3 Changing the clinical negligence compensation system

There has been since the second and third edition of this book a lot of soul-searching about our clinical negligence system.[14] This fourth edition maintains the discussion of the NHS Redress Scheme as it previously appeared in the third edition, as the discussion is still relevant. The tensions and challenges addressed then are still with us in 2013.

The tort system has not fallen to any no-fault-based compensation schemes such as those that exist in New Zealand and Sweden. These and other no-fault systems were discussed in *Making Amends*[14] and rejected largely on grounds of their likely expense. The *Making Amends* report was very thorough and provides an excellent real-time account of the clinical negligence litigation system and its issues. Among the 19 recommendations of the report, the major one was for the establishment of an NHS Redress Scheme, described in Recommendation 1:

> An NHS Redress Scheme should be introduced to provide investigations when things go wrong; remedial treatment, rehabilitation and care where needed; explanations and apologies; and financial compensation in certain circumstances.[14]

Recommendation 12 was also a key proposal:

> A duty of candour should be introduced together with exemption from disciplinary action when reporting incidents with a view to improving patient safety.[14]

The former CMO in *Making Amends* also invited views on whether the *Bolam* test should continue to be used for the NHS Redress Scheme:

> The NHS Redress Scheme
>
> – What should be the qualifying criteria: the 'Bolam' test currently used in assessing clinical negligence or a broader definition of sub-standard care?
> – If the latter, what would be the preferred formulation?[14]

5.3.1   History and context of the NHS Redress Act 2006

The NHS Redress Bill was introduced into the House of Lords on 12 October 2005 and had been subject to major amendments before passing into law. The Government was defeated when the Lords voted by 157 to 144 to allow apologies and offers of treatment or redress to be made without admission of liability.[16] The Bill provided for the establishment of a scheme to enable the settlement, without the need to commence court proceedings, of certain claims that arise in connection with hospital services provided to patients as part of the health service in England, wherever those services are provided. The applicable law to be applied was the common law of tort, and the *Bolam* and *Bolitho* principles would apply.

5.3.2   *Bolam* and *Bolitho*

The CMO at the time and the Government did not feel the need to depart from the traditional common law tort definitions of fault with its focus on peer-related reasonable practice, and this was a major criticism of the Bill. Action against Medical Accidents (AvMA) have suggested that a different, 'avoidability' test should have applied:

> An adverse event is compensatable except where it is the result of an unavoidable complication regardless of treatment or non-treatment . . . The onus would be on the NHS to demonstrate that it was an unavoidable complication, or offer redress . . .[17]

This AvMA proposal works in effect to switch the burden of proof from the claimant onto the defendant to disprove negligence. The test makes a lot of sense but it could and probably was viewed as too radical and perhaps too alien a construct to adopt in the context of a tort-based adversarial legal system. Lawyers and others are more comfortable and used to dealing with the *Bolam* and *Bolitho* framework for establishing fault. It is quite a bold step to say that as a trust, unless you can prove otherwise, you have to compensate the patient because he or she was treated in your hospital.

The tort system is, by its very nature, adversarial, and justice surely dictates that both claimant and defendant should be treated from a basis of equality and fairness and should start off from a level playing field. The patient clearly is the weaker party in the care equation, but then they would be if suing a commercial company for breach of contract or for faulty goods or services. Why should suing for clinical negligence fundamentally alter their status? The fact that they can access proper specialist professional legal advice corrects that power and knowledge imbalance, as it does in the other suing instances mentioned.

5.3.3   The NHS Redress Bill

When the Bill was going through Parliament it was thought that in order for it to work properly, it was important that patients have proper access to legal advice when entering the scheme and progressing through it as well as when considering any offer made under it.[18] The parameters of applicable cases to which any such scheme can apply, and which bodies can be members of a scheme, were stated and the Secretary of State given powers to set out in regulations the detailed rules that govern the scheme. These have still to be issued. The scheme covers people with claims in tort arising out of hospital treatment as part of the NHS, wherever that hospital treatment may be provided.[19] Not all tort claims are covered, but only those that are 'qualifying liabilities in tort'. These are defined as:

> liabilities in tort (a) in respect of personal injury or loss arising out of a breach of a duty of care in relation to the diagnosis of illness, or the care or treatment of any patient, and (b) arising as a consequence of any act or omission by a healthcare professional.[18]

The scheme will provide for financial compensation to be offered, and will specify an upper limit on the total amount of financial compensation that may be included in an offer under the scheme. It is currently intended that this limit will be set at £20,000 initially.[19] The DH states that the scheme will not cover systems negligence:

> A claim which alleges that a scheme member is directly liable in negligence for system failure or organisational error will not be within the scope of the scheme if the organisational error did not involve any act or omission by a health care professional. The reason for this is that the scheme is intended to cover low-level clinical negligence claims, which can be quickly investigated and resolved.[19]

The Bill did not have an easy passage through Parliament, and many believed that it was fundamentally flawed. AvMA states:

> AvMA, like most patients' organisations, welcomes the stated intentions of the NHS Redress Scheme which the Bill creates, but believes that, as currently designed, the scheme is fundamentally flawed and would have the opposite of the desired effects.[20]

Sixteen other patients' groups formally agreed with AvMA that improvements were needed to the Bill and signed up to the following statement:

The NHS Redress Bill should be improved to address:

- the need to have an independent means of deciding upon the merits of cases for redress under the scheme, rather than decisions being made by the NHS Trusts/the NHS Litigation Authority themselves
- the need for the advice and assistance to be provided to patients/their families during the scheme to be sufficiently expert in medico-legal matters and clinical negligence
- the need for more robust measures to ensure that lessons are learnt from medical errors identified through the scheme and action taken to improve patient safety.[20]

The Bill was notably thin on detail, and fundamentally, as *Bolam* and *Bolitho* remain the tests for deciding fault, the patient does need advice and assistance at the start, during and at the end of the claim. Clinical negligence litigation is generally notably complex, and the NHS Redress Scheme must not just be seen as a financially driven short-cut that compromises patient rights. The Government to its credit did not see it that way, and the roots of its thinking can be seen in *Making Amends*[14] and in the words of the Bristol Inquiry report.[15] The key is to make the scheme 'robust, independent and fair'.

The Bill improved as it progressed through Parliament and was amended significantly at the report stage debate in the House of Commons on Thursday, 13 July 2006, and changes made to make the scheme more independent, to give specialist advice and representation to patients, and for measures to ensure that patient safety lessons are learnt and implemented. The statutory duty of candour was also missing from both the Bill when it was originally published and eventually the Act. The softer option of leaving it to the NPSA to tell trusts to develop candour policies into patient communication strategies was adopted.[21] The duty of candour debate is still very much a live one, as AvMA state:

04.12.12: DoH Relegate Duty of Candour to Standard Clause in Hospital Contracts.

The Department of Health today announced that it will press ahead with its version of a Duty of Candour with patients when things go wrong – a mere standard clause in NHS contracts which will not cover GPs and dentists. This is in spite of widespread calls for a statutory duty as part of the 'Essential Standards of Quality & Safety' regulated by the Care Quality Commission, and an anticipated recommendation for a statutory duty from the Mid Staffordshire Public Inquiry. AvMA chief executive Peter Walsh described the move as an apparently cynical attempt to sidestep overwhelming support for a statutory duty and to pre-empt the public inquiry report. AvMA and other patients groups will continue to press for a full statutory duty of candour.[22]

Lord Justice Jackson is in favour of the NHS Redress Act and stated:[6]

The scheme envisaged by the 2006 Act is a sensible one, which will facilitate the early and economic resolution of lower value clinical negligence claims in respect of hospital treatment. An important factor is that, within the court system, clinical negligence claims of whatever value are assigned to the multi-track. This increases litigation costs. In my view, it would now be appropriate to draw up regulations in order to implement the 2006 Act. The proposed redress scheme is one which will promote access to justice at proportionate cost. The detailed content of any regulations made under the 2006 Act will require consultation. The regulations will cover matters such as the upper limit for financial compensation, what legal costs should be paid in respect of successful claims under the scheme, what legal work those costs should cover and so forth. I appreciate that drawing up draft regulations and then consulting AvMA, claimant solicitors, defendant solicitors, the NHSLA and others will take a little time. Nevertheless the Government has now had three years since the 2006 Act was drawn up. This matter should now be taken forward both in the interests of patients and (no less important) in the interests of saving the NHS from paying out unnecessary litigation costs.[6]

5.3.4   Progress towards developing an ingrained patient safety culture in the NHS

5.3.4.1   Patient safety initiatives

Since the second and third editions of this book appeared, a number of significant developments have occurred in the patient safety area within the NHS. A developing and pro-active patient safety infrastructure and culture can now be seen to be emerging. It is in this area that nurses and other health carers can make the most fundamental contribution to helping patients and securing their safety. There is a need for the individual nurse to be aware of the patient safety systems that exist, to understand why errors occur and then to guard against them. Participation in and promotion of patient safety strategies are vitally important if an ingrained patient safety culture is ever going to be developed in the NHS.

5.3.5   Tentative first steps

The Department of Health set the scene for the development of an NHS patient safety structure with *An Organization with a Memory*.[23] This report examined the key factors at work in organisational failure and learning. Practical experience from other sectors was analysed, and conclusions and recommendations drawn. One major recommendation was for the creation of a new national system for reporting and analysing adverse health incidents. The report noted that patient safety research and the knowledge of adverse incident rates in the United Kingdom were in their infancy:

> Yet the best research-based estimates we have reveal enough to suggest that in NHS hospitals alone adverse events in which harm is caused to patients:
>
> – occur in around 10 per cent of admissions – or at a rate in excess of 850,000 a year;
> – cost the service an estimated £2 billion a year in additional hospital stays alone, without taking any account of human or wider economic costs . . . Inquiries and incident investigations determine that 'the lessons must be learned', but the evidence suggests that the NHS as a whole is not good at doing so.[23]

The Health Foundation Research Scan[24] explores what is known about levels of harm in acute and primary care, the main causes of harm and whether or not harm is avoidable. The report reviewing more recent research suggests that levels of harm range between 3 and 25 per cent in acute care. It argues that the simplest definition of harm in health care is a negative effect, whether or not the effect is evident to the patient. The report states that there is very little published evidence from which to draw conclusions about levels of patient harm in primary care, but that the available evidence suggests that harm might be evident in 9 per cent of primary care records or around one in 48 consultations (25 per cent). This may include harms in both primary and secondary care.

The next stage was to take forward the recommendations made in *An Organisation with a Memory*, and this was done in *Building a Safer NHS for Patients*.[25] This report focused on the implementation strategies for developing a patient safety culture in the NHS, to ensure that patient safety lessons are learnt across the whole NHS. The foundation stones of the NPSA were laid in this document. The report placed patient safety within the context of the Government's NHS quality programme and highlighted linkages to other government initiatives. Central to the plan was the creation of a new national reporting scheme for adverse health care events and near-misses within the NHS, now known as the NRLS. The NPSA was set up in July 2001. The first NHS organisations were connected to the NRLS in November 2003, and all NHS organisations have had the capacity to report incidents to the NRLS since December 2004.

The Care Quality Commission (CQC)[26,27] state what health organisations must report to the NRLS:

5. Is it mandatory for NHS providers to report all patient safety incidents to the NRLS?

No. It is only mandatory to submit reports about the events and incidents shown in the tables above and described in detail in the Guidance about compliance: essential standards of quality and safety.

These reports are about the most serious of the incidents previously reported under voluntary arrangements. Reports about other kinds of events will continue to be made under the NRLS's voluntary arrangements.[26]

5.3.6   The state of play on patient safety incidents

The NPSA published its first NHS patient safety data analysis, which gave some indication of how patient safety matters are proceeding in the NHS, in 2005.[29] Until the end of March 2005, 85,342 patient safety incidents were reported. Most of these (68 per cent of the total) resulted in no harm to patients. Of the reported incidents, about one in 100 led to severe harm or death. In acute hospital settings, about three in every 1000 reported incidents resulted in death. Based on incidents and deaths reported over a three-month period by 18 trusts, the NPSA has estimated that each year there would be approximately 840 deaths and 572,000 incidents reported in acute trusts in England. The most common types of incidents reported are patient accidents (in particular, falls) and incidents associated with treatment, procedures and medication. Reporting levels are, according to the report, 'increasing rapidly'. These data, which have not been available before, are important as they provide a useful picture of patient safety in NHS trusts. The data can help inform the development of patient safety strategies at the individual health care, trust and NPSA levels. The Health Foundation[24] discusses errors in health care and states that the most common types are medication errors, administrative errors and diagnosis errors. The report discusses the factors thought to contribute to adverse events in health care. Factors include; human factors such as teamwork, communication, stress and burnout; structural factors such as reporting systems, infrastructure, workforce loads and the environment; and clinical factors such as complexity of care and length of stay. Most harm encountered is not severe. Older people are most likely to be effected. The report discusses preventability and states that though the most effective interventions remain a matter of debate, it is estimated that up to half of all adverse events are avoidable if good professional practice and evidence-based care are followed.

The NHS Commissioning Board have released figures of Organisation Patient Safety Incident reports[28]:

90 per cent of trusts in England submitted incident reports to the National Reporting and Learning System for this set of data. 53 per cent of organisations reported monthly during this period, compared with 59 per cent last time.

The data demonstrates that there is increased reporting of incidents to the National Reporting and Learning System, maintaining improvements in reporting culture. The data also shows that:

- 413,459 (68 per cent) of patient safety incident reports resulted in no harm to the patient;
- 154,681 (25 per cent) resulted in low harm;
- 39,039 (6 per cent) resulted in moderate harm;
- 5,235 (2 per cent) resulted in death or severe harm.

The most common types of incident reported were: patient accidents–slips, trips and falls (26 per cent); medication incidents (11 per cent); incidents relating to treatment and/or procedures (11 per cent). This trend remains consistent with previous data releases.[28]

5.3.7   The NPSA patient safety tools: resources

The NPSA has developed training support resources that include e-learning training modules, the incident decision tree (IDT), video-based training workshops, a safety culture survey, Root Cause Analysis (RCA) training and workshops.[29] (See the NHS Commissioning Board web site, Patient Safety section, http://www.commissioningboard.nhs.uk/ourwork/patientsafety/.) These can all help NHS health care staff and trusts develop a safer patient care environment. Key NPSA publications include *Being Open: Communicating Patient Safety Incidents with Patients and Their Carers*,[21] the *Manchester Patient Safety Framework (MaPSaF)*,[30] the *Patient Safety Bulletin*[31] and *Seven Steps to Patient Safety*.[32] *Seven Steps to Patient Safety* is a simple checklist for NHS staff to follow and to measure

---

Box 5.1   The seven steps to patient safety.

Step 1   Build a safety culture
Create a culture that is open and fair

Step 2   Lead and support your staff
Establish a clear and strong focus on patient safety throughout your organisation

Step 3   Integrate your risk management activity
Develop systems and processes to manage your risks and identify and assess things that could go wrong

Step 4   Promote reporting
Ensure your staff can easily report incidents locally and nationally

Step 5   Involve and communicate with patients and the public
Develop ways to communicate openly with and listen to patients

Step 6   Learn and share safety lessons
Encourage staff to use root cause analysis to learn how and why incidents happen

Step 7   Implement solutions to prevent harm
Embed lessons through changes to practice, processes or systems

Source: National Patient Safety Agency, *Seven Steps to Patient Safety: An Overview Guide for NHS Staff*, 2nd Print. London: NPSA, April 2004. © NPSA. Reprinted with permission.

---

their performance against so that they can help ensure a safe health care environment (Box 5.1).

The above NPSA publications and tools are all well written and contain straightforward and well-considered advice. If the advice is followed, an ingrained patient safety culture in the NHS may yet become a firm reality.

It is important to determine whether all this patient safety activity has worked. In order to find out, a number of possible performance indicators need to be considered. In doing this, it also needs to be accepted that in a complex health care environment such as the NHS, which treats over a million patients every day, some errors will be inevitable. In reality, the best we can hope to do is to try to minimise their occurrence as much as possible through adopting effective patient safety and clinical risk management strategies.

5.3.8   Some error statistics

The NHS 2005 staff survey (Table 5.1) shows that errors are still fairly endemic in the NHS.

Table 5.1   Statements about incident reporting

	% agree or strongly agree	% disagree or strongly disagree
My trust treats fairly those staff who are involved in an error, near miss or incident	40%	7%
My trust encourages us to report errors, near misses or incidents	75%	4%
My trust treats reports of errors, near misses or incidents confidentially	52%	6%
My trust blames or punishes people who make errors, near misses or incidents	9%	39%
When errors, near misses or incidents are reported, my trust takes action to ensure that they do not happen again	50%	8%
We are informed about errors, near misses and incidents that happen in the trust	30%	31%
We are given feedback about changes made in response to reported errors, near misses and incidents	33%	28%

Source: Healthcare Commission, *National Survey of NHS Staff 2005*, Summary of key findings (London, Healthcare Commission, March 2006). Reprinted with permission.

Errors and incidents:

- 40 per cent reported seeing at least one potentially harmful error, near-miss or incident that could have hurt either staff or patients in the previous month
- a fall in the number of staff witnessing at least one potentially harmful error, nearmiss or incident from 47 to 40 in 2003 to 2005
- generally employees feel that trusts are encouraging them to report errors, near-misses or incidents and 83 per cent said that the last potentially harmful error, nearmiss or incident they witnessed was definitely reported by them or a colleague
- but fewer staff are confident that their employer treats those involved fairly, handles reports confidentially and takes action to prevent recurrence.[33]

The National Survey of NHS Staff 2010 found on errors, near-misses and incidents:

Thirty-two per cent of staff said they had seen at least one error, 'near miss' or incident that could have hurt staff or patients in the last month (compared with 33% in 2009). Of front-line staff, 42% said that they had witnessed at least one such adverse event in the last month (43% in 2009). The number of ambulance staff witnessing errors, near misses or incidents has decreased from 37% in 2009 to 34% in 2010.[34]

5.4   Some patient safety performance indicators

5.4.1   Clinical governance

The concept of clinical governance is a central NHS quality improvement strategy. The concept incorporates clinical risk management and CNST compliance. If trusts have good clinical governance ratings, then they must be taking some positive steps in relation to risk management and patient safety. The Healthcare Commission used to be responsible for performance rating and monitoring trusts in regard to clinical governance compliance. The duty of regulation now falls to the Care Quality Commission (CQC). The CQC is the independent regulator of health and adult social care services in England. They also protect the interests of people whose rights are restricted under the Mental Health Act 1983.

According to the National Audit Office (NAO):

> The key principles of clinical governance . . . are: a coherent approach to quality improvement, clear lines of accountability for clinical quality systems and effective processes for identifying and managing risk and addressing poor performance. It involves putting in place the information, methods and systems to ensure good quality so that problems are identified early, analysed and action taken to avoid any further repetition. The Department of Health (the Department) expects clinical governance to integrate the previously rather disparate and fragmented approaches to quality improvement, such as clinical audit, risk management, incident reporting and continuing professional development into a single system and to ally it to accountability for quality.[35]

The NAO conclude in their report that the Government's clinical governance initiative has had many beneficial impacts. Clinical quality issues have been made more mainstream, and there is a greater or more explicit accountability of both clinicians and managers for clinical performance.[35]

The report notes[35] that there has been a change in professional cultures towards more open, transparent and collaborative ways of working. Evidence of improvements in practice and patient care was also noted, though it is stated that trusts lack robust means of assessing this and overall progress:

> However, our research and the outcome of the Commission for Health Improvement's reviews indicate that progress in implementing clinical governance is patchy, varying between trusts, within trusts and between the components of clinical governance. There is, not surprisingly, scope for improvement in: the support provided to trusts; putting in place overall structures and processes; communications between boards and clinical teams; developing a coherent approach to quality; and improving processes for managing risk and poor performance. There is also a need to improve the way that lessons are learnt both within and between trusts; and to put those lessons into practice. Overall, the key features of those organisations that have been better at improving the quality of care are quality of leadership, commitment of staff and willingness to consider doing things differently.[35]

The CQC state on clinical governance:

We have not specifically described what a system of clinical governance should look like in this guide, as clinical governance has several purposes beyond simply establishing the essential standards of quality and safety. However, it is important for providers of healthcare to have a strong system of clinical governance in place. While the guide as a whole supports the development of an effective clinical governance system, we believe that the outcomes and prompts for the following outcomes are of particular importance:

- Outcome 1: Respecting and involving people who use services
- Outcome 2: Consent to care and treatment
- Outcome 4: Care and welfare of people who use services
- Outcome 6: Cooperating with other providers
- Outcome 7: Safeguarding people who use services from abuse
- Outcome 8: Cleanliness and infection control
- Outcome 9: Management of medicines
- Outcome 10: Safety and suitability of premises
- Outcome 11: Safety, availability and suitability of equipment
- Outcome 12: Requirements relating to workers
- Outcome 14: Supporting workers
- Outcome 16: Assessing and monitoring the quality of service provision
- Outcome 17: Complaints
- Outcome 21: Records[27]

5.4.2   Patient safety initiatives

The NAO also looked at the Government's patient safety initiatives and found that progress is being made:

The safety culture within trusts is improving, driven largely by the Department's clinical governance initiative and the development of more effective risk management systems in response to incentives under initiatives such as the NHS Litigation Authority's Clinical Negligence Scheme for Trusts . . . However, trusts are still predominantly reactive in their response to patient safety issues and parts of some organisations still operate a blame culture.[36]

It was stated in the report that all trusts have established effective reporting systems at the local level, although under-reporting remains a problem within some groups of staff, types of incidents and near misses; also, most trusts pointed to specific improvements derived from lessons learnt from their local incident reporting systems, but these are still not widely promulgated, either within or between trusts. It was also found that the NPSA has provided only limited feedback to trusts of evidence-based solutions or actions derived from the national reporting system – a point emphasised and developed by the House of Commons Committee of Public Accounts.[7]

The House of Commons Health Committee also looked at patient safety, and stated:

Although reporting is useful for learning from incidents, it is not a reliable way of measuring the extent of harm. Judging the overall effectiveness of patient safety policy is made difficult because of the failure by the Department of Health (DH) to collect adequate data. Nevertheless, it is apparent that, for all the policy innovations of the past decade, there has been insufficient progress in making services safer. Underlying Lord Darzi's emphasis in the Next Stage Review on safety, there appears to be a tacit admission that not all services are safe enough yet. The perception that this is so is strengthened by the recent cases of disastrously unsafe care that have come to light in a small number of Trusts, such as Mid Staffordshire NHS Foundation Trust.[37]

The Committee made a number of recommendations and stated in summary:

The Government is to be praised for being the first in the world to adopt a policy which makes patient safety a priority. However, Government policy has too often given the impression that there are priorities, notably hitting targets (particularly for waiting lists, and Accident and Emergency waiting), achieving financial balance and attaining Foundation Trust status, which are more important than patient safety. This has undoubtedly, in a number of well documented cases, been a contributory factor in making services unsafe.

All Government policy in respect of the NHS must be predicated on the principle that the first priority, always and without exception, is to ensure that patients do not suffer avoidable harm. The key tasks of the Government are to ensure that the NHS:

develops a culture of openness and 'fair blame';
strengthens, clarifies and promulgates its whistleblowing policy;
provides leadership which listens to and acts upon staff suggestions for service changes to improve efficiency and quality and, by the provision of examples and incentives, encourages and enables staff to implement practical and proven improvements in patient safety.

In addition, the Government should examine the contribution of deficiencies in regulation to failures in patient safety.[37]

Another performance indicator of how well trusts are doing in patient safety and clinical risk management is the trust's CNST-achieved compliance level.[38]

If trusts have a low CNST rating, then probably not much is happening with patient safety; conversely, a high rating indicates a firm trust commitment to the concept.

5.4.3   The schemes managed by the NHSLA[39]

The NHSLA handles negligence claims on behalf of the NHS under a number of different schemes, as follows:

- The Clinical Negligence Scheme for Trusts (CNST) is a voluntary risk-pooling scheme for clinical negligence claims arising out of incidents occurring after 1 April 1995, funded out of members' contributions.
- The Existing Liabilities Scheme (ELS) covers clinical negligence claims arising out of incidents which occurred before 1 April 1995. It is not a contributory scheme: the costs of funding settlements made under ELS are covered centrally by the Department of Health.
- The Ex-RHAs Scheme covers any clinical liabilities incurred by the Regional Health Authorities before their abolition in April 1996, with the NHSLA itself acting as defendant.
- The Liabilities to Third Parties Scheme covers non-clinical 'third party' liabilities such as public and employers liability claims. Like CNST, it is a voluntary scheme funded through members' contributions.
- The Property Expenses Scheme covers 'first-party' losses by NHS bodies such as property loss or damage. Again it is a voluntary scheme, funded through members' contributions.[39]

5.5   How they work

Clinical risk management is a fundamental feature of the NHSLA schemes. Health organisations are assessed against a number of standards. These standards are good practice standards which are evidence-based. There is a set of risk management standards for each type of health care organisation incorporating organisational, clinical, and health and safety risks: acute, PCT & independent sector standards; mental health and learning disability standards; ambulance standards; and maternity standards.[40] The latest versions of these standards and the results of assessments are available on the NHSLA website at: http://www.nhsla.com/Pages/Home.aspx. Organisations which provide labour ward services are subject to assessment against both the acute (and PCT) standards and the maternity standards.[40] To help health organisations implement and sustain these standards the NHSLA maintains a programme of guidance and training. NHS bodies pay the NHSLA a financial contribution, a premium, which goes into a mutual pool. In return the NHSLA take over the negligence claim and will pay any compensation awarded by a court. The NHSLA may decide to defend or settle the claim without going to court. Most cases do not go to court and are settled. Currently, fewer than 2 per cent of the cases handled by the NHSLA end up in court, with the remainder settled out of court or abandoned by the claimant.[41] Discounts in contributions are available to those trusts that comply with the programmes of clinical risk management standards and to those with a good claims history. Discount levels are Level 1: 10 per cent; Level 2: 20 per cent; and Level 3: 30 per cent.[38] The maternity standards are also divided into three levels, and organisations successful at assessment receive a discount of 10 per cent, 20 per cent or 30 per cent from the maternity portion of their CNST contribution.[40]

Although scheme membership is voluntary, all NHS trusts (including foundation trusts) and PCTs in England currently belong. PCTs were abolished under the Health and Social Care Act 2012. The NHSLA state that these standards are assessed progressively and that each criterion has been allocated to one of three levels: Level 1 criteria represent the basic elements of a clinical risk management framework. Levels 2 and 3 are more demanding. Many are concerned with the implementation and integration into practice of policies and procedures, monitoring them and acting on the results. These levels also require staff to have a good understanding of clinical risk issues.[42]

The NHSLA state:

> The progression of organisations through the standards is logical and follows the development, implementation, monitoring and review of policies and procedures.
>
> Level 1 deals with establishing effective risk management systems and processes.
>
> Level 2 assesses whether the systems described at level 1 have been implemented.
>
> Level 3 concentrates on whether the organisation is monitoring its compliance with the systems and acting on the findings.[38]

Figure 5.1 lists the total number of reported CNST claims by specialty as at 31/03/12 (since the scheme began in April 1995, excluding 'below excess' claims handled by trusts).[43]

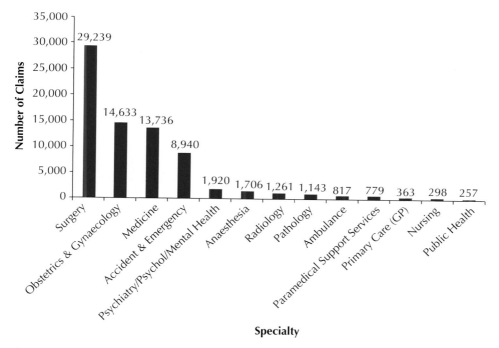

Figure 5.1   The total number of reported CNST claims by specialty as at 31/03/12. Reproduced with permission of The NHS Litigation Authority.

5.5.1   Most trusts are at level 1

The CNST was started in 1995 and while most trusts are still at level 1, it is fair to say that there has been a drift upwards towards a generally higher compliance level. In 2005/06 the gap narrowed between those trusts at level 1 and those at level 2. In assessing the success or otherwise of the CNST it is important to remember that level 1 shows that trusts maintain the basic elements of a clinical risk management framework. Looking at the criteria again, level 1 trusts have yet to implement, integrate and pro-actively work with the CNST standards, which is worrying.[38,42]

The reasonable man or woman in the street or, to borrow from the law of tort, the man or woman on the 'Clapham omnibus', would surely assume that after a good many years of the CNST (since 1995), most trusts would be at level 2, if not 3. What have the trusts being doing since 1995? How seriously have they taken clinical risk management and patient safety? According to the CNST levels, there has been only incremental developing interest over the period. The development of the NPSA patient safety infrastructure has brought about some discernible improvements here. The basic underlying problem is that good patient safety practices have yet to filter down properly to trusts and the workforce.

The NHLSA Report and Accounts 2011–12 has some trust assessment data which states:

'Assessments

. . . 54% (2010–'11 56%) of Trusts finished the year at Level 1; 33% (2010–'11 35%) at Level 2; and 11% (2010–'11 9%) at Level 3. A further 11 (2%) Trusts had no accreditation, in most cases because they were yet to be assessed.'[5]

Figure 5.2 shows the assessment picture.

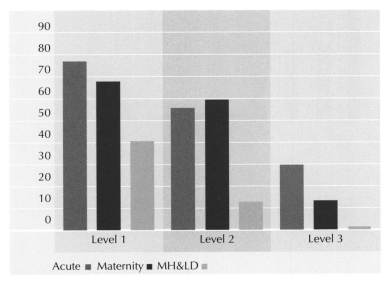

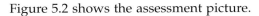

Figure 5.2   Number of trusts at each assessment level.[5] Reproduced with permission of The NHS Litigation Authority.

5.5.2   The Former CMO's view

In his annual report for 2004, the former Chief Medical Officer (CMO), Sir Liam Donaldson, stated, in the section on compliance with patient safety alerts, particularly with intrathecal chemotherapy guidance:

> In spite of all this, and of the continuing risk of another tragic death in their hospitals, NHS Trusts took 19 months to comply with the original guidance and 18 months to comply with revised guidance and, worse still, after a first round of peer review visits, 47 per cent of trusts were still not fully compliant with the latest up-to-date guidance. This case study reveals much about the safety culture of the NHS, which is clearly not yet focused or organized enough to reduce a potentially fatal risk to patients rapidly enough.[44]

Fair comment by the former CMO, which in a sense puts the less than satisfactory CNST trust attainment levels in some perspective.

5.5.3   Government 'overkill' and trust financial austerity: a defence for trusts?

Primary and secondary care in the NHS have been subject to many competing agendas over this last 15 years – certainly since the second edition of this book – and they continue to be so. The NHS is in a constant state of reform or revolution, as successive governments try to manage it effectively. It is a monolithic structure and by definition a high-risk and very technical enterprise. As we prepare new editions of this book, the NHS always seems to going through a period of financial austerity, and we pose the question whether the quality and safety agendas can survive in the not-so-new climate of thrift and financial austerity. Will the agendas remain at or near the top of trust agendas?

The patient safety agenda seems to have slipped from the top of agendas, and there is a vacuum left by the abolition of the NPSA that urgently needs filling.

There has been very little outcome measurement on whether risk management actually works and saves money. Our best guess is that it does. Common sense, however, would dictate that if you practise safely and more reflectively, then the risk of adverse incidents occurring should be reduced.

Sadly, in the past the Government has been guilty of 'overkill' in its health quality reform agenda and has exposed trusts to too much regulation in the field of health quality and patient safety. It has only recently started to consolidate overlapping arm's length agencies and policies that govern the area.

The Regulatory Impact Unit of the Cabinet Office in a joint report with the Department of Health said:

> A multitude of organisations undertake some form of inspection, accreditation or audit in the NHS. The bulk are statutory organisations or professional bodies, but a significant number are voluntary. Front-line staff and management

acknowledge the value added by inspection in driving up standards in health care, enhancing public accountability and ensuring patient safety. However, several recurring themes relating to review activity arose during the course of these interviews that were seen by staff to hamper effective delivery of health care. They were:

- Multiplicity, overlap and lack of co-ordination between reviewing organisations and their functions
- Duplication and inconsistency in requests for data and information
- Proportionality and transparency of reviews
- Burdens of preparation for reviews
- Benefits of review outputs.[45]

This report led to a concordat being published by the Healthcare Commission.[46] The concordat provides a code of objectives and practices for government and independent inspectorates to deliver more joined-up and appropriate inspection programmes that reduce the burden of inspection on health care staff.

This 'overkill' has, however, left its mark; there is now concern as to the responsiveness of NHS professionals to patient safety and quality initiatives. A fear is that the plethora of safety and quality initiatives have swamped the NHS in recent years. The 'overkill' may have desensitised staff that may see concepts such as clinical governance or clinical guidelines more as management tools designed to restrict professional autonomy and driven primarily by cost-cutting considerations.

The Health Foundation[47] have published a report which states that health professionals are generally reluctant to get actively involved in broader initiatives aimed at quality improvement. Many clinicians, the report states, are detached from, ambivalent about, hostile towards, or confused about, the concept of clinical governance. Some also do not regard such tools as clinical guidelines as being useful:

> ... although managers support greater systematization of clinical work through the use of such tools as clinical guidelines, the majority of clinicians do not always regard these guidelines and related initiatives as useful tools in providing quality of care. Clinicians may even resist them because they are perceived as hampering clinical freedom and impeding local practice. These perceptions and attitudes may be subtly changing over time, reflecting the greater integration of guidelines and EBP into organisations and quality initiatives or programmes.[47]

The Health Foundation canvass a solution to the problem of clinician engagement:

> The Health Foundation wants to inspire and build the will, enthusiasm and commitment among clinical communities to acknowledge and adopt system-wide quality improvement methods to enhance the patient experience and the quality of clinical care. The evidence from this review suggests that this goal will need a collaborative dialogue with healthcare professionals to explore what this means for the established model of professionalism.

We believe that an enhanced model of professionalism is required and one that has a number of components. It places a stronger emphasis on accountability, recognises the benefits of creating a different dynamic between patients and professionals, assumes a stronger sense of responsibility for how the wider health system works and for all dimensions of quality.[47]

A way forward might be to imbue patient safety and clinical quality with a human-rights dimension. By selecting and applying various United Nations conventions it will be possible to place patient safety and health care quality on a higher plane so that doctors, nurses and managers see the issue as a truly fundamental one.

5.6   Postcript

The NHS Commissioning Board name changed to NHS England on 1st April 2013.

The publication of the Mid Staffordshire NHS Foundation Trust Public Inquiry Report on 6 February 2013[48] has catapulted the issue of patient safety in NHS hospitals into the living room of every home in the United Kingdom. The report has been on the front page of daily newspapers across the country and has been the lead story on television news. *The Times* on 7 February had the banner front-page headline saying, 'NHS: No one is safe'.

The Francis report's finding have been well publicised, patients were let down by the Mid Staffordshire NHS Foundation Trust. There was a lack of care, compassion, humanity and leadership. The most basic standards of care were not observed, and fundamental rights to dignity were not respected. Elderly and vulnerable patients were left unwashed, unfed and without fluids. Some patients had to relieve themselves in their beds when they were offered no help to get to the bathroom. There were incidents of callous treatment by staff. Medicines were prescribed and not given. Patients who could not eat or drink without help did not receive it. There were insufficient staff on some wards and in the Accident & Emergency Department to deliver safe and effective care. There were also poor hospital discharge arrangements.

5.6.1   Some key patient safety recommendations

5.6.1.1   An integrated hierarchy of standards: common values: putting the patient first

The Francis report took the view that in relation to the CQC (Care Quality Commission), the current structure of standards, laid down in regulation, interpreted by categorisation and development in guidance, and measured by the judgement of a regulator, is clearly an improvement on what has gone on before, but it requires improvement. The report states that the standards to be enforced by the regulator should be a clear fundamental set of standards driven by the interests of patients, and devised by clinicians – a bottom up as opposed to a 'top down' system. The report states:

Unfortunately, for all its good intentions and its improvement on what went before, the current outcomes are over-bureaucratic and fail to separate clearly what is absolutely essential from that which is merely desirable.[48]

Recommendation 13 states the nature of standards.
Standards should be divided into the following:

Fundamental standards of minimum safety and quality – in respect of which non-compliance should not be tolerated. Failures leading to death or serious harm should remain offences for which prosecutions can be brought against organisations. There should be a defined set of duties to maintain and operate an effective system to ensure compliance.

Enhanced quality standards – such standards could set requirements higher than the fundamental standards but be discretionary matters for commissioning and subject to availability of resources.

Developmental standards – such standards would set out longer-term goals for providers, focus on improvements in effectiveness and be more likely to be the focus of commissioners and progressive provider leadership than the regulator. All such standards would require regular review and modification.

Recommendations 109–122 concern effective complaints-handling. Methods of registering a comment or complaint must be readily accessible and easily understood. Actual or intended litigation should not be a barrier to the processing or investigation of a complaint at any level. Provider organisations must constantly promote to the public their desire to receive and learn from comments and complaints; constant encouragement should be given to patients and other service users, individually and collectively, to share their comments and criticisms with the organisation. Comments or complaints which describe events amounting to an adverse or serious untoward incident should trigger an investigation.

5.6.1.2   The National Health Service Litigation Authority NHSLA

The report in its recommendations deals with the enhancement of the role of supportive agencies, and the NHSLA is discussed.

Recommendations 91–96 deal with the NHSLA. The report states that the NHSLA, through its risk management ratings, has made a contribution to the assessment of provider's governance, but the significance of this has been misunderstood and sometimes misapplied. The NHSLA should set more demanding levels for financial incentivisation, and arrangements should be made for the more effective sharing and recording of information. The NHSLA should make more prominent in its publicity an explanation comprehensible to the general public of the limitations of its standards assessments and of the reliance which can be placed on them.

5.6.1.3   Openness, transparency and candour

Recommendations 173–184 deal with openness, transparency and candour. The report states that for a common culture to be shared throughout the system, these three characteristics are required: openness – enabling concerns to be raised and disclosed freely without fear, and for questions to be answered; transparency – allowing true information about performance and outcomes to be shared with staff, patients and the public; candour – ensuring that patients harmed by a health care service are informed of the fact and that an appropriate remedy is offered, whether or not a complaint has been made or a question asked about it.

This requires, the report states, for all organisations and those working in them to be honest, open and truthful in all their dealings with patients and the public.

The report states that a statutory obligation should be imposed on health care providers, registered medical and nursing practitioners to observe the duty of candour; on directors of health care organisations to be truthful in any information given to a regulator or commissioner. There should be a criminal offence for any registered doctor or nurse or allied health professional or director of a registered or authorised organisation to obstruct the performance of these duties or dishonestly or recklessly to make an untruthful statement to a regulator. Enforcement of these duties should rest with the CQC, which should be supported by commissioners' and others' monitoring.

The report's recommendations have the potential to make the NHS a much safer place but another Mid Staffordshire NHS Trust crisis could well happen again unless our regulatory health care quality and patient safety infrastructure is changed dramatically.

The Government's initial response to the Francis report[48] was published on 26 March 2013.[49] The response is hard-hitting in terms of the Government's high expectations on NHS achievement of care quality, patient advocacy and patient safety in the NHS. Patient safety has been dramatically forced back on the agendas of hospitals and other health organisations by the Francis report and by the Government's initial response. Health carers and others have a clear government directive[49] to take make patient safety central to everything they do. The Government have appointed Professor Don Berwick, former adviser to President Obama, to review patient safety in the NHS and to propose a new improvement programme. He is to lead a National Patient Safety Advisory Group which is to report by the end of July 2013:

> The Group will also advise on how to bring about a genuine culture of change in the NHS so that staff at every level and across the entire healthcare system can take serious and profound action to make patient care and treatment as safe as it can possibly be.[49]

Other measures in the Government's initial response include:

- new Ofsted-style ratings for hospitals and care homes overseen by an Independent Chief Inspector of Hospitals and Chief Inspector of Social Care
- a statutory duty of candour for organisations which provide care and are registered with the Care Quality Commission
- a review by the NHS Confederation on how to reduce the bureaucratic burden on frontline staff and NHS providers by a third

- a pilot programme which will see nurses working for up to a year as a health care assistant as a prerequisite for receiving funding for their degree
- nurses' skills being revalidated, as doctors' are now, and health care support workers and adult social care workers having a *code of conduct and minimum training standards.*

The Health Foundation, a charity, commented on the Government's initial response:

> The government's response to Robert Francis QC's report is still unfortunately rooted in paternalism and the overriding ethos is of the patient being 'done unto' rather than being in active control. There must be a deep top-of-the-office commitment to the fully engaged patient to transform the NHS into a service that puts patients first and foremost.[50]

There is much good in the Government's response, such as the duty of candour and an Independent Chief Inspector of Hospitals. The Berwick patient safety review has the potential to bring important structural reforms to the NHS patient safety system. The overriding ethos may well be paternalistic, but the Government response is very forceful in terms of its commitment to bring about root-and-branch reform in care quality and patient safety and to put patients at the heart of the NHS. The Government's initial response is well articulated, practical, sincere and thoughtful.

The reforms proposed have a real potential to bring about effective change in the NHS. The response, however, is an initial one, coming only six weeks after the publication of the Francis report. There is a lot of consultation and other work that needs to be done before the definitive improvement infrastructure is in place. Much more details will need to emerge of the Government's proposals and then they will need to be seen in action. Some excellent first steps have been taken, though given the monolithic structure of the NHS bringing about these changes will be no easy task. It should also be noted that the NHS Commissioning Board name changed to NHS England on 1 April 2013.

5.7   Conclusion

There have been major changes in the NHS as regards risk, litigation and the patient safety field since the last edition of this book. Health care litigation and complaints are still with us, and perhaps always will be, given the nature of what the NHS tries to do. Everybody seems to agree that health care is an inherently risky and complex business. There has been a general acknowledgement that the tort-based common-law system is not the best way to compensate patients, but the Government has left the system largely intact. We have the NHS Redress scheme, which in its draft bill form was regarded by some as being fundamentally flawed. Properly amended, it does maintain an important potential to change things for the better for the injured patient. We have also seen the development of a new patient safety infrastructure system with the NRLS, and the work of the NPSA gave NHS staff some tools to deal with the patient safety problem. Nationally the NHSLA and CNST risk management standards do seem to have had a positive influence, and trusts can be seen to be moving, albeit slowly, towards higher levels of compliance. We have a developing NHS patient safety infrastructure, and there is more joined-up thinking about what needs to be done in order to achieve an ingrained patient safety culture in the NHS.

The NHS is probably a much safer place today than it was in the previous edition of our book in 2007, but as the Francis report[48] vividly shows, there is still a fair way to go before we can say that we have an ingrained patient safety culture in the NHS. The Government's initial response to the Francis Report[49] is very promising in terms of developing an ingrained patient safety culture in the NHS.

5.8   References

1. Department of Health, Liberating the NHS: Report of the arm's-length bodies review, 26 July 2010, Department of Health, London.
2. Better Regulation Taskforce, *Better Routes to Redress* (London, Cabinet Office Publications and Publicity Team, May 2004).
3. National Patient Safety Agency, Debate, 'Is there a growing litigation culture in the NHS?' NPSA Annual Review 2004–05 (London, NPSA), pp. 18–19.
4. M. Powers, *The Risk Management of Everything, Rethinking the Politics of Uncertainty* (London, Demos, 2004).
5. The National Health Service Litigation Authority, Report and Accounts 2011–12, HC 215, 28th June 2012, The Stationery Office, London.
6. The Right Honourable Lord Justice Jackson, Review of Civil Litigation Costs: Final Report, December 2009, The Stationery Office, London.
7. House of Commons, Committee of Public Accounts, *A Safer Place for Patients: Learning to Improve Patient Safety*, 51st Report of Session 2005–06, 6 July 2006 (London, The Stationery Office).
8. Marsh Ltd, Department of Health NHS Litigation Authority Industry Report, April 2011, Marsh Ltd, London.
9. Department of Health, NHS Litigation Authority Industry Review, Department of Health Response, 26 January 2012, Department of Health, London.
10. Patient Safety Curriculum Guide: Multi Professional Edition, WHO, Geneva, 2011.
11. Health Foundation, About US, Health Foundation, London. http://www.health.org.uk/public/cms/75/76/462/515/About%20us%20corporate%20publication%20leaflet.pdf?realName=8sMogx.pdf (accessed, 4 December 2012).
12. National Audit Office and the Audit Commission, *Financial Management in the NHS (England) Summarised Accounts 2004–05*, Report by the Comptroller and Auditor General, prepared jointly by the National Audit Office and the Audit Commission, HC 1092 – Session 2005–2006 (London, NAO, The Stationery Office, 7 June 2006).
13. *The NHS Litigation Authority Factsheet 2: financial information* (London, NHSLA) http://www.nhsla.com/CurrentActivity/Pages/FOIFactSheets.aspx (accessed 4 December 2012).
14. Department of Health, *Making Amends: A Consultation Paper Setting Out Proposals for Reforming the Approach to Clinical Negligence in the* NHS, A Report by the Chief Medical Officer (London, Department of Health Publications, June 2003).
15. Final Report, *Learning from Bristol: The Report of the Public Inquiry into Children's Heart Surgery at the Bristol Royal Infirmary 1984–1995*, Command Paper: CM 5207 (London, The Stationery Office).

16. Guardian Unlimited, *Yesterday in Parliament*, Compensation Culture (Press Association, 8 March 2006) http://politics.guardian.co.uk/commons/story/0,1726124,00.html (accessed 14 April 2006).

17. *Action against Medical Accidents*, Briefing on the NHS Redress Bill (Croydon, Surrey, 31 October 2005).

18. NHS Redress Bill [HL] Bill 137.

19. Department of Health, *NHS Redress: Statement of Policy* (Leeds, Department of Health, 2005).

20. *Action against Medical Accidents* (*AvMA*, NHS Redress Bill, Briefing for Report Stage, House of Lords (Croydon, Surrey, AvMA, February 2006).

21. National Patient Safety Agency, *Being Open: Communicating Patient Safety Incidents with Patients and Their Carers* (London, NPSA, 2005).

22. AvMa Latest News, *04.12.12: DoH Relegate Duty of Candour to Standard Clause in Hospital Contracts*. http://www.avma.org.uk/ (accessed 13 December 2012).

23. Department of Health, *An Organization with a Memory*, Report of an expert group on learning from adverse events in the NHS chaired by the Chief Medical Officer (London, The Stationery Office, 2000).

24. Health Foundation, The Health Foundation Research scan: Levels of Harm, January 2011, amended November 2011, Health Foundation, London.

25. Department of Health, *Building a Safer NHS for Patients: Implementing an Organization with a Memory* (London, Department of Health, 2001).

26. Care Quality Commission, *Statutory notifications: Guidance for registered providers and managers of NHS organisations* (London, CQC, July 2012) http://www.cqc.org.uk/sites/default/files/media/documents/20120621_100504_v5_00_guidance_on_statutory_notifications_from_nhs_bodies_for_external_publication.pdf (accessed 14 December 2012).

27. Care Quality Commission, *Guidance about compliance, essential standards of quality and safety, CQC* (London, CQC, March 2010) http://www.cqc.org.uk/sites/default/files/media/documents/gac_-_dec_2011_update.pdf (accessed 14 December 2012).

28. *NHS Commissioning Board Media Release* 13 September 2012 (NHS Commissioning Board, London) http://www.nrls.npsa.nhs.uk/news-cp/organisation-patient-safety-incident-reports-september-2012/ (accessed 13 December 2012).

29. National Patient Safety Agency, *Building a Memory: Preventing Harm, Reducing Risks and Improving Patient Safety*. The first report of the National Reporting and Learning System and the Patient Safety Observatory (London, NPSA, 2005).

30. National Patient Safety Agency, *Manchester Patient Safety Framework (MaPSaF) – Acute* (London, NPSA, 2006).

31. National Patient Safety Agency, *Patient Safety Bulletin 1* (London, NPSA, July 2005).

32. National Patient Safety Agency, *Seven Steps to Patient Safety: An Overview Guide for NHS Staff*, 2nd Print (London, NPSA, April 2004).

33. Healthcare Commission, *National Survey of NHS Staff 2005*, Summary of key findings (London Healthcare Commission, 2006).

34. Care Quality Commission, Media, *NHS staff have their say as the results of national survey are published*, The results of the eighth annual survey to collect the views of NHS staff across England are published today (16 March), by the Care Quality Commission (CQC), CQC, London. http://www.cqc.org.uk/media/nhs-staff-have-their-say-results-national-survey-are-published (accessed 13 December 2012).

35. National Audit Office, *Achieving Improvements through Clinical Governance: A Progress Report on Implementation by NHS Trusts*, Report by the Comptroller and Auditor General, HC 1055, Session 2002–2003 (London, The Stationery Office, 17 September 2003).

36. National Audit Office, Department of Health, A Safer Place for Patients: Learning to Improve Patient Safety, Report by the Comptroller and Auditor General, HC 456 Session 2005–2006, 3 November 2005 (London, The Stationery Office).

37. House of Commons, *Health Committee – Sixth Report*, Patient Safety http://www.publications.parliament.uk/pa/cm200809/cmselect/cmhealth/151/15103.htm Session 2008–09, Publications on the internet, Health Committee Publications. The published report was ordered by the House of Commons to be printed 18 June 2009.

38. National Health Service Litigation Authority, *Risk Management Standards for Acute Trusts* (derived from the former CNST and RPST Standards), Pilot Version (London, NHSLA, April 2006).

39. The NHS Litigation Authority, *Factsheet 2: Financial Information* (London, NHSLA, June 2012) http://www.nhsla.com/CurrentActivity/Pages/FOIFactSheets.aspx (accessed 13 December 2012).

40. The NHS Litigation Authority, *Factsheet 1: background information* (London, NHSLA, August, 2011) http://www.nhsla.com/CurrentActivity/Pages/FOIFactSheets.aspx (accessed 14 December 2012).

41. NHSLA, *How we handle claims* (London, NHSLA) http://www.nhsla.com/Claims/Pages/Handling.aspx (accessed 14 December 2012).

42. National Health Service Litigation Authority, *Clinical Negligence Scheme for Trusts General Clinical Risk Management Standards* (London, NHSLA, 2005).

43. The NHS Litigation Authority, *Factsheet 3: information on claims* (London, NHSLA) http://www.nhsla.com/CurrentActivity/Pages/FOIFactSheets.aspx (accessed 14 December 2012).

44. Department of Health, 'Learning how to learn, compliance with patient safety alerts in the NHS', *On the State of the Public Health*, Annual Report of the Chief Medical Officer 2004 (London, DH, 19 July, 2005).

45. Regulatory Impact Unit, Public Sector Team, *Making a difference, reducing burdens in health care inspection and monitoring* (London, Cabinet Office, 2003).

46. Healthcare Commission, Concordat, *Working in Partnership, Getting the Best from Inspection, Audit, Review and Regulation of Health and Social Care*, updated edition (London, Commission for Healthcare Audit and Inspection (Healthcare Commission), May 2006).

47. Health Foundation, Are clinicians engaged in quality improvement? May, 2011, Research/Evaluation report, Health Foundation, London.

48. (Francis Report 2013), *The Mid Staffordshire NHS Foundation Trust, Public Inquiry, Chaired by Robert Francis QC.HC 947*, Report of the Mid Staffordshire NHS Foundation Trust Public Inquiry, Executive summary (London, Stationery Office) http://www.midstaffspublicinquiry.com/report (accessed 11 February 2013).

49. Department of Health, *Patients First and Foremost, The Initial Government Response to the Report of The Mid Staffordshire NHS Foundation Trust Public Inquiry*, Cm 8576 (London, Stationery Office, 2013).

50. Health Foundation, *News, Patients absent in government response: the Health Foundation responds to the Government report*, 26 March (London, Health Foundation, 2013). http://www.health.org.uk/news-and-events/press/patients-absent-in-government-response-the-health-foundation-responds-to-the-government-report/ (accessed 1 April 2013).

Part Two: The Perspectives

6 Negligence

A   The Legal Perspective

Charles Foster

Barrister, Outer Temple Chambers, London, and Fellow of Green Templeton
College, University of Oxford

Lawyers use the word 'negligence', confusingly, in two ways. First, they use it
to describe a particular type of fault – a fault whose characteristics are defined
by a statute or past legal decisions. Negligence in this respect can be either criminal (leading to prosecution) or civil (leading to an action in the civil courts for
money). And second, they use it to describe that which must be proved in order
for a claimant to succeed in recovering money ('damages') in respect of damage,
if caused by that fault. When used in this second sense, lawyers are referring to
the tort of negligence. A tort is simply a legal wrong that does not involve a
breach of contract.

This chapter is concerned mostly with the tort of negligence. But criminal
negligence is important too. Medical manslaughter features commonly in the
newspapers. When a doctor is charged with killing a patient accidentally, he will
be convicted by the Crown court of manslaughter if the jury finds that he has
been grossly negligent – so negligent that his action or inaction deserves the

Nursing Law and Ethics, Fourth Edition. Edited by John Tingle and Alan Cribb.
© 2014 by John Wiley & Sons, Ltd. Published 2014 by John Wiley & Sons, Ltd.

penalty of criminal conviction.[1] This definition of gross negligence is, of course, circular: it comes down to saying someone should be convicted if he should be convicted. Precisely the same principles apply to the liability of a nurse for manslaughter, but as yet there are no reported English cases in which a nurse has been successfully prosecuted for manslaughter arising out of a breach of her professional duty to a patient.

The vast majority of medico-legal cases concern the civil law of negligence. They are tried in the County Court or the High Court (depending on their value and/or their complexity) by a judge sitting alone, without a jury. Only a tiny proportion will ever get to court. Most are settled or abandoned long before trial. Of those that do get to trial, many are decided in the defendant's favour. Clinical negligence cases are difficult for claimants to win. Some of the reasons for this will appear in this chapter.

It is very rare for nurses to be sued individually. If a nurse has been negligent, generally the employing health authority, NHS trust, private hospital or clinic will be sued. This is a consequence of the doctrine of vicarious liability, which states that employers are liable for the torts of their employees when the act or omission that constitutes the tort occurred in the course of the employment. This doctrine does not absolve the employee from responsibility: the claimant can sue the employee instead of or as well as the employer, but generally it would be foolish for a claimant to do so when the claimant knows that the issues in the action against the employer will be identical to those in the action against the employee, and that the employer will certainly be able to pay damages, whereas the employee may well not be able to do so.

Where an employee has been negligent, and the employer is successfully sued in relation to that negligence, the employer can sue the employee for an indemnity (*Lister* v. *Romford Ice and Cold Storage Co Ltd* (1957)), but in practice this is almost unheard of in nursing cases. With the rapid expansion of private medicine, however, it may become a contractual requirement of employment at a private hospital that the nurse has a policy of professional indemnity insurance which could pay an indemnity in the event of the hospital's liability. That fact, rather than any change in the substantive law of negligence, is likely in the future to lead to more actions against individual nurses.

6.1   The elements of the tort of negligence

To succeed in an action for clinical negligence, a claimant must show that:

(1)   the defendant owed the claimant a duty of care (i.e. a duty to do something that should have been done, or a duty not to do something that has been done); and
(2)   the defendant has breached the duty; and
(3)   the breach of duty has caused some injury, loss or damage to the claimant of a type which the law acknowledges.

6.2   The existence of a duty of care

A duty of care between a claimant and a defendant will exist if the following three criteria are satisfied (*Caparo Industries plc* v. *Dickman* (1990)):

(1)   the relevant damage was foreseeable; and
(2)   the relationship between the claimant and the defendant is sufficiently 'proximate'; and
(3)   it is 'fair, just and reasonable' to impose such a duty.

Foreseeability of damage is rarely an issue in clinical negligence cases, but the proximity of the relationship between the claimant and the defendant often is. The courts have been reluctant, in cases involving doctors, to say that the necessary proximity exists beyond the confines of the ordinary doctor–patient relationship, and have defined that relationship fairly narrowly. A good example is *Kapfunde* v. *Abbey National* (1998). Here the claimant applied for a job with the first defendant. The first defendant employed a doctor, the second defendant, to take a medical view of applicants, based on completed medical questionnaires. The second defendant told the first defendant that the claimant was, because of her history of sickle cell anaemia, likely to have unusually long absences from work. The court held that there was no doctor–patient relationship between the claimant and the second defendant, and that accordingly no duty of care existed.

Another example is *Goodwill* v. *BPAS* (1996), in which the defendant performed a vasectomy on his patient, and then advised him that he was sterile. Three years later the patient met the claimant, and he told her that he was sterile. They had unprotected sexual intercourse, and the claimant became pregnant. She sued the defendant for the cost of upkeep of the child.[2] The court held that the action must fail. There was no sufficiently proximate relationship between the relevant doctor and the claimant because the doctor could not know that his advice would be passed on to and relied on by the claimant.

A number of the cases on proximity were decided alternatively on the grounds of 'just, fair and reasonable'. It may now be that the question, 'is it just, fair and reasonable to impose a duty?' should be expanded to read, 'is it just, fair and reasonable to impose a duty to pay damages as big as those claimed?', and that in order for damages to be recoverable there has to be reasonable proportion between the damages claimed and the duty assumed.

The Compensation Act 2006, section 1, provides that:

[A] court considering a claim in negligence or breach of statutory duty may, in determining whether the defendant should have taken particular steps to meet a standard of care (whether by taking precautions against a risk or otherwise), have regard to whether a requirement to take those steps might (a) prevent a desirable activity from being undertaken at all, to a particular extent or in a particular way, or (b) discourage persons from undertaking functions in connection with a desirable activity.

6.3   Breach of duty

6.3.1   The general principles

A clinical professional will have discharged his duty to the patient if what that professional has done would be endorsed by a responsible body of practitioners in the relevant specialty at the material time. This is the famous and ubiquitous *Bolam* test.[3]

The *Bolam* test is a rule not only of substantive law (defining what amounts to adequate care), but also of evidence (indicating how a court determines whether adequate care has been given). Thus in *Maynard* v. *West Midlands RHA* (1984) Lord Scarman said:

> [A] judge's 'preference' for one body of distinguished professional opinion to another also professionally distinguished is not sufficient to establish negligence in a practitioner whose actions have received the approval of those whose opinions, truthfully expressed, honestly held, were not preferred . . . In the realm of diagnosis and treatment, negligence is not established by preferring one respectable body of professional opinion to another. (p. 639)

In the past the *Bolam* test has been caricatured as asserting that a professional escapes liability if he can get someone who at some stage has qualified in the relevant specialty and avoided utter professional disgrace to stagger into the witness box and say that he or some of his (unspecified) friends would have acted as the defendant did. This was never the case in theory, although it may, in some more outlandish county courts, have worked like that.

That caricature was laid finally to rest in a case before the House of Lords called *Bolitho* v. *City & Hackney Health Authority* (1997). *Bolitho* underlined the word 'responsible' in the *Bolam* test. The central passage reads:

> [I]n cases of diagnosis and treatment there are cases where, despite a body of professional opinion sanctioning the defendant's conduct, the defendant can properly be held liable for negligence . . . In my judgment that is because, in some cases, it cannot be demonstrated to the judge's satisfaction that the body of opinion relied upon is reasonable or responsible. In the vast majority of cases the fact that distinguished experts in the field are of a particular opinion will demonstrate the reasonableness of that opinion. In particular, where there are questions of assessment of the relative risks and benefits of adopting a particular medical practice, a reasonable view necessarily presupposes that the relative risks and benefits have been weighed by the experts in forming their opinions. But if, in a rare case, it can be demonstrated that the professional opinion is not capable of withstanding logical analysis, the judge is entitled to hold that the body of opinion is not reasonable or responsible. I emphasise that in my view it will very seldom be right for a judge to reach the conclusion that views genuinely held by a competent medical expert are unreasonable. The assessment of medical risks and benefits is a matter of clinical judgement which a judge would not normally be able to make without expert evidence . . . it would be wrong to allow such assessment to deterio-

rate into seeking to persuade the judge to prefer one of two views both of which are capable of being logically supported. It is only where a judge can be satisfied that the body of expert opinion cannot be logically supported at all that such opinion will not provide the bench mark by reference to which the defendant's conduct falls to be assessed . . . (p. 243)

Bolitho said nothing new, but caused a lot of unnecessary hysteria.[4] It was dubbed a 'claimant's charter'. It was feared that it would encourage medically illiterate judges to substitute their own uninformed views of what was medically reasonable for the views of distinguished practitioners. It is unlikely, as the cited passage clearly states, to have that effect in many cases. But it will have the effect of making experts look more critically at the practices they are defending. It will not lead to a proliferation of litigation, but it might lead to a proliferation of footnotes in expert reports.

The requirement that practice, to be defensible, has to be 'responsible' begs the question of whether, in a clinical world increasingly dominated by evidence-based medicine, a practice that the literature clearly shows leads to statistically worse results than another economically comparable practice can sensibly be said to be 'responsible'. It is likely to be found irresponsible not to adopt an evidence-based approach, and irresponsible not to adopt an intelligent strategy in deciding which evidence-based approach to use. The Nursing and Midwifery Council (NMC)'s own code of professional conduct states: 'You have a responsibility to deliver care based on current evidence, best practice and, where applicable, validated research when it is available'.[5] It may be that the clinical negligence cases of the future will be battles between statisticians, with the issue to be decided by the judge being whether the published results that are said to justify a particular clinical approach really do justify it.

The standard that the law expects of practitioners is the standard that is appropriate to a person undertaking the relevant task. Thus a nurse undertaking the work that normally (and appropriately) a senior house officer would do, undertakes to do it as well as a senior house officer would and cannot complain if she is judged by that standard.[6]

The standard of care expected is decided by reference to the post occupied by the person giving the care, rather than to the rank or status of that person or to the individual characteristics or training of that person. Thus, for instance, where the performance of work of a type reasonably done by staff nurses is criticised, the question of whether the work has been done negligently will be answered by reference to the standard expected of responsible staff nurses, not by reference to the standard that might normally be expected of that particular staff nurse with her particular experience.[7]

Liability for negligent prescribing by nurses is likely to be approached by the courts, at least for the next few years, by reference to the standard of prescribing expected of those doctors who originally performed the task that the nurse has taken on. Public policy considerations make it inconceivable that nurses will have less expected of them.

There is a legal duty to keep reasonably up to date,[8] but the courts do not expect practitioners to read every relevant article that appears in the professional press.[9] Of course, the duty to keep up to date includes a duty to know about guidelines affecting the profession: it is far less excusable not to know of a relevant NICE guideline than it is not to have read an editorial in an immensely obscure specialist journal.

It is clear that one does not decide that a particular practice is or is not responsible by counting the number of practitioners who do or do not do it. This principle is important in cases involving super-specialists doing pioneering work (*De Freitas* v. *O'Brien* (1995)).

For some reason section 2 of the Compensation Act 2006 felt it necessary to declare that 'an apology, an offer of treatment or other redress, shall not of itself amount to an admission of negligence or breach of statutory duty'.

6.3.2   Obtaining properly informed consent

In the past the *Bolam* test has been held to apply to the issue of obtaining consent from patients. Thus a clinician would not be negligent if what he had told a patient about a procedure would be what a responsible body of practitioners in the relevant specialty would have told that patient (*Sidaway* v. *Board of Governors of the Bethlem Hospital and the Maudsley Hospital* (1985)).

This extension of *Bolam* to the realm of consent has recently been doubted by some commentators, although the *Sidaway* case, which asserted it (a House of Lords case), has certainly not been overruled. The doubts arise firstly from an increased acknowledgment by lawyers that there are several speeches in *Sidaway*, not all of which can be boiled down to the simple comment '*Bolam* applies to consent', and from an off-the-cuff comment in *Bolitho* to the effect that the remarks there about the *Bolam* principle were made in the context of 'cases of diagnosis and treatment',[10] not in the context of consent to treatment. In inserting this caveat the House of Lords might have had in mind the Senate of Surgery's document *The Surgeon's Duty of Care*,[11] which has subsequently been extended to all registered medical practitioners by the GMC's guidelines: *Consent: Patients and doctors making decisions together*.[12] The details of these guidelines do not matter for present purposes. It is enough to say that they state categorically how consent must be obtained. If the ruling body of medical practitioners states that particular procedures must be followed, can it seriously be argued that there is a responsible body of medical practitioners that would not follow those procedures? The point is a moot one: it has yet to be tested in the courts.

The relevant guidelines on consent for nurses are in the NMC Standards of Conduct, Performance and Ethics for Nurses and Midwives.[13] They are much more sensible and general, and far less prescriptive than those imposed by the Senate of Surgery and the GMC, and nurses are unlikely to find that these guidelines deprive them of their *Sidaway* shield (*Sidaway* is discussed in Chapter 7). The guidelines read:

13. You must ensure that you gain consent before you begin any treatment or care

14. You must respect and support people's rights to accept or decline treatment and care

15. You must uphold people's rights to be fully involved in decisions about their care.

16. You must be aware of the legislation regarding mental capacity, ensuring that people who lack capacity remain at the centre of decision making and are fully safeguarded

17. You must be able to demonstrate that you have acted in someone's best interests if you have provided care in an emergency.[13]

6.3.3   The relevance of protocols to civil liability

The points above about guidelines raise the general question, important to nurse practitioners, of the relevance of protocols to issues of breach of duty. Clinicians from all medical and nursing specialties worry about protocols because they think that failure to follow them will necessarily connote negligence. In legal theory, of course, this is nonsense: *Bolam* does not cease to apply simply because a protocol has been drafted.

In the context of nurses failing to follow protocols, two situations have to be distinguished. The first is where a nurse has carelessly failed to do what the protocol says. An example might be failure to give the prescribed regime of post-operative antibiotics because of forgetfulness or ignorance of the regime. Here, *Bolam* will not protect, because *Bolam* never applied: there is no responsible body of nursing opinion that forgets or is ignorant of protocols. The second situation is where a nurse has failed to do what a protocol says because she exercised her own independent clinical judgement and decided to do something other than what the protocol says. Here, *Bolam* would excuse the nurse if there were a responsible body of nursing opinion that would, in the relevant circumstances, have acted in the way that the nurse did.

As a general rule, adherence to local or national protocols is likely to protect, because the courts are likely to find that those protocols represent responsible practice (if not embodying the only responsible practice).[14] Departure from local protocols may be *Bolam*-justifiable if the departure was made in the exercise of clinical judgement for responsible clinical reasons. Departure from national protocols, such as those imposed by NICE, may create problems, even if the departure is endorsed by other members of the same profession because the courts will tend to think that nationally endorsed protocols definitively circumscribe acceptable practice.

Note that *Bolitho*'s endorsement of the propriety of looking at the reasoning that leads to clinical decisions is likely to bring greater judicial readiness to look at the research and consultation that led to the formulation of the relevant guidelines. It is therefore important that the formulation process is well documented.

6.4 Causation

6.4.1 The conventional rule

The claimant has to show that but for the defendant's negligence he would probably have avoided the injury and loss claimed. Thus lawyers often talk about the '51 per cent test' or 'proof on the balance of probabilities'. In the context of causation they simply mean that the claimant will succeed if he shows that it is more likely than not that the defendant's default caused the injury/loss.

Causation is an essential element of the tort of negligence. Beware of confusing questions about whether causation has been established with questions about how much compensation should be awarded.

6.4.2 Loss of a chance

It is often asserted that damages for loss of a chance are not recoverable in the English law of tort. This is untrue. In some commercial fields such damages are regularly recovered.[15] But whether they can be or should be recoverable in clinical negligence cases is contentious. The authority generally cited for the proposition that such damages are not recoverable in tort is the House of Lords case *Hotson* v. *East Berkshire Health Authority* (1987). But *Hotson* says nothing of the sort. The Court of Appeal in *Hotson* decided that loss of a chance was damage that the law recognised, and that accordingly to prove that one had lost a chance was to prove causation. The Court of Appeal was anxious to avoid treating claimants who sued in tort and in contract differently. Damages are uncontroversially recoverable for loss of a chance in contract.[16] Why, the Court of Appeal said, should an NHS patient who is deprived by a doctor's negligence of a chance of recovery be unable to recover damages, whereas the same patient, treated identically but privately (and therefore under a contract) by the same doctor, be successful? The court said that such an anomaly would be monstrous. The House of Lords never decided the question of recoverability of damages for loss of a chance: it merely decided that on the facts of that case it did not need to decide.

The question was considered again by the House of Lords, in the context of failure to diagnose cancer, in *Gregg* v. *Scott* (2005).[17] The House there rejected the loss of chance analysis in clinical negligence cases (at least those relating to failure to diagnose), adopting the straightforward balance of probabilities test. Lost chances have probably not left medical law completely, but the arguments that invoke them will have to be more complex than before.[18]

6.4.3 Causation: material contribution

Sometimes it will be impossible for the experts to say that the defendant's default has, on the balance of probabilities, caused the damage, but they may be able to say, on the balance of probabilities, that the default has materially contributed to the damage. Where this is the case, the claimant is entitled to succeed in full.

An example is *Bonnington Castings* v. *Wardlaw* (1956). The claimant there was a steel dresser. In the course of his work he was exposed to silica dust from two sources. The exposure to dust from one source was a consequence of the defendant's breach of statutory duty; the exposure to dust from the other was not. He developed pneumoconiosis. It was impossible to determine the contribution that the 'guilty dust' and the 'innocent dust' had made to his disease. All that could be said was that the contribution made by the 'guilty dust' was not *de minimis*. Those facts, said the House of Lords, meant that the claimant was entitled to judgment for damages representing all his illness and its financial consequences. Lord Reid said:

> I cannot agree that the question is: which was the most probable source of the [claimant's] disease, the ['innocent dust'] or the ['guilty dust']? It appears to me that the source of his disease was the dust from both sources, and the real question is whether the ['guilty dust'] materially contributed to the disease. What is a material contribution must be a question of degree. A contribution which comes within the exception de minimis non curat lex is not material, but I think that any contribution which does not fall within that exception must be material. I do not see how there can be something too large to come within the de minimis principle but yet too small to be material. (p. 621)

The House of Lords appeared to extend this principle in *McGhee* v. *National Coal Board* (1972). They said there that where the defendant's default had materially increased the risk of the injury that in fact occurred, the claimant succeeded in full. This case produced uproar among practitioners and academics. It was pointed out that if all you could do was to prove a material contribution to risk, you had failed to prove that there was anything causative about the defendant's default at all. Judges were extremely reluctant to follow *McGhee*, but it haunted the law of tort until it was exorcised by the House of Lords in *Wilsher* v. *Essex AHA* (1988). In *Wilsher* Lord Bridge said:

> *McGhee* . . . laid down no new principle of law whatever. On the contrary, it affirmed the principle that the onus of proving causation lies on the [claimant]. Adopting a robust and pragmatic approach to the undisputed primary facts of the case, the majority concluded that it was a legitimate inference of fact that the [defendant's] negligence had materially contributed to the [claimant's] injury. The decision, in my opinion, is of no greater significance than that . . . (pp. 881–2)

Whenever the House of Lords describes the decision of a differently constituted House as 'robust and pragmatic', it is clear that there is deep intellectual embarrassment. The fact is that the House thought that *McGhee* was plainly wrong. But *McGhee* has been rehabilitated – at least in the context of industrial disease litigation.

In *Fairchild* v. *Glenhaven Funeral Services Ltd* (2003) several defendants negligently exposed the claimant to asbestos. But which defendant was responsible for the development of the disease? Was the disease caused by a single exposure? Or was the exposure for which several defendants were responsible cumulatively causative?

Fairchild smiled on Lord Wilberforce's test in *McGhee*. Lord Bingham said: 'It seems to me just and in accordance with common sense to treat the conduct of A and B in exposing C to a risk to which he should not have been exposed as making a material contribution to the contracting by C of a condition against which it was the duty of A and B to protect him' (para. 34).

Lord Nicholls noted that in such cases the court would apply 'a different and less stringent test' than the normal but-for test.

There has been a good deal of discussion about the practical effect of this. In *Barker* v. *Corus UK Ltd* (2006) the House of Lords addressed the question of what, in *Fairchild*-type situations, is the liability of each defendant. Is it the total loss, or a loss proportionate to degree of fault? It was held that it was the latter. *Fairchild* was interpreted as saying that the damage is not the disease itself, but the increased risk of contracting it.

Exactly how this will pertain to clinical negligence litigation is unclear. Can *Fairchild* be exported to the wards? We don't yet know.

What is clear is that material contribution is back, and already having a significant effect on the way that clinical negligence cases are litigated. It is potentially extremely helpful to claimants in cases where experts cannot be pressed to agree with the artificial speculations about biological processes that lawyers love so much.

Material contribution came of age in a medical negligence context in *Bailey* v. *Ministry of Defence* (2008).[19] There, material contribution was clearly said to be different from the but-for test. Waller LJ observed that: 'In a case where medical science cannot establish the probability that "but for" an act of negligence the injury would not have happened but can establish that the contribution of the negligent cause was more than negligible, the "but for" test is modified and the claimant will succeed' (para. 46).

Bailey was applied in *Conan-Ingram* v. *Williams* (2010), where it was also said that the effect of *Bailey* is to entitle the claimant to recover the full value of the claim. There is likely to be a good deal of litigation about this. If apportionment is factually possible, there is scope for arguing that *Bailey* is to do with causation solely as an element of liability, rather than as a determinant of quantum.

6.4.4   Causation: multiple competing causes

Often in clinical negligence cases there will be a number of candidates for the post of 'cause' of the injury. That was the case in *Wilsher*. The claimant there suffered from retrolental fibroplasia. It was said that this was a result of the negligent administration of hyperbaric oxygen. But there were several alternative explanations, and it could not be said that the negligent explanation was probably correct. Accordingly the claimant failed to establish causation.

6.4.5   The requirement that the loss is legally recoverable

Not everything a claimant might justifiably complain of is recognised by the law as 'loss or damage' sufficient to ground liability. The most obvious examples relate to psychiatric harm. If the only harm suffered is psychiatric, the claimant will have to show, in order to obtain judgment, that a recognisable psychiatric illness has been suffered. Mere distress and shaking-up are not enough.[20] A good example was *Reilly* v. *Merseyside RHA* (1994). The claimants were trapped in a hospital lift for 1 hour 20 minutes. They suffered fear and claustrophobia but no physical injury. They were not entitled to any damages.

6.5   The assessment of quantum

6.5.1   General

'Quantum' is simply the value of a case. There are a number of possible 'heads of claim' in clinical negligence cases. They are divided up as follows:

- pain, suffering and loss of amenity
- special damage
- future loss
- hybrid heads of claim.

Damages in negligence cases are almost always intended to be simply compensatory – to put the claimant into the position he would have been in had the defendant not been negligent in so far as money can do that. In rare circumstances damages can be awarded that are intended to represent the court's disapproval of the defendant's oppressive or otherwise immoral conduct. These are referred to as aggravated damages. A good example of aggravated damages in a clinical negligence case is *Appleton* v. *Garrett* (1995). There, a dentist who was sued in negligence and trespass for doing unnecessary dental work on patients in order to enrich himself, was ordered to pay aggravated damages, calculated as 15 per cent of the compensatory damages for pain, suffering and loss of amenity that he also had to pay.

The claimant is under a duty to 'mitigate' his loss. That means that he has to take reasonable steps to reduce the total sum of damages payable. Thus he is not entitled to buy in extravagantly priced care, or go to his hospital appointments in a chauffeur-driven Rolls-Royce. If non-dangerous medical treatment would alleviate his condition, he may be obliged to have it: if he does not, he may forfeit that part of his claim that relates to the difference between the condition he is in fact in and the condition he would have been in had he had the treatment. All the comments below about damages have to be read subject to this caveat about mitigation.

6.5.2   Damages for pain, suffering and loss of amenity

These are exactly what they say. They are inevitably quantifications of the intrinsically unquantifiable. In trying to assess this head of claim, lawyers rely on guidelines that prescribe broad brackets of awards for particular types of injury and disability,[21] and on reported cases.

The Law Commission criticised awards of damages for pain, suffering and loss of amenity as being too low. That is a common complaint. Certainly the disparity between such awards and awards of damages in libel cases for injury to reputation can often be insulting to claimants who have suffered personal injuries. In *Heil* v. *Rankin and Others* (2000), the Court of Appeal decided that where the conventional award of damages for pain, suffering and loss of amenity was £10,000 or less, there should be no change, and that above that there should be a gradual tapering-up of awards so that the largest awards would be about one-third higher than they had previously been. Insurers were generally happy with this decision, since the vast number of cases they face attract awards of less than £10,000. The NHS will be hit particularly hard, since damages for pain, suffering and loss of amenity in clinical negligence cases are very often over the £10,000 threshold. In 2012 the Court of Appeal said that damages for pain, suffering and loss of amenity would be increased by 10 per cent for all claims resulting in judgment from 1 April 2013: see *Simmons* v. *Castle* (2012).[22] This is intended to compensate to some degree for one of the changes brought about by the 'Jackson Reforms' of costs in civil litigation. This change is the (general) non-recoverability of the 'success fee' from a losing party. When a claim is brought under a Conditional Fee Agreement (a 'no-win no-fee' agreement), the 'success fee' (the uplift payable to the successful claimant's lawyers to compensate them for the risk they have assumed of getting no fee at all) is no longer, from 1 April 2013, recoverable from a losing defendant.

6.5.3   Special damages

These, broadly, are the financial losses that have accrued between the time of the negligence and the time of the trial. They can only be described broadly this way because they include heads of claim (for instance, the cost of care) that relate to work that has been done free for the claimant, and it is rather artificial to describe these as 'financial losses'.

They typically include the cost of travel (both of the claimant and of visiting relatives) to and from hospital, prescription and other medical expenses, the cost of care, lost earnings and the cost of equipment needed to cope with disability. In relation to each claim, the court will ask itself whether the claimant has proved that the loss has in fact occurred; whether the loss was caused by the negligence; and in relation to expenditure, whether it was reasonable in principle to spend money on whatever the head of claim is, and if so whether it was reasonable to spend the amount of money that is claimed.

If care has been given free by relatives or friends, the court values the cost of buying in that care and then reduces this sum by about 25 per cent to take account of the fact that no tax or National Insurance has been paid, as it would have been, had the care been bought.

In practice, special damages are often agreed. Judges rightly shout at barristers who ask them to decide whether the travelling expenses were, say, £250 as opposed to £275.

6.5.4   Future loss

Because this involves speculation about future events, it is much more difficult to calculate. The basic system used is the multiplier–multiplicand system. The multiplier relates to the number of years over which the particular loss runs; the multiplicand represents the annual loss under that head.

Obviously the multiplier cannot simply be the number of years over which the loss runs. If a claimant will lose £1000 per year for ten years, he would be overcompensated if the court were to award him £10,000 because it has to be presumed that he will invest the award of damages. The amount of investment income has to be taken into account if the award is to represent the actual loss. The court in fact presumes that the award will be invested in index-linked government securities (*Wells* v. *Wells* (1998)). Exactly what the discount should be to take account of this presumption is controversial. Defendants said that it should be 3 per cent per annum; claimants pointed out that the rate of return on these securities has fallen over the last couple of years, and often contended for a rate of around 2 per cent. There is a statutory power to fix the discount rate.[23] Since 28 June 2001 it has been fixed at 2.5 per cent.

There are calls for this to be reduced downwards. It is hard to get a rate of return of 2.5 per cent on the open market, and accordingly the present figure of 2.5 per cent may mean that claimants getting lump sum payments with a significant element of compensation for future loss are being undercompensated. At the time of writing, the question of amendment of the return rate was being reviewed, but no decision had been reached.

The multiplier also needs to take into account future contingencies such as the possibility that the claimant would in any event have died, or (in the case of a future loss of earnings claim) have been unable to work in any event. The calculation of multipliers is becoming a sophisticated science in its own right – a science led by actuaries.

Significant heads of future loss often include future loss of earnings, future care, future accommodation requirements and the cost of equipment. Obviously in relation to equipment costs there needs to be expert evidence about the lifetime of each item of equipment. In the case of accommodation costs, claimants are given the costs of any necessary conversion and the costs associated with moving to the required accommodation, plus the court's valuation of the financial disadvantage resulting from the additional money tied up in the new property being unavailable. This is calculated, very roughly, in relation to the income that would have been earned had that sum been available for investment (*Roberts* v. *Johnstone* (1988)).

Sometimes it will be impossible to use the multiplier–multiplicand system to calculate future loss. It may be, for instance, that because of an injury a claimant would be at a disadvantage on the labour market were he to be made unemployed, but at the time of trial he is employed and that employment is expected to continue. Here, the court may make a (rather arbitrary) award to represent the disadvantage, and will assess in doing so the prospects of that claimant finding himself adrift on the labour market as well as the level of disadvantage once he is adrift (*Smith* v. *Manchester Corporation* (1974)).

6.5.5   Hybrid heads of claim

Some heads of claim do not fall neatly within the above categories. The best example is damages for loss of congenial employment – an award to compensate the claimant for not being able to continue doing a particularly satisfying job (*Hale* v. *London Underground Ltd* (1992)). Nursing is one of the classically cited examples of satisfying employment.

6.5.6   Structured settlements

The court most commonly awards, or the defendant agrees to pay, a lump sum of damages. That lump sum or part of it may then be invested in such a way that it produces an annuity that meets the claimant's assessed needs at various stages through his life. This form of investment is called a structured settlement. This may have tax advantages or be otherwise advantageous – for instance, if there are concerns that a claimant, or whoever would be managing the money, might fritter it away. The court now has power to order that the whole or part of the compensation due to a claimant should be paid by way of periodical payments.[24] At the moment, with multiplier discount rates being so out of sync with the commercial rates actually recoverable, periodical payments are particularly attractive to claimants.

6.6   Proving the case

6.6.1   General

It is for the claimant to prove the case. Proof is on the balance of probabilities. The general rule is that things are proved by adducing evidence or by getting the other side to agree to them. If something is blindingly obvious and common knowledge, the judge may 'take judicial notice' of it, thus dispensing with the formal requirement of proof or agreement. But this is an extremely limited and in practice unimportant exception to the general rule.

Evidence is a highly technical branch of the law in its own right, and cannot be dealt with in this chapter. It is important to remember that evidence includes evidence not only of fact but also of opinion from appropriately qualified experts.

6.6.2   The maxim *res ipsa loquitur*

Although Lord Woolf hated Latin tags, lawyers still use them because they are convenient shorthand. One of the most common is *res ipsa loquitur*: 'the thing speaks for itself'. It refers to the situation where the mere facts of a case shout loudly and unequivocally 'negligence, and nothing but negligence'.

A lot of mystique has sprung up around this maxim. It has at various times been suggested that where the maxim applies, the burden of proof shifts from the claimant to the defendant. It has now been established that this is wrong: the burden of proof never moves.[25]

6.7   Clinical negligence: the future

Clinical negligence claims are big business. The numbers of claims brought has increased very rapidly over the last few years. The loss of legal aid for clinical negligence claims might stop the trend. Such claims are now increasingly funded by 'no win, no fee' arrangements, and obviously such arrangements concentrate the mind of the claimant's lawyers harder on the merits than an unlimited legal aid certificate previously did.

The issue of costs in civil litigation was reviewed by Lord Justice Jackson. His recommendations, which will have a tectonic effect on clinical negligence claims, were set out in his report, *Review of Civil Litigation Costs: Final Report.*[26] Many of his most significant recommendations have been adopted, and will come into effect in April 2013.[27] The changes include: a general rule that the success fees of successful lawyers on Conditional Fee Agreements cannot be recovered from the losing side (see section 6.5.2 above); a fixed costs regime for all lower value personal injury claims; contingency fees (whereby the fees recoverable are a fixed percentage of the total damages); and costs management (whereby there is judicial agreement of a costs budget for litigation, with a presumption that the recoverable costs will not be greater than that budget).

The Jackson reforms were, broadly, welcomed by insurers and defendant lawyers. It is not surprising. The reforms make the courts less accessible to claimants, particularly in complex clinical negligence litigation. It is often not possible to determine whether or not a clinical negligence claim has any merit without detailed and costly investigation. Claimant lawyers are likely to shy away from those investigations. That means that many high-value and meritorious cases will never get going.

Comparisons are often drawn between the rise in clinical negligence cases in England and the situation in the litigation-mad USA. The comparison is not a good one. In the USA juries generally assess damages, and are much less scientific, much more generous, and much less strictly compensatory about it than are the professional judges who assess damages in England. If irrationally large awards of damages are not going to become available, irrationally large numbers of clinical negligence actions are unlikely.

It is sometimes said that a lot of litigation is launched by litigants wanting an apology and an explanation rather than damages. This is true. Increasingly, procedures for investigation (and, if appropriate, compensation) that bypass the courts are available. These include informal mediation. Arbitration and mediation are increasingly common in clinical negligence cases. They seem to work. It may seem unfair that a claimant's entitlement to damages should depend on proving fault. The claimant's need for compensation is just as great whether or not fault can be proved. This consideration has led some to advocate no-fault liability schemes for clinical negligence. The basic problem is cost, and it seems highly unlikely that any British government in the foreseeable future will be prepared to finance such an initiative. In the case of National Health patients injured by National Health negligence, it is arguable that there is a de facto no-fault liability scheme in place anyway in relation to many of the costs claimed in clinical negligence actions. This is because much of the medical treatment and nursing care and many of the appliances that NHS negligence makes necessary are themselves provided by the NHS.

There have been some urgent calls for reform of the system of compensation for clinical negligence, notably in the Chief Medical Officer's paper *Making Amends*.[28] Many of the Chief Medical Officer's proposals have been embodied in the NHS Redress Act 2006. This may change radically the way that clinical negligence claims are handled. It allows for the establishment of redress schemes whereby certain categories of case were dealt with entirely outside the court system. It is too early to say what effect it will have. Many of its most significant effects will be through as yet undrafted secondary legislation. For the moment, the liability of NHS bodies and of individual practitioners will remain governed by the principles set out above.

6.8   Notes and references

1. See *R* v. *Adomako* [1994] 5 Med LR 277; *R* v. *Misra (Amit)* [2005] 1 Cr. App R. 21.
2. For actions in relation to the birth of an unwanted child now, see *Macfarlane* v. *Tayside Health Board (HL)* [2000] 1 Lloyds Rep. Med. 1.
3. Arising from Mr Justice MacNair's direction to the jury in *Bolam* v. *Friern Hospital Management Committee* [1957] 1 WLR 582.
4. For a discussion of this issue, see C. Foster, Medical negligence: the new cornerstone (*Bolitho* v. *City & Hackney HA*), *Solicitors' Journal*, 5 December 1997, p. 1150; C. Foster, *Bolam*: consolidation and clarification, *Health Care Risk Report*, **4** (5) (1998), p. 5.
5. Nursing and Midwifery Council, *NMC Code of Professional Conduct: Standards for Conduct, Performance and Ethics* (London, NMC, 2004), para. 6.5.
6. See *Wilsher* v. *Essex Area Health Authority* [1986] 3 All ER 801; *Djemal* v. *Bexley Health Authority* [1995] 6 Med LR 269; and *Nettleship* v. *Weston* [1971] 2 QB 691. The NMC *Standards of Conduct, Performance and Ethics for Nurses and Midwives* (2008) states, at para. 38: 'You must have the knowledge and skills for safe and effective practice when working without direct supervision', and at para. 39: 'You must recognise and work within the limits of your competence'.
7. See *Wilsher* v. *Essex Area Health Authority* [1986] 3 All ER 801, per Lord Justice Mustill at pp. 810–3.
8. There is also an obligation in professional ethics: the NMC *Standards for Conduct, Performance and Ethics for Nurses and Midwives* (2008) states at para. 35: 'You must deliver care based on the best available evidence or best practice', at para. 36: 'You must ensure any advice you give is evidence based if you are suggesting healthcare products or services', at para. 40: 'You must keep your knowledge and skills up to date throughout your working life', and at para. 41: 'You must take part in appropriate learning and practice activities that maintain and develop your competence and performance.
9. See *Crawford* v. *Charing Cross Hospital* (1953) *The Times*, 8 December; *Gascoine* v. *Ian Sheridan and Co.* [1994] 5 Med LR 437.

10. *Bolitho* v. *City & Hackney Health Authority* [1998] AC 232, per Lord Browne Wilkinson at p. 243.
11. The Senate of Surgery, October 1997.
12. General Medical Council, 2008. Available on the GMC website at http://www.gmc-uk.org/guidance/ethical_guidance/consent_guidance_index.asp
13. Nursing and Midwifery Council, *The Code: Standards of conduct, performance and ethics for nurses and midwives* (London, NMC, 2008), paras 13–17.
14. See *Re C (a minor) (medical treatment)* [1998] Lloyds Rep Med 1; *Airedale NHS Trust* v. *Bland* [1993] 4 Med LR 39; *Early* v. *Newham HA* [1994] 5 Med LR 214; *Penney, Palmer and Cannon* v. *East Kent Health Authority* [2000] 1 Lloyds Rep. Med. 41.
15. See, for instance, *First Interstate Bank of California* v. *Cohen Arnold & Co.* [1996] 1 PNLR 17; *Allied Maples Group Ltd* v. *Simmons & Simmons (a firm)* [1995] 1 WLR 1602.
16. See, for instance, *Chaplin* v. *Hicks* [1911] 2 KB 786.
17. [2005] 2 WLR 268.
18. See the discussion in C. Foster, Last chance for lost chances, *New Law Journal*, **155** (7164) (2005), pp. 248–9. Note, too, the curious and much criticised case of *Chester* v. *Afshar* [2005] 1 AC 134, in which it was held by the House of Lords that where (a) there has been a negligent failure to warn about an entirely randomly occurring risk; and (b) the patient would, if warned, have still undergone the procedure at the hands of the same operator and in identical circumstances, but at a different date; and (c) the randomly occurring risk in fact eventuates, without any intra-operative negligence at all on the part of the operator, the claimant succeeds in establishing causation.
19. EWCA Civ 883. There were early signs of a return in, e.g., *Tahir* v. *Haringey HA* [1998] Lloyds Rep Med 105, in which the court laid down guidelines indicating when the *Bonnington Castings* analysis would be the correct one in a clinical negligence context.
20. See *Nicholls* v. *Rushton*, *The Times*, 19 June 1992.
21. *The Judicial Studies Board Guidelines for the Assessment of General Damages in Personal Injury Cases*, 4th edn (London, Blackstone Press, 1999).
22. [2012] EWCA Civ 1039.
23. Damages Act 1996, section 1.
24. See Damages Act 1996, section 2(1)(a), inserted by Courts Act 2003, section 100.
25. See *Ratcliffe* v. *Plymouth & Torbay HA and Exeter & North Devon HA* [1998] PIQR P170.
26. London, HMSO, 2009.
27. The Legal Aid, Sentencing and Punishment of Offenders Act 2012 provides the necessary statutory authority for those parts of the reforms that require primary legislation.
28. Department of Health, June 2003.

B   An Ethical Perspective – Negligence and Moral Obligations

Harry Lesser

Honorary Research Fellow in Philosophy, Centre for Philosophy, University of Manchester, Manchester

In a broad sense the legal and ethical uses of the term 'negligence' are the same: negligence is the failure to exercise the appropriate level of care. But there are some important differences between what is required legally and what is required ethically, not as a rule because they are in conflict (though as we shall see this can occasionally happen), but because the level of care required by ethics is higher than that required by the law, and goes beyond it in several different ways. To see what these are, we need to examine various parts of the NMC code: *Standards of Conduct, Performance and Ethics for Nurses and Midwives* (2008), which has already been quoted in Part A, and in particular the section on the management of risk (32–34).

6.9   Harm and risk

The first point to be noted – one which is made very clear in Part A – is that the courts come into operation only if harm has occurred. Failure to meet the legal duty of care, whether by nurses, midwives or specialist community public health nurses, concerns the law only if harm or damage appears to have resulted. The law then has to decide a number of things: whether there has in fact been harm or damage, how great it is and of what sort, whether and to what extent it was the result of a failure of care, who is responsible for the failure of care, how much compensation is appropriate, and whether the negligence was criminal. But, as Charles Foster says in Section 6.1, for an action for clinical negligence to succeed there must be 'injury, loss or damage to the claimant of a type which the law recognises'. Ethics is different: a professional who exposes a patient or client to serious and unnecessary risk is still morally to blame even if by good fortune no harm is done. The law is concerned essentially with redressing, and sometimes with punishing, the harm done by negligence; ethics is concerned with the obligation to avoid negligence, whether harm in fact results or not. To make a very obvious point, a professional who has subjected a patient to unnecessary risk of this kind but without any harm resulting is in no danger of legal action, but ought nevertheless to have a 'bad conscience', and (more importantly) to resolve that this should not happen again.

6.10 The Code of Professional Conduct

The section of the Code concerned with the management of risk forms the final part of the section headed 'Work with others to protect and promote the health and wellbeing of those in your care, their families and carers, and the wider community', the other three parts of which deal with sharing information with colleagues, working as part of a team and effective delegation. The section runs:

32. You must act without delay if you believe that you, a colleague or anyone else may be putting someone at risk.
33. You must inform someone in authority if you experience problems that prevent you working within this code or other nationally agreed standards.
34. You must report your concerns in writing if problems in the environment of care are putting people at risk.

Now this is appreciably wider than what is required by the law, and not only because it is dealing with risk rather than actual harm. The law requires a nurse or midwife to avoid causing harm of a type recognised by the law (section 6.1) to those to whom they owe a duty of care (section 6.2) by failing to give care of a standard 'decided by reference to the post occupied by the person giving the care' (section 6.3). The ethical code requires them to take action, either by correcting the situation themselves or by reporting it to the appropriate authority, if there is a risk of harm, of any sort, to any person, whether or not they are a patient, being caused by the actions of anyone in the working team of which they are part, whether or not this is connected with their particular duties. It requires them also to report problems in the 'environment of care' that may not be being caused by the actions of any particular person but by the physical conditions in which they work, or by features of the environment which are not physical, such as the team ethos or what is taken to be acceptable standard practice. We may thus say that the Code goes beyond the law in five ways: it seeks to prevent all forms of harm; it is concerned not only with the patients or clients, but also with 'their families, and carers, and the wider community'; it makes all members of the team responsible for preventing harm; it is concerned with a safe environment as well as safe action; and it is concerned with 'managing risk', whether or not harm actually results. It is particularly important to note that managing risk is the responsibility of all members of the team, and not only those in charge.

6.11 The problem of avoiding risk

However, there is a problem in deciding how risk is to be managed. Even in ordinary life it is impossible absolutely to avoid causing some risk to oneself or others. One might try to deal with this by saying that risks should always be minimised. But if one invariably tried to minimise risk, as the top priority, one would be able to do nothing worthwhile at all: after all, switching on the electric light, crossing the road, travelling in any vehicle, all involve some risk to oneself and others. This could be dealt with, it might be argued, by simple common sense in assessing which risks are so low, and which costs of not taking a risk so high, that the risk should obviously be taken. But this is not always so easy to assess, and there is a particular problem with medical care. The problem is that, while not to care for a patient would very often result in harm or the risk of harm, most, perhaps all, forms of care and treatment involve some level of discomfort, harm or risk. To decide when the likelihood of a cure or an improvement outweighs the risk, or the actual pain or harm, for a particular patient or client is not always easy.

Often, of course, the likelihood of a cure is very high, and the side-effects of the medication a short-term discomfort clearly worth enduring for the sake of the cure: the nurse administering the medication is clearly safeguarding both the health and the well-being of the patient. But sometimes matters are much less simple, and it is by no means clear how to balance the risks and possible benefits of a particular kind of treatment. Where possible, this can be dealt with by explaining matters to the patient and accepting their decision. Indeed the Code says (12): 'You must share with people, in a way they can understand, the information they want or need to know about their health', and (13): 'You must ensure that you gain consent before you begin any treatment or care'. When this happens, the patient has taken an informed decision to face the risk in the hope of getting a cure: the risk is still there but it has been correctly 'managed'.

Indeed, it is entirely right that the Code speaks of 'managing risk' rather than simply avoiding it. 'Managing risk' involves three parts of the Code. There is the section actually called 'Managing risk', quoted in full above, which in effect, though this is not actually stated, involves not exposing a patient or client, or indeed a member of the wider public, to any risk that is not essential to the treatment or to the carrying out of necessary tasks, and which indicates what is to be done if this happens (see above). There are provisions 12 and 13, which require informed consent before treatment which carries a risk begins (indeed before any treatment begins). And there are provisions 16 and 17, which concern patients or clients who lack mental capacity or who are admitted in an emergency, and may for example be unconscious, and so unable to give consent, and with no family member around to give consent for them. Thus (17): 'You must be able to demonstrate that you have acted in someone's best interests if you have provided care in an emergency' – or, presumably, if for whatever reason you have had to take a decision on their behalf, because they were unable to make it for themselves.

With regard to the first of these, the previous section indicates in what ways the Code requires more from the nurse than the law does. With regard to consent, this is also true, though less obviously. If the patient has had the risks and possible benefits of the proposed treatment explained to them, and has given consent, the nurse is covered, as far as the law is concerned. But ethics requires that the explanation be a proper one, in plain language, 'in terms they can understand', and, one might add, without either exaggerating or minimising the risks – which means not only telling the truth but also putting it over in a way that is neither needlessly alarmist (e.g. by listing all the things that could go wrong but are very unlikely to do so, with the result that the treatment sounds much more risky than it is) nor too optimistic (e.g. by ignoring a genuine danger because the risk is low). This is something that is by and large done much better now than it was a generation ago, and something that, again by and large, nurses did, and perhaps still do, though the gap has narrowed, better than doctors. But it is still something which requires careful thought and choosing of one's words, if the demands of ethics are to be met as well as those of the law.

Again, in those cases where the nurse has had to make a decision on the patient's behalf, the law will be satisfied if the decision is among those that could reasonably be made. Thus, if the pros and cons are finely balanced, the nurse is probably legally covered whichever decision he or she takes. But ethically the nurse is still obliged (insofar as time permits) to consider carefully what is the best thing to do. It is perhaps worth pointing out – though this is largely drawing attention to the obvious – that these problems cannot be solved by a demarcation of the duties of the nurse and the doctor. There has been a tradition of seeing medicine and nursing as clearly divided, with the functions of the nurse being, for example, to keep the patient as comfortable as possible and to carry out the doctor's instructions. It may be questioned whether this ever corresponded to what went on in practice; and it seems now to be agreed that no such exact demarcation of duties is either possible or desirable.

One may sum all this up by saying that in this field ethics differs from law by being concerned with avoiding potential harm rather than redressing actual harm; with all forms of harm that nurses are able to prevent; and with not only doing one's duty, but with thinking out (time permitting) the best thing to do in the given circumstances. The ethical standards are thus higher than the legal ones, and the Code requires more than compliance with the law. This raises a further question, whether the personal ethics of the individual nurse ought to be even more exacting than the Code. Personal ethics, unlike formal codes, needs to be concerned not only with meeting standards but also with pursuing ideals. Professionals, such as nurses, need to be concerned to maintain a level of care above the minimum required by the law and the Code, and to remember that in one sense duty is never completely done.

However, as soon as one says this, one must at once use common sense to qualify it. On the one hand, one needs an ethics that goes beyond duty; on the other, one must remember that nurses, like other people, have been issued with one pair of hands and feet and live through days with 24 hours in them, that hospitals are understaffed, and that even meeting the standards of the Code can take all the time available. Not only would it be unjust to nurses to expect more than is possible or reasonable: if the standards are set too high, the practical result will be worse rather than better. What seems to be required here is a combination of a resolution to maintain a standard of care at least a little above what is required by the law and the Code, with an aspiration to achieve more when time, energy and opportunity permit. What is also required is a sensible use of one's personal feelings, so that they help to maintain the standard rather than weakening it. To recognise that one sometimes fails in one's duty and to resolve not to repeat those failures are both useful; but guilt feelings that are inappropriate (for example, feeling guilty about a failure of aspiration which is not a failure of duty) or excessive (for example, guilt feelings which persist after the resolution not to repeat the failure has been made) often, like the setting of excessively high standards, have the effect of making actual practice worse rather than better.

6.12   The ethical duty of care

These considerations, the concern of ethics with potential as well as actual consequences, the way in which the Code requires more than mere compliance with the law, and the way in which personal ethics should, if possible, consider aspirations as well as duties, are in the main concerned with the duty of care to patients and clients, and with ways in which the Code imposes a stronger duty than does the law. But, as has already been mentioned, the Code imposes a duty not just to do one's best for patients and clients, but to 'protect and promote the health and wellbeing of those in your care, their families and carers, and the wider community.' This raises two further issues.

One such issue concerns the nurse who just happens to be at the scene of an accident, or to be around when someone is taken ill. Legally, there is no obligation to offer help: nurses, midwives and health visitors are under no legal obligation to stop and assist, unless they are already under a duty to help the person in question because of their contract of employment. Moreover, the current version of the Code, unlike the previous version, imposes no specific duty to stop and help, perhaps because it is in the main concerned with the nurse's work as part of a team. Nevertheless, it is hard to see how, under such circumstances, the general duty to the wider community could be carried out other than by providing the care which 'could reasonably be expected from someone with your knowledge, skills, and abilities', to quote the previous version of the Code. This is also in line with the preamble to the Code, in which the Nursing and Midwifery Regulator declare that, 'We exist to safeguard the health and wellbeing of the public.' The Code also says (17): 'You must be able to demonstrate that you have acted in someone's best interests if you have provided care in an emergency', which seems to imply that this is something which will happen, since there is no suggestion that this refers only to emergencies in the hospital. And the very last provision of the Code (61) is: 'You must uphold the reputation of your profession at all times', which it would be hard to do if nurses withheld their skills when they were especially needed.

Interpreted in this way, the Code is very much in line with ordinary morality, which holds both that one ought to help those in need if one can, and that in the particular case of a medical emergency the obligation on health professionals to stop and help is greater than that on other people, because they have the relevant knowledge and skills. There is one problem here: although there is no legal obligation to offer care, once it is offered it is subject to legal obligations, and the victim has a legal claim if they suffer harm as a result: hence the importance of provision 17, quoted above. The existence of this legal paradox, that a nurse cannot be sued for not offering care at all but can be sued for negligence once it is offered, does not remove the moral obligation to offer care. But it is to be hoped that the law of negligence will not, as it has in some countries, develop in such a way that people will be afraid to offer help because the legal risk is so great.

A second area in which moral duty goes beyond legal duty concerns unborn children. Midwives and other health professionals have no legal duty to care for unborn children, and are not legally liable for pre-natal injuries to the child if they have cared properly for the mother. But ethically it would seem that, as long as the interests of mother and child are compatible, the duty of the nurse or midwife must be to both, so that whatever benefits the child should be done, even if it does not directly benefit the mother. In any case, this will normally benefit the mother, in the sense that it will be strongly in accordance with her wishes. There is here an issue of ethical theory, as to whether a fetus/unborn child is a kind of being to which duties can be owed. But this is, unlike some other theoretical issues, a purely linguistic matter: it seems clear that there is a moral duty on the midwife to care for the unborn child as well as the mother, and nothing of substance turns on the question whether this duty is actually owed to the child, owed to the mother, or simply a moral obligation on the midwife: what is actually required will be the same. So, if doing or refraining from doing certain things will benefit the unborn child, or keep it safe, but have no effect on the health of the mother, there seems to be no legal duty on the midwife to do them, or even to inform the mother about them or to recommend them. But there is nevertheless a very clear moral duty to look after both mother and child.

6.13   Conflicts between law and ethics

So far, we have been dealing with various ways in which the moral duty to promote and safeguard the interests and safety of patients and clients goes beyond the legal duty to avoid negligence, but is not incompatible with it. However, there are two areas in which there can be an actual conflict between legal and ethical duties, or rather, in which there are conflicting ethical duties, and, though the law comes down on one side, it is not clear that ethically this is the side that should always prevail. One area concerns the mother and unborn child: if the legal duty is to the mother, but, as was argued in the preceding section, the moral duty is to both, then a conflict is possible, if the needs of the mother and child do not coincide. Very often, of course, either what will benefit one will also benefit the other, or the mother strongly wants to put the child first. The most striking instance in which there is a conflict of needs or of interests occurs when the mother is having an abortion. This conflict of needs could lead to a conflict between legal and moral duties, since the law puts the needs of the mother first, once permission for an abortion has been given, but some nurses would hold either that abortion is always morally wrong or that it is wrong in this instance, because, for example, the mother has no morally serious reason for wanting it. In fact, conflict is usually avoided, because the law specifically allows a nurse with conscientious objections not to take part in providing an abortion. It is true that conscientious objection is no longer mentioned in the Code, perhaps because of the increased emphasis on working as part of a team, but provision 49 says that 'You must adhere to the laws of the country in which you are practising', and to deny to a nurse the right to conscientious objection would be a clear breach of the law.

However, there are two possible problems here. The nurse who has a conscientious objection to abortion as such is covered by the law, but not the nurse who has an objection to a particular abortion, or a particular class of abortions, such as those carried out for social reasons. It would seem, though, that expecting scruples of this sort to be respected is incompatible with being a member of a team. To be excused from a general category of work, because of one's moral scruples, is practicable and just, but to expect to be excused from particular tasks as and when they arise is impracticable and unreasonable: a nurse must decide at the outset whether they are or are not prepared to take part in the provision of abortions. Thus the earlier version of the Code, while specifically recognising the possibility of conscientious objections, required them to be reported 'at the earliest possible time' and also emphasised that the nurse or midwife with these objections had a duty 'to provide care to the best of your ability until alternative arrangements are implemented'.

Second, a very determined opponent of abortion might take the view that it could be the duty of a nurse or midwife not merely to refuse to take part but actually to try to sabotage the whole process. But given that there is no obvious way of doing this, and, more importantly, given that this is incompatible with being a member of a team, there seems to be no way in which this could be ethically justified. It would in any case be a clear breach of provision 49 (see above). To campaign for a change in the law would be a citizen's right, and perhaps they would see it as a duty: to sabotage legal activity cannot under normal conditions be either. It is true that one can conceive of actions carried out in hospitals or by medical practitioners that it would be the duty of a decent and humane person to prevent if they could: female genital mutilation would be an example. But in the United Kingdom at the present time all such actions are illegal, so that, in the unlikely event of their taking place in supposedly reputable surroundings, and so coming to the attention of a nurse, there would be no conflict of duties but a clear duty to prevent illegal activity.

So in the case of abortion the conflict between the legal and ethical duty of care to the mother and the ethical duty of care to the child can be dealt with by the nurse either opting for conscientious objection or accepting the situation. But more complex situations can occur. Suppose, as sometimes happens, that a Caesarean section would be very advisable to prevent harm (e.g. brain damage) to the child, but the mother is refusing to have the operation, on the ground that she will not herself suffer any harm if she gives birth naturally, whereas any operation involves some risk, however slight. Legally, it seems, the midwife should support the mother's decision; ethically, she might well feel that she should bring all reasonable pressure to bear to get the mother to agree. What she should actually do is a disputed matter: it might, for example, be argued that since the mother, however she feels now, clearly does not want to have a brain-damaged child, the duty to both mother and child is to bring the pressure to bear. Whatever decision the midwife takes, the important point here is that it is possible, though hopefully rare in practice, for a health professional to decide that they have an ethical duty to an unborn child which conflicts with their legal duty to the child's mother. What they should then do – and different courses of action may be appropriate in different circumstances, depending on the choices available and the likely consequences of each choice – is a matter for the person involved rather than the academic theorist: it does not seem that any general rule could be made.

The second kind of ethical conflict concerns the tension between provisions 24 and 32 of the Code. These say, respectively, that 'You must work cooperatively within teams and respect the skills, expertise and contributions of your colleagues' and 'You must act without delay if you believe that you, a colleague or anyone else may be putting someone at risk.' In principle, these do not conflict: the nurse is required to respect what her colleagues do when it is right, but to take action when it puts someone at risk. The problem arises when the nurse believes that someone is being put at risk and the colleague does not. This could arise with regard to a particular patient or client, or with regard to general policy or what provision 34 calls 'the environment of care'.

Certainly, both the law and the Code require the nurse to take action under these circumstances; but what kinds of action do they require or support? The law requires a nurse to question orders that they believe to be wrong or mistaken, such as orders which put a patient at risk; but if the orders are confirmed by a doctor or by higher authority, the nurse is not regarded as legally negligent if they then act on them. The Code goes much further than this, requiring the nurse to 'act without delay' if they believe someone is being put at risk. Some of the ways of doing this, though not required by the law, are supported by it. The law will support and safeguard 'whistleblowing', reporting the matter to the appropriate authority. It will also support a nurse who refuses, on professional grounds, to carry out instructions, or a policy, which they believe to be dangerous. And it will support a nurse who for good clinical reasons exempts a particular patient from the established hospital policy. Thus far there are no problems, since what the Code requires and the law does not, the law will nevertheless support.

But there are two possible, though rare, situations in which support from the law is lacking. One would be if the grounds for believing someone was being put at risk were other than professional, being based on something one was told, or had derived from one's experience, which was at variance with current professional opinion. This, though unlikely, is possible and could be justified, if, for example, the patient did not conform to the normal pattern and this was known to their family. Thus a nurse who was told by a patient's brother or sister that they knew a certain treatment was dangerous could well be justified, if the family were sensible people, in withholding the treatment; but it is not absolutely clear that this would be supported by the law, though it would probably be morally right.

The other thing the law will not support is the actual prevention of treatment being carried out, as opposed to refusing to do it oneself. It would be very rare for this to be justified, but not totally impossible. If the consequences of administering a drug were sufficiently terrible, there could be a moral duty not only to refuse to administer it, and/or to report the matter, but even to prevent its being administered, despite the lack of support from the law.

What is much less rare than these situations is, as indicated above, the tension between acting as a cooperative member of a team and objecting to what the team is currently doing, if it is putting someone at risk. There is an important ethical change in the way this tension is now regarded. The previous version of the Code viewed it as a tension between the personal accountability of the nurse and the obligation to carry out instructions from doctors or senior colleagues. The new Code regards the nurse as always part of a team, and the tension is between two things that belonging to a team requires, one being that the members of the team cooperate and the other that each member of the team is responsible for making sure, as best they can, that what the team is cooperating on is in fact the right thing to do, or at least is not obviously wrong. So the nurse who objects to a particular treatment on good grounds is being more loyal to the team than the person proposing the treatment, since they are making sure that the team is doing its job correctly.

This change in attitude is healthy in a number of ways. It makes the Code accord much better with the actual situation and feelings of nurses. It may be a useful corrective to the increasing individualism of the past generation or so, which has its merits but also has encouraged selfishness. If the patient is included in the team, and encouraged as part of the team to work towards their recovery, there is a potentially more useful model of the nurse–patient and doctor–patient relationship than either the paternalistic model (in which they are there to do what they are told) or the consumerist model (in which they are commissioning a service). And, even when things go wrong, the nurse who objects or blows the whistle is still carrying out their duty as a member of the team: there is a problem in deciding what, in this situation, supporting the team requires, but there is no requirement to withdraw support.

One must, though, emphasise that the decision not to cooperate, however much in line with one's responsibilities to the team, should not be taken lightly. The running of any institution requires that individuals make some sacrifice of their personal judgement to the decisions of the team or of those in charge: life would be impossible if these decisions were constantly prevented from being carried out. Even the questioning of orders or decisions, though sometimes very necessary, has to be kept within strict limits, if activities are not to grind to a halt. Also, anyone taking the most drastic step, of actually trying to prevent a decision from being acted on, may well face disciplinary action, and then find that, even if they are morally right, the law and the Code do not in practice adequately protect them. Even whistleblowers, who, if they are reporting genuine instances of risk, are obeying both the law and the Code, may find that, whatever the theory, in fact they are in real trouble. But, despite the need to keep institutions running, and despite the importance of not encouraging people to put themselves on the line when it is not necessary, we must always remember the terrible harm that can be done if no steps are taken to prevent wicked or mistaken actions or policies.

Each health professional will have to decide for themselves when responsibility for team decisions and actions requires that they put themselves on the line.

One hopes that most people will never have to make such a decision. The only guideline one can offer is that this should be considered only if the alternative is clearly seriously harmful. If one's moral duty conflicts with one's legal duty, or if two moral duties conflict, it has to be a matter of individual conscience as to which should be given precedence; and there has also to be awareness that there may be a price to pay.

6.14   Conclusion

A carer has both a legal and a moral duty to avoid negligence. The ethical duty differs from the legal one in the following ways:

(1) It operates whether or not any harm actually follows from the negligence, and whether or not it is a kind of harm recognised by the law or affects people for whom the law regards the nurse as responsible.
(2) Ethically, all members of the team are responsible for making sure that the team's activities do not expose anyone to needless risk, and for taking the appropriate action to prevent this.
(3) The NMC Code requires a higher standard than the law, and requires the carer, on occasion, to weigh up likely harms and benefits in order to decide what it is best to do.
(4) The carer should try to have a personal ethical standard a bit higher than that of the Code, including ideals as well as duties, in so far as time and energy make this possible.
(5) There are ethical duties of care to unborn children and to accident victims, if one can help them, although this is not required by the law.
(6) Ethics may occasionally require someone to go against their legal duty, for example, by actively preventing something harmful being done, or giving preference to someone they are not obliged to care for over someone they are obliged to care for. (These situations are rare but not impossible.)

7 Consent and the Capable Adult Patient

A The Legal Perspective

Jean McHale

Professor of Health Care Law, Director of the Centre for Health Law, Science and Policy, Birmingham Law School, University of Birmingham, Birmingham

Obtaining the consent of a patient to treatment is a crucial part of health care practice. It fosters the bond of trust between practitioner and patient by according the patient respect for his autonomy of decision-making. The Nursing and Midwifery Code provides that:

13. You must ensure that you gain consent before you begin any treatment or care.
14. You must respect and support people's rights to accept or decline treatment and care.
15. You must uphold people's rights to be fully involved in decisions about their care.
16. You must be aware of the legislation regarding mental capacity, ensuring that people who lack capacity remain at the centre of decision making and are fully safeguarded.
17. You must be able to demonstrate that you have acted in someone's best interests if you have provided care in an emergency.[1]

Nursing Law and Ethics, Fourth Edition. Edited by John Tingle and Alan Cribb.
© 2014 by John Wiley & Sons, Ltd. Published 2014 by John Wiley & Sons, Ltd.

Obtaining consent before undertaking treatment is also part of the health professional's legal obligation. If treatment is given without consent, she runs the risk of being sued for damages in the civil law courts or prosecuted in criminal law.

The nurse has two main roles in the consent process. First, when she is acting as the primary carer, providing the patient with treatment, she has the task of obtaining the patient's consent. The expansion in the role of the nurse means increasingly that it is the nurse herself who will be taking on this role. Second, even if a doctor obtains the patient's consent, a patient may be confused or uncertain about his treatment choice and may turn to the nurse for clarification. When complying with her legal obligations in relation to consent to treatment the registered nurse needs also to be aware of her professional ethical obligations, including her role as advocate for her patient. Here, as in other areas of her practice, the nurse may find herself torn between what she believes are the obligations required of her under the Nursing and Midwifery Council Professional Code and her obligations under the contract of employment.

Consent to treatment is one area of health care practice in which the courts may be invited to consider the application of the European Convention of Human Rights through the Human Rights Act 1998.[2] Issues that concern consent to treatment can be found in relation to the debates concerning many areas of health care, and this is reflected in many of the other chapters of this book. This chapter discusses consent to treatment and the competent adult patient. First, the general nature of consent in law and capacity to consent to treatment is discussed. Second, the liability of the nurse in both civil and criminal law if she fails to provide the patient with information regarding his treatment is considered. Third, it examines the situation in which a nurse believes that the doctor has provided her patient with insufficient information with which to make a treatment decision. Some of the difficulties that can face the nurse in attempting to act as an advocate for her patient are examined, particularly in the context of inter-professional conflicts of disclosure.

It should be noted that while this chapter does give an introduction to the issues, it is obviously not possible to explore the full breadth and range of complex issues that arise consequent upon consent to treatment; for a fuller exploration readers are referred to other sources.[3]

7.1   Consent to treatment: Some general issues

7.1.1   The consent form

One of the most frequent cries to be heard in a hospital is: 'Have you got his consent form?' All nurses are familiar with the consent forms given to patients to sign before they go in for an operation. But the fact that the patient has signed a consent form does not necessarily mean that consent is valid. It depends upon the circumstances; simply signing a form does not by itself mean that the implications of that consent have been explained. Equally, consent given orally may be perfectly valid if the patient has been properly informed. However, while it is not strictly required, written consent has the advantage of drawing a patient's attention to the fact that he is consenting to a clinical procedure, and it may provide some evidence of his consent should there be any future dispute as to whether consent was given.

7.1.2   Express and implied consent

While consent may be given expressly, whether in writing or orally, in some situations even express oral consent is not required. If a patient proffers his arm for a bandage to be applied, although she may say nothing, his actions imply that she has consented to the procedure. But there are dangers in too readily assuming that a patient has given implied consent.

7.1.3   Capacity to consent

In order for consent to be valid in law a patient must be capable of making that treatment decision. Adult patients are presumed to have capacity to consent or to refuse consent to a particular treatment, although this refusal can be rebutted.[4] But what is meant by 'capacity'?[5] Obviously, the patient will require some understanding of the implications of the decision that he or she is to make, but how much? Today the law concerning decision-making relating to persons who lack mental capacity is governed by the Mental Capacity Act 2005. The Act itself drew upon an extensive consideration of this area by the Law Commission.[6] Interestingly, the case law from the publication of the Law Commission's report in 1995 and the Mental Capacity Act itself coming into force in 2006 drew upon many of the principles and statements made in that report. The Law Commission's proposals constituted a comprehensive review of capacity over the whole area of care and treatment of the mentally incompetent adult, including such issues as advance directives (see Chapter 10A) and powers of attorney. This chapter focuses upon those provisions which relate to the issue of consent to treatment.

7.1.4   The Mental Capacity Act 2005

The Mental Capacity Act 2005 provides a statutory framework for decision-making concerning adults lacking mental capacity.[7] Like the common law, the Act roots decision-making in a 'best interests' test. It does not automatically provide for a third-party decision-maker to act on behalf of an adult lacking capacity, although in contrast to the common law it does allow for the appointment of a person to make treatment decisions on behalf of the person lacking capacity through a 'lasting power of attorney'.[8]

Section 1 of the Mental Capacity Act 2005 sets out a series of 'principles' that are to underpin decision-making. There is a statutory presumption in favour of decision-making capacity. In addition, there is a requirement that all reasonably practicable steps are to be taken to ensure that the individual makes the decision. Furthermore, as at common law, decisions must be reached on the basis of the 'best interests' of the individual. Section 2(1) states that a person will lack capacity where they are unable to make the decision themselves owing to 'an impairment of or a disturbance in the functioning of the mind or brain'. As at common law, the capacity test is decision-specific. A person may have the capacity to make one decision, while at the same time being incapable of making another.

Prior to the Act the test for capacity was considered by the courts. In *Re C (adult: refusal of treatment)* (1994) the court upheld the right of a 68-year-old paranoid schizophrenic who had developed gangrene in his foot to prevent his foot being amputated in the future without his express written consent. Mr Justice Thorpe suggested a three-part test to determine capacity, as follows:

> first, comprehending and retaining treatment information, secondly, believing it and thirdly, weighing it in the balance to arrive at a choice.

At the hearing it was claimed that C was not competent because of his delusions that he was a doctor and that whatever treatment was given to him was calculated to destroy his body. But despite these claims Mr Justice Thorpe held that he was satisfied that C was capable of giving or refusing consent because he understood and had retained the relevant treatment information, and believed it and had arrived at a clear choice. One potential problem with the test in *Re C* is that it makes capacity dependent on the information that the patient is actually given. If the nurse provides a patient with a great deal of complex information he or she may be unable to understand it and as a result lack capacity. In contrast, if a basic explanation is given, the very same patient may possess the capacity to consent.

This approach was developed in the later case of *Re MB (medical treatment)* (1997), in which a woman with a needle phobia, while agreeing to a Caesarean section that was clinically required, repeatedly refused the anaesthetic prior to the Caesarean section (this case is discussed further below in section 7.2.5). Lady Butler-Sloss held that a person is not capable of making a decision where:

(a)   the person is unable to comprehend and retain the information which is material to the decision, especially as to the likely consequences of having or not having the treatment in question; and

(b)   the patient is unable to use the information and weigh it in the balance as of the process of arriving at a decision.

Section 3(1) of the Mental Capacity Act 2005 now in effect codifies the *Re C* test and sets out the circumstances in which a person is unable to make a decision. It states that a person is unable to understand the information that is necessary in relation to this decision; unable to retain it; unable to use or weigh up the information as part of the decision-making process or unable to communicate the decision by any means (this includes talking and sign language). Information here includes information regarding the foreseeable consequences of the necessary decision.[9] The fact that a decision may be perceived as being irrational does not necessarily mean that it will be held to be unlawful.

Lack of capacity may be permanent or may be temporary in nature; this may be a considerable practical problem, if a patient has fluctuating capacity. The Act in many ways can be seen as maximising capacity in such a situation. Section 3(2) provides that:

> The fact that a person is able to retain the information relevant to a decision for a short period only does not prevent him from being regarded as able to make the decision.

Statutory safeguards are given to those caring for the person who lacks mental capacity, thus removing any legal uncertainty as to their actions. Section 5 provides that where a person acts in the best interests of an adult lacking capacity, they will not be subject to legal liability as long as, first, they have undertaken reasonable steps to ascertain that the adult lacks capacity; second, that they reasonably believe that the person lacks decision-making capacity; and third, the decision that has been made is in the person's best interests.

If a person lacks capacity, then treatment may be given where it is in their best interests to do so. The best interests test that exists at common law is codified and structured under the Mental Capacity Act 2005. Section 4 of the Act sets out some guidance as to what constitutes a person's best interests. The person must not simply take into account age or appearance or condition/aspect of behaviour which could lead to unjustified assumptions about his best interests. In addition relevant circumstances should be taken into account, such as whether it is likely that the person will at some time have capacity in relation to this issue. Factors that should be taken into account 'as far as is reasonably practicable' include an individual's past and present wishes and feelings, any beliefs and values that would have been taken into account if they had capacity and any 'other factors that he would be likely to consider if he were able to do so'.[10]

The legislation makes provision for the appointment of an independent mental capacity advocate under sections 35–7 to provide representation and support for a person who lacks capacity. Such a person should be appointed in a situation in which there is no close friend or family member who can be consulted and it is necessary to give 'serious medical treatment' to the adult.

Further guidance as to the operation of the legislation is contained in the Mental Capacity Act Code of Practice issued to accompany the legislation.[11]

7.1.5   Criminal law and consent to treatment

As a general rule, if a patient gives consent to a medical procedure being undertaken, then no criminal liability will result. But the fact that consent has been given does not automatically mean that the treatment itself is lawful. The individual does not have absolute freedom in English law to do what he or she wishes with his or her body.[12] Some medical procedures such as female circumcision are expressly prohibited by statute.[13] Uncertainties surround the legality of certain other medical procedures. For example, while it appears that as long as organ transplant operations do not constitute an unjustified risk to the life of the donor, they will not be held to be unlawful,[14] the lawfulness of animal to human transplantations is still to be resolved.[15] Where a major operation is undertaken without consent, there is the possibility of a prosecution under section 18 of the Offences Against the Person Act 1861. This section makes it an offence to 'unlawfully and maliciously' cause grievous bodily harm to a person with the intention of causing grievous bodily harm. However, it is more likely that a nurse who has given treatment without the patient's consent will be prosecuted for the less serious crime of battery. This makes unlawful any non-consensual touching.[16]

7.2   Civil law liability

7.2.1   Battery

While treating without obtaining the patient's consent may lead to a criminal prosecution, it is far more likely that absence of consent will lead to an action in the civil courts. First, an action may be brought in the tort of battery. An action in battery arises if a patient is touched without his consent. Not every touching will lead to liability: for example, an action is unlikely to result from the nurse accidentally brushing a patient's shoulder as she passes in a corridor. There is no need to prove that the touching caused damage – the fact that it took place is sufficient for an action to be brought. In *Chatterton* v. *Gerson* Mr Justice Bristow held that no liability would arise as long as the patient was informed and understood in broad terms the nature of the procedure that it was proposed to undertake, and she had given consent.[17] If a broad general consent is given, then any further claim that a patient has been given inadequate information should be brought not in battery but in negligence.[18]

7.2.2   Treating in an emergency where no consent can be obtained

There may be some situations in which it is lawful for the nurse to go ahead and treat a patient without obtaining his consent, most notably in an emergency situation as in the patient brought bleeding and unconscious into casualty. In such situations treatment can be given on the basis of necessity. In addition, if a patient has given initial consent to an operation but then, later, during the operation it is discovered that he is suffering, for example, from a life-threatening condition such as a cancerous tumour, then this may be removed. But while necessity may justify the performance of a medical procedure in an emergency, exactly what is necessary is a matter of degree.[19] The nurse should ask herself if this particular procedure is immediately necessary or could it be postponed until the patient recovers consciousness and can make his own decision.

7.2.3   Consent and refusal

The patient has the right both to consent to and to refuse medical treatment. An action in battery may be brought if treatment is given in the face of an explicit refusal of consent. A well-known case often quoted as a warning to those who may be tempted to treat in the face of refusal is the Canadian case of *Malette* v. *Schumann*.[20] The claimant was brought into hospital following a road accident. A nurse found a card in the claimant's pocket that identified her as being a Jehovah's Witness and that requested that she was never to be given a blood transfusion. Despite the card the doctor performed the transfusion. On recovering her health, the patient brought an action in battery. She succeeded and was awarded $20,000 damages. In a later English case, that of Ms B, continuation of treatment against the patient's wishes was held to be a battery. Ms B was quadriplegic. She was supported on a ventilator but wanted this support withdrawn.[21] The hospital refused to accede to her wishes. She went to court and ultimately her claim was successful. She was held to have decision-making capacity and she thus had a right to refuse treatment – which included the right to refuse ventilation. Nominal damages were awarded against the hospital for continuing to treat her. Subsequently the ventilator support was removed, and she died. (See also Chapter 10.) The Mental Capacity Act now specifically sets out the procedure which enables individuals to execute an 'advance decision' or so-called 'living will' which enables persons over the age of 18 to refuse treatment in sections 24–26. In addition sections 9–11 of the Act enable persons over 18 to authorise the creation of a lasting power of attorney to give another person power to make decisions about such matters as health and social care when they lack decision-making capacity. These powers are considered further in this book in relation to end-of-life decision making (see Chapter 13).

A further reason why patients may argue that their decision to refuse treatment should be upheld is because this is a fundamental human right, one that is now safeguarded under the Human Rights Act 1998. A number of the rights contained in the European Convention of Human Rights may be relevant in this context: for example, Article 3, because imposition of treatment upon a competent patient against their wishes may be held to constitute inhuman or degrading treatment or punishment. In addition, Article 8, which concerns the right to respect for privacy of home and family life, may be applicable – but as this right is not absolute, it can be argued that there will not be an infringement of Article 8 where the patient is not in a position to give informed consent.[22] Article 9 of the Convention – freedom of religion – may also be used to support the refusal of treatment in a situation in which the reason why the individual is refusing treatment is because of a tenet of their particular religious belief. In the past in a number of cases refusal of treatment on religious grounds has been overruled by the courts, particularly in the context of refusal by child patients.[23] It will be interesting to see how these issues are considered in the future.

7.2.4   Overruling a refusal of treatment

7.2.4.1   Free not forced consent

A patient must reach his decision whether to consent or refuse treatment freely and without pressure being applied by relatives or by carers. In *Re T* in 1992 an important factor in the decision to authorise a transfusion was that T's refusal came after she had spent time alone with her mother, a confirmed Jehovah's Witness. Ensuring that a patient gives free and full consent may be practically very difficult for a nurse working on a busy ward. Inevitably, the amount of time that can be spent with a patient discussing the implications of a decision is subject to the time constraints of practice, but the patient must not be browbeaten by relatives or by medical staff into making the decision. In determining whether consent has been given in a particular situation, the court will look to the circumstances. The fact that a patient is, for example, a prisoner does not mean that he is unable to give free consent. In *Freeman* v. *Home Office* the court held that whether the prisoner/patient had, in fact, consented was a question of fact for each individual case.[24] But in this type of situation it is of particular importance that when information is given to the patient, it is made clear to him that he has a free choice.

7.2.5   Pregnant women refusing care

A midwife is faced with a pregnant woman in difficulties in labour who is refusing even to contemplate a Caesarean section. By rejecting treatment she is placing her life and that of the fetus in jeopardy. Should her refusal of treatment be respected? This issue came before the English courts in a series of cases during the 1990s. In *Re S* the case concerned a woman six days overdue giving birth where the medical team sought to undertake a Caesarean section.[25] To attempt a normal birth would have caused a very grave risk of rupture to the uterus because the fetus was in transverse lie, placing the lives of mother and child in grave danger. S, a born-again Christian, refused the operation because it was against her religious beliefs. The hospital went to court to obtain a declaration, which was controversially granted by Sir Stephen Brown. The judge made reference to the rights of the fetus, but English courts have in the past consistently rejected claims that the fetus has such rights.[26]

Sir Stephen Brown placed some emphasis on a US case, *Re AC*.[27] In a number of cases, courts in the USA were prepared to order pregnant women to be given a Caesarean section despite their refusal of treatment.[28] In *Re AC* the court initially ordered a Caesarean section on a woman dying of cancer. This order was overturned on appeal after AC had died. The court said that in 'virtually all cases' a refusal could not be overridden; they did admit there may be exceptional circumstances in which a Caesarean may be ordered. An example given in discussion in the case was very similar to the facts in *Re S*. Nevertheless, *Re AC* is widely seen as the case that curtailed judicially ordered Caesarean sections in the USA.[29] In many ways *Re S* can be regarded as an exceptional case – an aberration. After the decision the Royal College of Obstetricians and Gynaecologists (RCOG) published a consultation paper stating: 'It is inappropriate and unlikely to be helpful or necessary to invoke judicial intervention to overrule an informed and competent woman's refusal of a proposed medical treatment even though her refusal may place her life and that of her foetus at risk.'[30]

Despite this, in a number of subsequent cases judicial intervention was sought and the courts authorised the performance of Caesarean sections upon women who had refused such procedures.[31] The Court of Appeal was given an opportunity to rule on this issue in *Re MB*.[32] MB had a fear of needles. This had led her to refuse to have blood samples taken during pregnancy. In the late stages of pregnancy it was discovered that the fetus was in the breach position. A Caesarean section was proposed. MB initially agreed; however, she was opposed to administration of anaesthetic by needles. MB then went into labour. She agreed to a Caesarean section and the administration of anaesthetic by mask, but at the last moment refused the anaesthetic. The hospital then sought a court order, which was given by Mr Justice Hollis. He found that MB was incompetent because of the effects of the needle phobia on her decision-making powers. She asked her lawyer to appeal. She then herself agreed to the Caesarean section, and the operation was carried out the following day. MB challenged the legality of the procedure. On appeal to the Court of Appeal the right of the competent patient to refuse treatment was confirmed. However, it was also recognised that, in an emergency, treatment could be given where a patient lacks capacity, as long as this was on the basis of necessity, the procedure not extending beyond what was reasonably required by the patient. Lady Butler-Sloss noted the judgment of Lord Donaldson in *Re T* where he stated that the doctor must assess carefully whether in that case the patient had the capacity 'commensurate with the gravity of the decision' she purported to make. The Court of Appeal referred to the three-stage test for capacity set out by Mr Justice Thorpe in *Re C* discussed above. Lady Butler-Sloss commented:

> A competent woman who has the capacity to decide may, for religious reasons, other reasons, for rational or irrational reasons or for no reason at all, choose not to have medical intervention, even though the consequence may be the death or serious handicap of the child she bears, or her own death.

She went on to state:

> Irrationality is here used to connote a decision which is so outrageous in its defiance of logic or of accepted moral standards that no sensible person who has applied his mind to the question to be decided could have arrived at it . . . Although it might be thought that irrationality sits uneasily with competence to decide, panic, indecisiveness and irrationality in themselves do not as such amount to incompetence, but they may be symptoms or evidence of incompetence. The graver the consequences of the decision the commensurately greater the level of competence is required to take the decision.

Capacity may be eroded owing to temporary incompetence, as indicated by Lord Donaldson in the earlier case of *Re T* as 'confusion, shock, pain and drugs'. The Court of Appeal on the facts of this particular case upheld the decision of the judge at the first instance that MB had lacked capacity. She was competent to consent to the Caesarean section. However, she did not have competence to refuse as she was 'at that moment suffering an impairment of her mental functioning which disabled her. She was temporarily incompetent'. Her phobia of needles impaired her ability to decide.

Two points arise here. First is the extent to which the circumstances of pregnancy itself served to erode the woman's capacity. In view of the fact that temporary factors may erode capacity, Kennedy is surely right to argue that '. . . there is an urgent need to establish the boundaries of the permissible' in this area.[28] Second, Butler-Sloss makes an important statement confirming that the law sanctions 'irrational' refusals. Nonetheless, the judgment leaves unclear where the boundary can be drawn between 'acceptable' irrationality, which will not impact on respect for the patient's right to decide, and an 'irrational' decision, which may impact on capacity in such a way that an individual's competence to make that decision is affected.

Having found MB to be temporarily incompetent, the Court of Appeal then considered whether the procedure itself could be authorised. The House of Lords in *Re F* had confirmed that medical procedures may be undertaken on adults lacking mental capacity where it is in his or her best interests.[33] The Court of Appeal held that the treatment was in MB's best interests in this emergency situation. But in whose best interests was this procedure? The Court of Appeal took into consideration the fact that agreement had initially been given by MB for the Caesarean section. Furthermore, evidence from the consultant psychiatrist was to the effect that if the child had been born disabled or had died, MB herself would have suffered long-term harm. In contrast, little harm would be caused by the administration of the anaesthetic against her wishes. What of the interrelationship between the best interests of both the fetus and the woman? The Court of Appeal upheld earlier cases such as *Paton v. British Pregnancy Advisory Service*[34] in confirming that the fetus has no independent status in English law. They were of the view that Sir Stephen Brown in *Re S* had reached an incorrect conclusion. The Court of Appeal stated:

> Although it may seem illogical that a child capable of being born alive is protected by the criminal law from intentional destruction, and by the Abortion Act from termination otherwise than as permitted by the Act, but is not protected from the (irrational) decision of a competent mother not to allow medical intervention to avert the risk of death, this appears to be the present state of the law.[35]

Thus even at the point of birth itself, the court could not intervene in the face of refusal of medical intervention by a competent woman with the aim of safeguarding the position of the fetus.

Re MB also recognises that there may be circumstances (beyond the Mental Health Act 1983) when the use of forcible treatment may be justifiable. Lady Butler-Sloss stated:

> The extent of force or compulsion which may be necessary can only be judged in each individual case and by the health professionals. It may become for them a balance between continuing treatment which is forcibly opposed and deciding not to continue with it. This is a difficult issue which may need to be considered in depth on another occasion.[36]

One of the most important aspects of the decision in *Re MB* is that it provides guidance for future cases in this area by setting out procedures that should be undertaken. This includes the requirement that the woman should be represented in all cases save where, in exceptional circumstances, she does not wish to be so. This recommendation goes some way to meet concerns as to the manner in which such proceedings have been brought. This guidance was considered further in *St George's NHS Trust* v. *S*, discussed below.

7.2.6   Caesarean sections and the Mental Health Act

There have also been a number of cases in which the Mental Health Act 1983 was used to sanction the performance of Caesarean sections upon mentally incompetent women. Section 63 of the Act provides that:

> [T]he consent of a patient shall not be required for any medical treatment given to him for the mental disorder from which he is suffering.

The boundaries of section 63 – what amounted to medical treatment for mental disorder – came before the courts in *Tameside and Glossop Acute Hospital Trust* v. *CH*.[37] CH was detained under section 3 of the Mental Health Act 1983. She was suffering from paranoid schizophrenia. She was then discovered to be pregnant. It was held that as she lacked capacity to consent to or refuse treatment, a Caesarean section could be authorised, as the performance of a Caesarean section was treatment for 'mental disorder' and thus fell within the scope of section 63 of the Mental Health Act 1983. This was because if a stillbirth had occurred, her health would have deteriorated, and she needed strong antipsychotic medication which could not be given to her when she was pregnant. The court followed the approach in *B* v. *Croydon HA* that section 63 of the 1983 Act encompassed matters that related to the 'core treatment' (in that case including force-feeding).[38] Such a broad interpretation of this provision has been criticised. For example, as Grubb has argued, section 63 does not cover any physical condition that impedes treatment of mental disorder. As he notes: 'The Government saw section 63 in far more limited terms covering perfectly routine, sensible treatment.'

A contrasting approach was taken by the Court of Appeal in the case of *St George's NHS Trust* v. *S*.[39] S was diagnosed as suffering from severe pre-eclampsia. She was advised that she should have an early delivery. S, who had intended a home delivery, refused treatment. She asserted that nature should take its course, although she was informed as to the risk of death and disability to herself and the fetus. Her GP initiated steps that led to her detention in hospital under section 2 of the Mental Health Act 1983. She was subsequently transferred to another hospital. While she persistently refused treatment and sought legal advice, the hospital authority, without her knowledge, made an *ex parte* application to the High Court for a declaration to the effect that it would be lawful to undertake treatment, including a Caesarean section. Meanwhile, S had been in touch with solicitors with the intention of making an application to a Mental Health Review Tribunal. The declaration was granted. It appears that the judge was under an incorrect impression that S had been in labour for 24 hours. S gave birth to a daughter. The detention under the Mental Health Act was terminated. S discharged herself. While detained in hospital, S was not offered treatment for her mental disorder. An action was subsequently brought for judicial review to challenge the legality of the action taken. The Court of Appeal again emphasised the fact that the competent adult is entitled to refuse treatment.[40] Lord Justice Judge stated:

> In our judgment while pregnancy increases the personal responsibilities of a woman it does not diminish her entitlement to decide whether or not to

undergo medical treatment. Although human and protected by the law in a number of different ways as set out in the judgment in Re MB . . . an unborn child is not a separate person from its mother. Its need for medical assistance does not prevail over her rights.

These words are indicative of the tensions in drawing the boundaries between moral acceptability and legal enforcement in this area. While some may regard a pregnant woman as possessing moral responsibilities to the fetus in the latter stages of pregnancy, this still does not limit her legal rights. The orthodoxy of *Paton* and subsequent cases was again confirmed by the court. The court held that a battery had been committed on S. Lord Justice Judge stated:

how can an enforced invasion of a competent adult's body against her will even for the most laudable of motives (the preservation of life) be ordered without irredeemably damaging the principle of self-determination?

The court examined the provisions of section 2(2) which provide that:

An application for admission for assessment may be made in respect of a patient on the grounds that (a) he is suffering from a mental disorder of a nature or degree which warrants the detention of the patient in a hospital for assessment (or for assessment followed by medical treatment) for at least a limited period; and (b) he ought to be so detained in the interests of his own health and safety or with a view to the protection of other persons.

The Court of Appeal emphasised that the criteria for detention under the section were cumulative. In this case the doctors had been justified in their assessment that the woman was suffering from depression that constituted 'mental disorder'. However, S was not being detained in order that treatment be given for her mental disorder. It was stated that:

For the purposes of section 2(2) a detention must be related to or linked with the mental disorder. Treatment for the effects of pregnancy does not provide the necessary warrant.

Thus the courts have affirmed that, for treatment to be lawful under section 63, it must be crucial to the mental disorder. While here the treatment was not treatment for mental disorder within the provisions of the statute, as Bailey Harris notes, questions regarding the connection between the disorder and the treatment proposed are likely to arise in the future.[41] Finally, there had been irregularities in the documentation used by the hospital. Forms had not been completed when the woman was transferred between hospitals, as was required by regulations made under section 19 of the Mental Health Act. This would, in any event, have entitled S to discharge herself from hospital. While some might regard her decision as unjustifiable or even irrational, this did not mean that it was of no legal validity. The Mental Health Act cannot be used as a means of circumventing the competent woman's right to refuse a Caesarean section.

The decisions of the Court of Appeal in *Re MB* and *St George's NHS Trust* v. *S* are in many respects welcome. The autonomy of the patient is confirmed. Judicial guidance is also given as to the correct procedures that should be adopted when making an application for a declaration and the need for pregnant women and their advisers to be provided with adequate information. Referring what appear to be insurmountable differences between the parties to the courts constitutes recognition that there are certain decisions that, because of their inherently difficult nature, may not be suitable for resolution by the parties alone because of their multifaceted nature and because there are broader issues of public policy that may arise. A conflict between the patient and her midwife or doctor over the conduct of childbirth may in fact be well suited to the involvement of an independent arbiter. It also provides safeguards for the patient. There are dangers in low-visibility of 'hard case' treatment decisions as evidenced by the concern of the courts to be involved, for example, in sanctioning certain invasive procedures on adults (lacking mental capacity) such as sterilisation or decisions at the end of life.[42]

Nonetheless, these controversial Court of Appeal decisions leave many issues to be resolved, in particular around the interpretation of 'capacity' to decide. The test for capacity is decision-relative. The graver the consequences of the ultimate decision, the more careful the scrutiny given to the capacity of the patient to make that decision. This is inevitable. The more serious the consequences of the refusal, the more important it is to ensure that the patient possesses the necessary competence to make the treatment decision. It is also the case that as temporary incompetence may invalidate capacity, it is important to ensure that the notion of capacity is not manipulated to deny individual autonomy. Nurses and midwives as patient advocates are likely to play important roles in this process.

7.2.7   Consent and civil law liability: Negligence

For a general discussion of the law of negligence, see Chapter 6. Obtaining a broad general consent to medical procedures being performed is sufficient to avoid liability in battery. But in addition, for a patient to give full and effective consent, she must have some appreciation of the risks that the medical procedure in question may go wrong. If a patient is not informed of the risk of complications and if one or more of these complications arises, then she may bring an action in negligence. The basis of her claim is first that those who are treating her are under a duty to provide her with information about the risks of the treatment; second, that this duty has been broken; and third, that she has suffered harm because had she known of the risk (which did in fact materialise), she would not have consented to the treatment.

The leading House of Lords case is *Sidaway* v. *Bethlem Royal Hospital Governors*.[43] Mrs Sidaway underwent an operation after having suffered for some time from a recurring pain in her neck, right shoulder and arm. The operation was performed by a senior neurosurgeon at the Bethlem Royal Hospital. Even if the operation were carried out with all due care and skill, there was a 1–2 per cent risk of damage to the nerve root and the spinal column. Although the risk of damage to the spinal column was less than that to the nerve root, the consequences were more severe. The plaintiff was left severely disabled after the operation. She brought an action in negligence claiming that she had not been given adequate warning of the risks of the operation. During the hearing it was revealed that while the surgeon had told her of the risks of damage to the nerve root, he had not told her of the risks of damage to the spinal column. In acting in this way he was conforming to what in 1974 would have been accepted as standard medical practice by a responsible and skilled body of neurosurgeons. The House of Lords rejected the claim that the surgeon had acted negligently. An 'informed consent' approach was rejected by all the Law Lords – except Lord Scarman. Some support was given to the suggestion that the test that a court should use in deciding whether the advice given was negligent was the same as that used in deciding whether medical treatment was negligent – the *Bolam* test.[44] This test provides that a health care practitioner:

> is not guilty of negligence if he has acted in accordance with a practice accepted as proper by a responsible body of medical men.

This approach was followed by Lord Diplock in the House of Lords. This obligation of disclosure applies to all types of medical procedure. A broader approach was taken by Lord Bridge, who said that a judge could disagree with the evidence given to him:

> I am of the opinion that the judge might in certain circumstances come to the conclusion that disclosure of a particular risk was so obviously necessary to an informed choice on the part of the patient that no reasonably prudent medical man would fail to make it.

He commented:

> The kind of case I have in mind would be an operation involving a substantial risk of grave adverse consequences, as for example, [a] 10 per cent risk of stroke from the operation . . . In such a case, in the absence of some cogent clinical reason why the patient should not be informed, a doctor . . . could hardly fail to appreciate the necessity for an appropriate warning.

Where the risk of an adverse effect was slight or insignificant, the information could be withheld where this was an accepted practice within the community of medicine. The risks disclosed must be reasonably foreseeable. Lord Templeman distinguished between general risks that would normally be known to the patient and special risks that might be required to be disclosed. Lord Templeman stressed that it was for the court to decide whether the practitioner had acted negligently or not. No distinction is drawn between therapeutic and non-therapeutic forms of care.[45] While the courts have traditionally been hesitant to scrutinise the responsible body of professional practice in the years following *Sidaway*, one example of a case in which they did do so was *Smith* v. *Tunbridge Wells*.[46] Mr Smith, a 28-year-old married man with two children, suffered a rectal prolapse. Surgery was proposed and was undertaken. While the operation was successful, the plaintiff suffered nerve damage during surgery and was left impotent. He brought an action claiming that he should have been informed of the risk of impotence. His claim was upheld by Mr Justice Morland who stated:

In my judgment by 1988, although some surgeons may still not have been warning patients similar in situation to the plaintiff of the risk of impotence, that omission was neither reasonable nor responsible.

Until relatively recently this case could be regarded as very much the aberration. However, over the last few years there have been indications that the courts are prepared to scrutinise the body of professional practice, and we return to this a little later.

7.2.7.1   'Informed' consent

An alternative approach to the professional practice standard which has been adopted in a number of other countries such as Australia, Canada and the USA is that of 'informed consent'.[47] Several states in the USA now require a standard of disclosure based upon the information that a 'prudent patient' would expect to receive. In *Sidaway* Lord Scarman, who delivered a dissenting judgment, supported this approach, saying that the patient should be given such information as a prudent patient would wish to know. While at that time the majority in the House of Lords rejected such an approach, subsequently both in law and in practice there has definitely been a move towards its adoption. Health care professionals are now being directed to give patients more information about certain types of treatment. There is a perceived need for enhanced frankness and openness by health care professionals. One of the issues emphasised in the debate around the unauthorised retention of human material, including organs, at Alder Hey and at a number of hospitals up and down the country has been the failure to obtain adequate consent from relatives for the retention of such material.[48] The Inquiry Report into Bristol Royal Infirmary suggested a number of ways in which the provision of information could be improved.[49] It emphasised the need for 'respect and honesty' in health care and for the health care professional–patient relationship to be seen as one of partnership. Consent is also to be seen as a process:

> Trust can be only sustained by openness. Secondly, openness means that information be given freely, honestly and regularly. Thirdly, it is of fundamental importance to be honest about the twin concerns of risk and uncertainty. Lastly informing patients and in the case of young children their parents must be regarded as a process and not as a one-off event.[50]

The report recommended that 'Patients must be given such information as enables them to participate in their care.' It suggested processes for improving the conveyance of information such as ensuring that information is evidence-based, and that, importantly, 'information should be tailored to the needs, circumstances and wishes of the individual'. The Government committed itself to taking this report further and this led to the production of informed consent guidance by the Department of Health.[51]

While professional practice seemed to become increasingly responsive to an 'informed consent', as opposed to 'professional practice standard', this issue was not subject to scrutiny by the courts for several years. Gradually in the 1990s indications emerged that the judiciary were prepared to question the 'profes-sional practice' standard of the *Bolam* test. The decision of the House of Lords in *Bolitho* v. *City and Hackney HA* signalled a different approach.[52] In this case Lord Browne Wilkinson stated that:

> if in a rare case, it can be demonstrated that professional opinion is not capable of withstanding logical analysis, the judge is entitled to hold that the body of opinion is not reasonable or responsible.[53]

Admittedly this judgment was limited in scope and, despite some suggestions made at the time, it does not at all mean that the *Bolam* standard in negli-gence – the standard of the responsible body of professional practice – is dead. In addition, these comments relate to diagnosis and treatment. *Bolitho* itself did not address the question of disclosure of risk. However, it can be seen as being indicative of an increasing judicial willingness to take a 'hard look' at the view expressed by a body of professional opinion. The application of *Bolitho* to diag-nosis and risk disclosure was considered in the decision of *Pearce* v. *United Bristol NHS Trust*.[54] Here the Court of Appeal looked at the decisions in *Bolitho* and in *Sidaway*. Lord Woolf held that:

> if there is a significant risk which would affect the judgement of a reasonable patient then in the normal course it is the responsibility of a doctor to inform the patient of that significant risk, if the information is needed so that the patient can determine for him or herself as to what course she should adopt.[55]

On the facts of the case the woman was advised against a Caesarean section and the child was delivered stillborn. There was a small risk of 1–2 in 1000 that the child would be stillborn. The claimant was unable to establish that this was 'significant'. Nonetheless, although the claimant was unsuccessful in this par-ticular case, the judgment itself can be seen as another step towards a patient-based approach to consent to treatment.[56]

The movement towards judicial recognition of enhanced disclosure was con-firmed by the House of Lords in *Chester* v. *Afshar*.[57] Miss Chester, who suffered back pain, consulted a rheumatologist. She was found to have a significant dete-rioration of the spinal discs. She was referred to Mr Afshar, a consultant neuro-surgeon, who advised her that surgery was needed to remove three discs. Miss Chester asked Mr Afshar about the 'horror stories' of such operations. At trial there was a dispute as to the information that actually had been given. Mr Afshar stated that he had informed her that there was a small risk of lower spinal cord nerve root disturbance, haemorrhage and infection. However, Miss Chester stated that she had not been given this information but rather had been told by the consultant that he 'hadn't crippled anybody yet'. Miss Chester stated that if she had been given the information as to the risk of treatment, she would not have gone ahead with the information at the time, and she would have sought further opinions as to the best course of treatment.

At trial Miss Chester's evidence was preferred. The trial judge held that 'the defendant's failure to advise the claimant adequately was negligent'. In the House of Lords the discussion fundamentally concerned the causation point, which is discussed below in section 7.2.7.4. However, there was consideration 'obiter' of the risk disclosure issue by Lord Steyn. Importantly, he cast the issue of disclosure in terms of 'autonomy'.

> A surgeon owes a legal duty to a patient to warn him or her in general terms of possible serious risks involved in the procedure. The only qualification is that there may be wholly exceptional cases where objectively in the best interests of the patient the surgeon may be excused from giving a warning. This is, however, irrelevant in the present case. In modern law medical paternalism no longer rules and a patient has a prima facie right to be informed by a surgeon of a small, but well established, risk of serious injury as a result of surgery.[58]

> Secondly, not all rights are equally important. But a patient's right to an appropriate warning from a surgeon when faced with surgery ought normatively to be regarded as an important right which must be given effective protection whenever possible.

> Thirdly, in the context of attributing legal responsibility, it is necessary to identify precisely the protected legal interests at stake. A rule requiring a doctor to abstain from performing an operation without the informed consent of a patient serves two purposes. It tends to avoid the occurrence of the particular physical injury the risk of which a patient is not prepared to accept. It also ensures that due respect is given to the autonomy and dignity of each patient.[59]

Judicial willingness to scrutinise the information given to a patient was demonstrated further in the subsequent case of *Birch* v. *University College London Hospital NHS Foundation Trust*. Mrs Birch had consented to a cerebral catheter angiogram to be performed to see if there was an aneurysm in the brain.[60] She suffered a stroke. While she had been informed of the risk of the stroke, what she had not been informed of was that there was an alternative procedure (namely, non-invasive magnetic resonance imaging) which could have been undertaken. The judge Cranston J held that she should have been informed of these alternatives. He said that

> The duty to inform a patient of significant risks will not be discharged unless she is made aware that fewer or no risks are associated with another procedure. In other words, unless the patient is informed of the comparative risks of different procedures she will not be in a position to give her fully informed consent to one procedure rather than to another.[61]

The judgments in *Pearce, Chester* v. *Afshar* and *Birch* can be seen as a broad 'patient-centred approach'. It thus appears that it is likely to become increasingly difficult to justify withholding information regarding the risks of treatment from patients. This may also be reflective of the fact that there is a tendency towards enhanced disclosure today on a routine basis in health care and that in many cases the responsible body of professional practice is likely to favour broader disclosure. Nonetheless, it does not mean that the duty of information disclosure extends always to comprehending the information given. In the subsequent case of *Al Hamwi* v. *Johnston and Another* the action failed.[62] The trial judge, Mr Justice Simon, drew a distinction between giving information and ensuring that the patient understood that information. He stated that it was 'too onerous' to impose on the doctor a duty to ensure that the patient understood the information that had been given.[63]

7.2.7.2   Therapeutic privilege

While in the majority of cases providing a patient with information about her treatment can be seen as a positive step enhancing her autonomy, there may be some situations in which those caring for her believe that information may be withheld under what is known as the 'therapeutic privilege', where this is in the best interests of the patient. In *Sidaway* Lord Templeman said:

> [S]ome information may confuse, other information may alarm a particular patient . . . the doctor must decide in the light of his training and experience and the light of knowledge of the patient what should be said and how it should be said.[64]

The application of this principle may be questioned in the light of recent medical practice with the movement towards providing a patient with full information and also in respect of what appears to be enhanced judicial willingness to scrutinise the provision of information to patients. Certainly if a therapeutic privilege exception remains it needs to be exercised with extreme caution in the light of earlier judicial dicta in cases such as *Chester*.

The courts, as indicated above, appear to be increasingly prepared to scrutinise the standard of disclosure proffered by health care professionals.[65] It may also be the case that in the future, should information be withheld from patients, claims will be brought under the Human Rights Act 1998. The trend is towards disclosure, and this should be welcomed as part of the nurse's partnership in clinical practice with her patient. Cooperation rather than conflict will surely facilitate better patient care.

7.2.7.3   The questioning patient

The nurse may give the patient some explanation of the procedures and potential risks of the treatment but the patient may later approach the nurse and ask for further information. How should the nurse respond? In the House of Lords in *Sidaway* some of the members of the court indicated that there might be an obligation to provide a full reply, if questions are asked. Lord Bridge said:

> [W]hen questioned specifically by a patient of apparently sound mind about the risks involved in a particular procedure proposed, the doctor's duty must, in my opinion be to answer both truthfully and as fully as the questioner requires.[66]

But these statements were 'obiter' and not binding. Subsequently in *Blyth* v. *Bloomsbury AHA* (1987), Lord Justice Kerr said that there was no obligation to disclose all information when a question was asked; it was sufficient if the information given was that which would be given by a responsible body of medical practitioners – the *Bolam* test. He stressed that the response of health care professionals to the patient's questions should depend on factors such as the circumstances, the nature of the information, its reliability and relevance and the condition of the patient. That case was, however, decided in 1987 and needs now surely to be placed in its historical context: recent judicial statements indicate a move towards willingness to recognise an obligation to answer questions.[67] Failure to answer patients' questions today is unlikely to be supported by a responsible body of professional practice. Today, it is submitted, a nurse should consider very carefully indeed before she decides to withhold information from a questioning patient, and any refusal will require very clear justification.

7.2.7.4   Causation

Even if a patient can establish that she should have been given more information, that by itself is not sufficient for an action in negligence to succeed (Chapter 6). The patient must go on to show that the failure to provide information caused the harm suffered. The test developed by the courts was subjective: would the patient have chosen differently, had she been given more information? The effect of this test was that in practice a patient may find it very difficult to prove causation since in many cases they would have taken the decision to choose the treatment even if provided with more information. However, a different approach was taken in the House of Lords in *Chester* v. *Afshar* discussed in section 7.2.7.1. Miss Chester was not informed of the risk. However, she did indicate that there was a possibility that had she been informed of the risk she would ultimately have decided to go ahead. The House of Lords still held that the failure to inform was negligent. The decision of the House of Lords followed the approach taken in the Australian case of *Chappel* v. *Hart* in finding that disclosure here was necessary in order to safeguard the patient's autonomy.[68] Lord Hope held that unless such an approach was taken, it 'would render the duty useless in the cases where it is needed the most'. If Miss Chester's claim had been rejected, the consequence would have been that those persons who admitted that they would still have gone ahead with the surgery were placed in a worse position than those who were less straightforward.[69] This means that the courts are prepared in principle to take a more generous approach to the causation test in some informed consent cases.

7.3   Conflicts in disclosure

There has been considerable debate in nursing surrounding the concept of the nurse as patient advocate.[70] One part of the role of the nurse as advocate is in helping her patients to exercise their rights. The ability to make a free choice regarding one's treatment is perhaps one of the patient's most important rights. If the nurse is acting as a member of a health care team and she believes that the information given by a doctor in the team to a patient is insufficient, what should she do? Does the law require her to advocate for her patient? There is no express recognition in English law at present of the role of the nurse as patient advocate, but there may be situations in which she would be held liable for failure to disclose.

The nurse may decide not to participate in a clinical procedure on the grounds that the patient has been inadequately informed, or she may decide to provide the patient with more information herself. But in taking either step she risks disciplinary proceedings and ultimate dismissal for disobeying orders.[71] In addition, in deciding to go ahead and disclose, the nurse runs the risk that her assessment of the amount of information the patient requires may be wrong. What if the patient is unable to cope with the information given and suffers a nervous breakdown? An action may be brought against the nurse claiming that she was negligent in disclosure. Whether such an action would succeed would depend on the test employed by the court. It is submitted that a court would assess whether she had acted negligently in disclosing, by reference to a professional body of nursing opinion.

A nurse may protest to a doctor that a patient has not been given sufficient information, but on being told by the doctor to obey orders, she may decide not to give the patient more information about treatment risks. But what if the treatment risk materialised and the patient suffered harm? Any negligence action for failure to provide adequate information would probably be brought against the doctor rather than the nurse. If an action was brought against the nurse, it might not succeed. In the past the courts have held that as long as a nurse is following a doctor's orders, she will not be held liable.[72] But with the development of the role of the nurse as an autonomous practitioner and as advocate for her patient, the situation may be very different today. If such an action were brought, a court would have to consider whether, in remaining silent, she had acted in accordance with a responsible body of professional nursing opinion. It has been suggested that a nurse may be found liable if she undertakes a task under instructions that she believes to be 'manifestly wrong', following comments made by the House of Lords in *Junor* v. *McNichol*.[73] It is possible that participation in treatment of a patient who has not been told of a very high risk of death or serious injury would come within this category. However, this would presumably only arise in the most exceptional case.

7.4   Conclusions

Over the last quarter of a century the law in relation to consent to treatment has evolved towards what may be seen as a more overtly 'autonomy-based' approach. But in many respects the movement towards an 'informed consent' approach in relation to the provision of care and treatment has been driven by factors other than law. Greater provision of information has become an accepted part of clinical practice. Professional norms themselves have changed – driven by scandals and controversies such as the Bristol Royal Infirmary and Alder Hey inquiries. Moreover, the provision of information today is no longer simply in the control of the professional. Today's patients have far greater access to information about diagnosis and treatment – the advent of the internet impacted considerably on the power dynamic of the health practitioner–patient relationship. Today it is comparatively easy to discover information about possible treatment options. Patients are consequently likely to be far more likely to be able to be engaged in treatment decisions and indeed far more questioning than was the case in the past.

The law in this area poses considerable challenges for the nurse. The nurse must confront the same difficult questions of disclosure as her medical counterpart when treating the patient as a sole practitioner. Determining whether the patient possesses capacity and what risks should be disclosed will be assessments for the nurse much as for her medical counterpart. Guidance in determining capacity today again is very different compared to the past. Here the law has evolved considerably and today the Mental Capacity Act 2005 places consent on a clear statutory footing with helpful guidance in the form of the Code of Practice to the legislation. But the legal process is simply the tip of the iceberg of clinical practice in the area of consent to treatment. The law itself can only go so far. Many of these decisions involve considerable degrees of assessment and discretion, as, for example, in the operation of the capacity test. Nurses have a vital role to play in the actualisation of the reality of respect for consent to treatment on the ward and in the community, whether as independent practitioners or when treating as part of a team. One huge practical challenge here of course is that of time. Proper and effective dialogue with patients takes time. Provision of information by itself may not be enough – a patient may need time and opportunity to return to the health care practitioner and discuss the treatment options further. The law may provide the structure for ascertaining how capacity and information provision may be determined but it is only one part of a much more complex dynamic. These issues are examined further in Part B of this chapter, 'An Ethical Perspective – Consent and Patient Autonomy'.

7.5   Notes and references

1. Nursing and Midwifery Council, The Code, Standards of Performance, Ethics and Conduct for Nurses (2008).
2. See, for example, E. Wicks, The right to refuse medical treatment under the European Convention on Human Rights, 8 Med LR 17 (2001).
3. See, for example, General Medical Council, *Consent, Patients and Doctors Making Decisions Together* GMC (2008); D. Lock, Consent to treatment. In A. Grubb, J. Laing & J. McHale (eds), *Principles of Medical Law*, 3rd edn (Oxford, OUP, 2010); J.K. Mason & G. Laurie, *Mason and McCall Smith's Law and Medical Ethics*, 8th edn (Oxford, OUP, 2010) chapter 4; A. McLean Autonomy, *Informed Consent and Medical Law: A Relational Challenge* (Cambridge, Cambridge University Press, 2008).
4. *Re T (adult: refusal of treatment)* [1992] 4 All ER 649.
5. See generally M. Gunn, The meaning of incapacity, 2 Med LR 8 (1994).
6. Law Commission Mental Incapacity Report (1995).
7. See further P. Bartlett, *Mental Capacity Act 2005* (Oxford, OUP, 2005).
8. Sections 9–11.
9. Section 3(4).
10. Section 4(6).
11. Department of Constitutional Affairs, *Mental Capacity Act Code of Practice* (2007).

12. See *R* v. *Brown* [1993] 2 All ER 75.
13. Female Genital Mutilation Act 2003.
14. This was suggested by Lord Edmund Davies in a statement made extra judicially – see *Proceedings of the Royal Society of Medicine*, **62** (1969), pp. 633–4.
15. See M. Fox & J. McHale, Xenotransplantation, 6 Med LR 42 (1998).
16. P.D.G. Skegg, *Law, Ethics and Medicine* (London, Clarendon Press, 1984), p. 32.
17. [1981] QB 432.
18. See the comments of Mr Justice Bristow in *Chatterton* v. *Gerson*, and M. Brazier, Patient autonomy and consent to treatment: the role of the law, *Legal Studies*, **7** (1987), p. 169.
19. *Devi* v. *West Midlands HA* (1981) (CA Transcript 491).
20. (1990) 67 DIR (4th) 321 (Ont CA).
21. *Re B (adult: refusal of medical treatment)* [2002] 2 All ER 449.
22. See discussion in E. Wicks, The right to refuse medical treatment under the European Convention on Human Rights. 8 Med LR 17 (2001), and J. McHale & A. Gallagher, *Nursing and Human Rights* (Oxford, Butterworth Heinemann, 2004).
23. See, for example, *Re L (medical treatment; Gillick competency)* [1998] 2 FLR 810.
24. [1984] QB 524.
25. [1992] 4 All ER 671.
26. *Paton* v. *British Pregnancy Advisory Service* [1978] 2 All ER 987. Balcombe LJ: 'The foetus cannot, in English law, in my view, have any right of its own at least until it is born and has a separate existence from its mother.'
27. [1990] 573 A 2d 1235.
28. See further I. Kennedy, A woman and her unborn child; rights and responsibilities, In P. Byrne (ed), *Ethics and Law in Health Care and Research*(Chichester, John Wiley, 1990).
29. In *AC* itself an enforced Caesarean was rejected. The court did indicate that they may be used in suitable cases and mentioned a court decision very similar to *Re S*. However, they did not express an opinion on that case.
30. Royal College of Obstetricians and Gynaecologists, *A Consideration of the Law and Ethics in Relation to Court-Authorised Obstetric Interventions* (1994), and see also the revisions in *Supplement to a Consideration of the Law and Ethics in Relation to Court-Authorised Obstetric Interventions* (RCOG, 1996).
31. *Rochdale NHS Trust* v. *C* [1997]; *Norfolk & Norwich NHS Trust* v. *W* [1996] 2 FLR 613.
32. [1997] 2 FLR.
33. [1990] 2 AC 1.
34. [1979] QB 276.
35. [1997] 2 FLR 441.
36. *Ibid* at 439.
37. See also A. Grubb, Treatment without consent: pregnancy (adult), *Medical Law Review*, **191** (1996).
38. [1995] 1 All ER 683.
39. [1998] 3 All ER 673.
40. Reference was made to the judgment of Lord Mustill in *Airedale NHS Trust* v. *Bland* and to Lord Reid in *S* v. *Mc* [1972] AC 24.
41. R. Bailey Harris, Pregnancy, autonomy and refusal of medical treatment, *Law Quarterly Review*, **550** (1998), p. 554.
42. For example, *Re B* [1987] 2 All ER 206 and the discussion in the Law Commission Report *Mental Incapacity* as to the involvement of judicial scrutiny of such treatment decisions, e.g. Part VI of the Report.
43. [1985] 2 WLR 503.
44. See *Bolam* v. *Friern Hospital Management Committee* [1957] 2 All ER 118.

45. *Gold* v. *Haringey Health Authority* [1987] 2 All ER 888.
46. [1994] 5 Med LR 334.
47. See, for example, in the context of Australia *Rogers* v. *Whittaker* [1993] 4 Med LR 79 and Canada *Reibl* v. *Hughes* (1980) 114 DLR (3d) 1; also see A. Maclean, The doctrine of informed consent: does it exist and has it crossed the Atlantic? *Legal Studies*, **24** (2004), p. 386.
48. *Report of the Inquiry into the Royal Liverpool Children's Hospital (Alder Hey)* (2001) http://www.rclinquiry.org.uk and *Bristol Inquiry Interim Report Removal and Retention of Human Material* (2000) http://www.bristol-inquiry.org.uk
49. See discussion in A. Gallagher & J. McHale, After Bristol: the importance of Informed Consent, *Nursing Times*, **97** (2001), p. 32.
50. Bristol Royal Infirmary Final Report, p. 286.
51. *Learning from Bristol: The Department of Health's Response to the Report of the Public Inquiry into Children's Heart Surgery at Bristol Royal Infirmary 1984–1995*. Cm 5363 (2002), pp. 139–40.
52. [1997] 3 WLR 1151.
53. *Op cit.*
54. PIQR P53. (CA) and see further M. Jones, Informed consent and fairy stories, *Medical Law Review*, **7** (1999), p. 103.
55. *Op cit.*
56. See further the discussion of this issue by A. Grubb, 7 Med LR 61 (1997).
57. [2005] 1 AC 134.
58. *Ibid*.
59. *Ibid* at paras 16–18.
60. [2008] EWHC 2237.
61. *Ibid* at para. 74.
62. [2005] EWHC 206.
63. See further J. Miola, Autonomy rued OK? Al *Hamwi* v. *Johnston and Another*, *Medical Law Review*, **14** (2006), p. 108.
64. *Op cit.*
65. See also discussion in A. McLean, From Sidaway to Pearce and Beyond: Is the legal regulation of consent any better following a quarter of a century of judicial scrutiny, *Medical Law Review*, **20** (1) (2012), p. 108.
66. *Op cit.*
67. For example, *Pearce* v. *United Bristol Healthcare NHS Trust* (1998) 48 BMCR 118 CA.
68. [1998] HCA 55.
69. For criticism of this case, see M. Stauch, Causation and confusion in respect of medical non-disclosure, *Nottingham Law Journal*, **14** (2005), p. 66.
70. See generally, G.R. Winslow, From loyalty to advocacy: a new metaphor for nursing, *Hastings Centre Report*, **32** (1984); E.W. Bernal, The nurse as patient advocate, *Hastings Centre Report*, **33** (1992).
71. See further as to the extent of the obligation of a nurse to obey a doctor's instructions, J. Montgomery, Doctors' handmaidens: the legal contribution. In S. McVeigh & S. Wheelar (eds), *Law and Medical Regulation* (Aldershot, Dartmouth, 1993).
72. *Pickering* v. *Governors of United Leeds Hospitals* (1954).
73. [1959], *The Times*, 26 March, House of Lords.

B   An Ethical Perspective – Consent and Patient Autonomy

Bobbie Farsides

Professor of Clinical and Biomedical Ethics, Brighton and Sussex Medical School, University of Sussex, Brighton

Consent is a moral and legal cornerstone of contemporary health care, just as it is important in the proper functioning of so many human relations and interactions.

Interventions which proceed without the consent of the patient immediately require moral scrutiny, and even where it is claimed that consent has been given, we want to ensure that this means much more than the mere fact that a form has been signed and witnessed. It is important to show that far from being a protective mechanism for health care professionals, the primary role of consent is to protect patients. In the society we inhabit it is particularly important to protect a patient's status as an autonomous individual who has an interest in remaining in control of his own life, even when he feels at his most vulnerable or when he finds himself in a potentially challenging environment such as a hospital.

In part A of this chapter, Jean McHale has given a full account of consent in a legal context.[1] Clearly, the law is very important in this area, and it is true that legal change in recent years has been significant. However, it is crucial to understand why consent is important ethically and why that would be the case whatever the law said on the matter. In ethical terms consent is important because it demonstrates respect for persons, it protects the autonomous individual from certain harms, and through participating in a consent process the person's autonomy may be further enhanced.

Autonomy is both a prerequisite for consent and a product of it. The call to place consent at the heart of the health care encounter arises in part from the wish to develop a relationship between a patient and a health care professional which has the potential to be contractual rather than hierarchical, egalitarian rather than paternalistic, and patient-centred rather than medically determined.

Consent, when properly conceived, will look something like the concept defined by Raanon Gillon in his book *Philosophical Medical Ethics* '. . . a voluntary un-coerced decision made by a sufficiently autonomous person on the basis of adequate information to accept or reject some proposed course of action that will affect him or her.'[2]

This definition offers what we might call an ideal type model, but Gillon is confident that it can be embraced by health care professionals and translated into practice. For this to happen, the health care professional must adopt a particular attitude to patients, and take seriously the duties implied by the definition. Acquiring proper consent might turn out to be a time-consuming process, but this is no reason to argue against its importance. In fact it might be a basis upon which to argue for more of that most basic of resources – time.

7.6   Consent and autonomy

Before going any further it is important to define our terms, and then if not defend at least explain the emphasis placed on autonomy when discussing consent.

According to Gillon's definition, consent is the domain of 'sufficiently autonomous people'.[2] This immediately requires two things of those requesting consent from a patient. First, an understanding of what is meant by 'autonomy' and second, the ability to judge someone sufficiently autonomous to give consent on a particular occasion. What should *not* happen is the blanket exclusion of classes of individuals from the consent process (e.g. children, people with cognitive impairments, those with addiction problems) on the grounds of lack of autonomy. In many ways Gillon's approach to autonomy is entirely in step with the legal landscape as set out in the Mental Capacity Act 2005[3] and outlined in the preceding chapter.

Autonomy is a fundamentally significant concept in Anglo-American bioethics, and the importance of respecting patient autonomy is clearly highlighted in the codes of ethics governing the main health care professions. There are many reasons why autonomy has become such a dominant concept, some historical, some cultural, and some to do with the success of particular models of analysis within bioethics.[4]

To quote Beauchamp and Childress, 'respect for the autonomous choices of other persons runs as deep in common morality as any principle, but little agreement exists about its nature and strength or about specific rights of autonomy'.[5]

Here are just a few frequently quoted accounts of what it means to be autonomous, demonstrating the range of ideas theorists have seen in the concept:

> I am autonomous if I rule me and no one else rules I.[6]
>
> A person is autonomous to the degree that what he thinks and does cannot be explained without reference to his own activity of mind.[7]
>
> [A]cting autonomously is acting from principles that we would consent to as free and equal rational beings.[8]
>
> I and I alone am ultimately responsible for the decisions I make and am in that sense autonomous.[9]

The word 'autonomy' is derived from the Greek *autos* and *nomia*, and means self- rule. Most definitions remain true to this root, and include ideas of self-governance, sovereignty, control and quite often independence. To be autonomous is to be in control of one's life in a very particular way, referring as it does to rationality as opposed to mere freedom. Responsibility is quite appropriately seen as a closely related concept, and the autonomous person may be free or unfree to act upon their autonomous choices, but in doing so must accept some responsibility for the consequences. More extreme definitions sometimes appear to suggest that one can only enjoy full autonomy if the choices one makes are completely unaffected by others. However, this is not the only way to think about autonomy, and more recently theorists have attempted to offer definitions which do not commit them to the substantive independence seen as necessary by some of the philosophers quoted above.

Gerald Dworkin, who quotes all the preceding definitions in his own work, characterises autonomy as 'the capacity of a person critically to reflect upon, and then attempt to accept or change his or her preferences, desires, values and ideals.'[10]

To explain himself more fully he states:

> Putting the various pieces together, autonomy is conceived of as a second-order capacity of persons to reflect critically upon their first-order preferences, desires, wishes, and so forth and the capacity to accept or attempt to change these in the light of higher-order preferences and values. By exercising such a capacity, persons define their nature, give meaning to their lives and take responsibility for the kind of person they are.[11]

Despite the variety in these definitions it is possible to glean the essence of the concept, and it is obvious that valuing and respecting autonomy entails respecting the person's right to give or withhold their consent to interventions which will affect them. By participating in the consenting process the autonomous person has the opportunity to judge the choice within the larger context of their life, goals and projects and make a decision consistent with the values they hold and the path they wish to pursue. This is why consent and autonomy are so inextricably linked at a personal level, and why personal choice is important in a medical setting where very important decisions with far-reaching implications often need to be made.

7.6.1   The 'political' context

It is also possible to argue that consent and autonomy at an individual level are important because they fit well within the broader political context within which health care is provided. In this, the early part of the second millennium, we find ourselves facing great changes in our national health care system. Changes which some would argue are driven by an ideology that has been challenging the welfareist assumptions of the NHS throughout the latter part of the 20th century.

We have seen a growing emphasis on individual choice as a driver of decisions within a number of public services, and in a political climate which appears to have favoured individualism over collectivism, personal effort over state welfare, and the power of the consumer over that of the bureaucratic machine, it is hardly surprising that autonomy is what the advertising executives call a positive buzz word.

However, we need to be careful and recognise that placing autonomy at the centre of things is suggestive of a Northern European and/or American cultural perspective with its emphasis on such notions as privacy, individual initiative and consumerism. To be autonomous is to fit the picture of what it is meant to be an effective and successful member of society in these societies, but it is possible to challenge the supremacy of this value from other cultural perspectives.[12] It is also important to once again acknowledge that the flip-side of the coin when discussing autonomy is responsibility, and while patients might welcome greater choice and control over their health care choices, it is less clear that they are rushing to take greater responsibility for their health and well-being.

In terms of professional culture within the health service there have also been interesting shifts which have meant the patient's voice is now louder and more significant. The pendulum has swung against medical paternalism, and there has been a sustained chipping-away at the medical model of care which has led to a re-characterisation of the classic relationship between doctor and patient, and doctor and nurse.

Instead of the all-powerful doctor and his (sic) handmaiden the nurse ministering to the sick patient, the relationship between carers and patient is now presented as a contractual model, with each party having rights, duties and even responsibilities. The patient has become the client, and in some senses at least has become indistinguishable from any other type of consumer. At the same time the nurse has been encouraged to develop her own professional autonomy and, where necessary, act to promote that of the patients if it is under threat from the doctor.[13] It could be argued nurses and patients have both witnessed the gradual breakdown of well-established patterns of medical paternalism.

I have referred to 'autonomy' as a positive buzz word, conversely 'paternalism' is often treated as a bioethical example of a dirty word.[14] Hard paternalism is defined as acting or choosing on another's behalf because you feel qualified to do so, and because you believe it to be in their best interest that you do so irrespective of their past or future consent, and irrespective of their belief that they are perfectly able to act on their own behalf. So, for example, if I decided to quickly grab a person's arm and give them a therapeutic injection which they do not want but in my opinion need, my actions would be classed as paternalistic in the strong sense. Such paternalism is difficult to justify (and legally very unsafe behaviour), and by underlining the importance of acquiring-consent circumstances, we protect against paternalistic practices of this type being widespread.

Soft paternalism, on the other hand, involves acting on another's behalf and in their best interest because you believe them to be temporarily unable to exercise their autonomy, which could translate into a temporary inability to participate in the consenting process. In such cases one might protect against the unacceptable excesses of paternalism by introducing another notion of consent often referred to as 'hypothetical consent'. In such a case one might choose in the patient's best interest and with reference to ideas about what they might or might not consent to, were they able to participate. Thus we intervene only because we consider them to be unable to consent for themselves, and in deciding for them we attempt to make a choice that they will ultimately accept. So, we could say that if the person does not want the injection because they are scared of jabs but does want the therapeutic benefits, our decision to quickly give the injection while they are distracted might be justifiable (although even here the absence of consent makes the professional vulnerable and the situation unstable). If the patient is pleased with the outcome and gives retrospective approval for the action, then the paternalism is of a softer nature.

The nursing profession has played a significant role in challenging anachronistic models of medical intervention that were particularly prone to hard paternalism. However, in recent years it has become clear that some patients find the burdens associated with non-paternalistic models of health care quite difficult to bear. It is also true that in certain areas medicine practices which were seen as paternalistic have been replaced with very different practices which may nonetheless be open to the same description. One could think of provision of information, where in the past the paternalist was understood to withhold painful truths in the interest of not upsetting the patient. Some would claim that now we impose painful truths on some patients who would 'rather not know' because we feel it is better for them to do so. Clearly clinicians will refer to an evidence base that tells them the advantages and disadvantages of disclosure of diagnosis and prognosis in particular conditions, but to avoid a new variant of paternalism they also need to ascertain what an autonomous person is telling them about what they wish to know and when.

Clearly, people will differ in their evaluation of these changes in the political and professional landscape, but what is clear is that we now operate in a system where theoretically at least great emphasis is placed upon the issue of personal choice within the health care system. This means it is particularly important to assess whether consent is playing the part it is meant to play, and if so whether this is to the benefit or detriment of particular patients.

7.6.2   Information provision

As clearly stated in Gillon's definition, the moral and legal requirement to acquire consent commits the health care professional to providing sufficient information to allow that consent to be given, therefore the room for negotiation is sometimes limited. However, as I began to suggest above when discussing paternalism, there are contexts within which the autonomous patient must be allowed to determine the amount of information they are given. On the issue of prognosis, for example, a health care professional might have good reason to assume that it is in the interests of the patient to know their predicted future, but it would be difficult to justify imposing the information upon an autonomous individual who has clearly stated that they do not wish to know.[15] Thus the autonomy of the patient and the need to respect it might have to trump the health care professional's commitment to fuller disclosure and their own beliefs about what is in the patient's best interest.

Just as Jean McHale requires the nurse to justify withholding information, the nurse must also have valid reasons for imparting information that the competent patient does not wish to receive.[16]

The term 'adequate information' calls for judgement to be applied, and since at least the early 1990s there has been a great deal of debate around the issue of what counts as sufficient, with some commentators suggesting that the standards required in some contexts force doctors to be 'needlessly cruel' in imposing information upon people.[17] One area of concern relates to clinical experimentation, where we have come to believe that the information sufficient for consent must be particularly detailed. As a research nurse will often be the person involved in the process of providing information and acquiring consent, she must contribute to the complex decisions about how much information is sufficient, and when more information is unnecessary and maybe even harmful because it goes beyond that which would be imparted in a clinical setting.[18]

7.7   Voluntariness, coercion and consent

Consent, Gillon tells us, is a 'voluntary and un-coerced decision'.[2] By making this explicit, he is not implying that health care professionals are ever in the business of directly coercing patients or forcing them into involuntary choices, but rather that the context within which decisions are made might not always enhance the voluntariness of the decision, and might sometimes be coercive. By definition patients have concerns about their health, and being a patient might be linked to very particular forms of vulnerability. Furthermore, despite ever greater access to medical information, the health care professional is still the expert upon whom a patient depends, not just for treatment but also for basic care, and importantly maintenance of dignity.

As already mentioned, many would agree that being in hospital, or maybe even just attending an outpatients appointment, can be a very difficult experience – however autonomous one is in other areas of life. Hospitals can be intimidating and alien environments within which people are stripped of many of their usual props and supports, and where those aspects of their identity which give them confidence can be undermined.

Furthermore, we become a patient against the background of the life we already lead and the broader context within which the patient operates might have limiting effects on their ability to consent.

Patients do not shed their other social identities when they enter the hospital setting, but these are not always that visible. For some individuals their ability to consent may be compromised by their position within their cultural group. For example, women within certain cultures might have the capacity to consent, but would not expect to have *the right* to determine what happens to them due to cultural norms and expectations. Individual women might therefore be unpractised in exercising choices of the type involved in consenting within a health care setting.[19] This could pose difficulties when they are faced with ethically fraught choices, such as whether to accept an offer of pre-natal screening for genetically inherited diseases common to their ethnic group.[20,21] It might also lead to concerns about their ability to refuse courses of action proposed by others, and this is important given that the right not to agree to something is an essential component of Gillon's definition of consent.

When talking about vulnerability and the potential for coercion, it is of course important to avoid stereotypical assumptions and to determine in the particular case whether an individual is subject to such pressure.

However, given that communication is key to effective consent, in terms of both imparting information and ascertaining a patient's wishes, beliefs and goals, it is surely appropriate to be mindful of the ways in which barriers to communication might make consent more challenging and the patient more vulnerable.

The nurse can play an important role in this respect, and it is no coincidence that doctors often call upon senior nursing colleagues to be present when imparting particularly complex news and presenting treatment options. The nurse is there as a support to the patient but also as an independent verifier of the doctor's success in setting up a situation where the patient has the tools with which to consent.

7.8   Sufficient autonomy to consent

As suggested above, by making part of the criteria for valid consent the need for the patient to be 'sufficiently autonomous', Gillon demands that we judge the capacity of an individual to act autonomously in a given situation, rather than label groups and individuals capable of giving consent or otherwise. While it is important to remember that the Mental Capacity Act requires us to start from an assumption of capacity and puts the onus upon professionals to demonstrate that capacity is lacking, if they wish to deem the patient incompetent to make a particular decision, this is not to deny that some human beings fall outside the category of competent autonomous being – examples being the fetus, the neonate, the person with advanced dementia and the person in persistent vegetative state.[22]

We now understand and accept that groups such as children[23] and the cognitively impaired benefit from closer attention and careful discrimination between individuals, when it comes to their capacity to consent across a range of issues.

It is incumbent upon those dealing with these groups to judge each individual in relation to the capacity required in a particular situation.[24]

People with quite severe learning disabilities or mental health problems could be seen as autonomous in certain respects and circumstances, and therefore able to give or withhold their consent.

In some types of case there will be heated debate over the extent to which people can be autonomous and thereby capable of consenting. Examples differ in kind but might include the interesting cases of people with eating disorders or people with non-mainstream religious views such as the Jehovah's Witness cited in part A of this chapter.

In the case of people with eating disorders there may be a real difficulty in ascertaining the extent to which the underlying illness affects a person's autonomy, but the fact that it is an illness rather than a chosen way of life will be seen to make a difference in terms of their responsibility for their choices. Just as the substance abuser's or alcoholic's first-order desire for their drug impairs their autonomy, the person with an eating disorder is disproportionately determined by the relationship they have with food. Having said this, it is important to remember that even those who find aspects of their life dominated by illness or addiction might remain capable of making autonomous choices in other areas of their life. So, for example, the young woman with bulimia nervosa might be unable to control her compulsions, but she might be perfectly capable of seeking and consenting to dental treatment for the problems associated with her condition.

7.9   Insufficient autonomy to consent

The question of how to proceed morally in the absence of consent is a difficult one. Now at least the legal position is clear, and we have the power to appoint a medical proxy to make decisions on our behalf when we are no longer able to do so. However, proxy consent is not unproblematic: for example, one has to establish *how* to decide for another.

One option is to attempt to choose as you believe the person would have chosen had they been able to do so, often referred to as substituted judgement. This route was not advocated in the legislation, instead the proxy is advised to choose in the person's best interest. Naturally the hope is that the proxy will adopt a broad concept of best interest which will go beyond the physical needs of the patient to also address and incorporate some sense of what would be in keeping with the person's values and preferences.[25]

This wider concept of best interests would hopefully mean that in deciding for the person their proxy would make reference to what had been important to them. In the vast majority of cases there will be no conflict between medical best interests and best interests more widely understood, but this might not always be the case. So, for example, if a patient had always been a passionate antivivisectionist, their proxy decision-maker might consider it in their best interest to avoid, where possible, drugs tested on animals, even if this would not serve the patient's medical best interests. A more conventional example would be in the case of organ donation where a dying patient might no longer benefit directly from further medical intervention, but their organs might be in a better condition for donation if certain treatments are administered. It could then be argued that the treatment is justified as being in their best interests if it is clear that it is important to them that their wish to be a donor be fulfilled.

As discussed earlier in the chapter, the Mental Capacity Act also clarifies the law regarding advance statements. Even when their legal status remained ambiguous, the ethical principle behind such documents was clear, in that they attempt to extend the ability to make choices beyond the point at which a person's lack of capacity would usually exclude them from doing so. In practical terms advance decisions are a form of treatment refusal, and in order to ensure their legal validity they need to be carefully drawn up to adequately capture the context within which they could be used. One of the criticisms levelled at very medically oriented advance statements is that their enforcement is dependent on the patient finding themselves in the clinical situations they have anticipated.

For these reasons it is probably more productive to think about extending one's ability to make choices, or at least have reference made to your prior choices through the concept of advance care planning, a process managed by nurses, as opposed to lawyers. In response to the limitations of the formal advance decision some end-of-life care projects have begun to work with a rather different type of document which concentrates more on the issue of values, goals and priorities which the patient would wish to see reflected in the decisions made on their behalf when they are being cared for at the end of life.

Another important advance decision relates to the donation of organs after death, and here the nature of the consent given is treated rather differently. As this chapter goes to press the law is about to be changed in Wales, and there is a consultation under way in the rest of the United Kingdom regarding the basis for consent to become a donor after death.

At present a patient may have clearly stated their wish to donate (opted in) and taken the trouble to register those wishes with the appropriate bodies and individuals. In this case the Human Tissue Act 2004[26] gives primacy to these wishes, and in formal legal terms the decision cannot be overridden by relatives. However, in practice, we still operate a system where family agreement to postmortem donation is sought, and few, if any, clinicians would even consider overriding the objections of a grieving family.

Some would argue that this undermines the individual's right to choose what happens to their body after death and denies them the opportunity to act in accordance with their values. In response to this claim even a strong advocate of organ donation might accept the implied criticism but say that in this situation the wishes of the family and the commitment to the greatest good trump those of a person now dead in order to maintain trust in and commitment to the programme as a whole. Once again, we find a situation where the fact that someone has consented may not be able to do all the work in establishing the ethical way forward.[27]

7.10   Deliberation

The requirement that a patient should have the time and opportunity to deliberate before making a choice appeals to common sense. Health care choices often have far-reaching effects, some of which will only become apparent upon reflection. Even in the most straightforward of decisions a patient will probably benefit from believing that they had been given time to decide rather than being rushed into a decision. Admittedly there will be emergency situations in which this will not be possible. For example, if an event occurs within the course of childbirth which threatens the safety of the woman and the unborn child, a decision might have to be made with great haste. Furthermore, the practicalities of outpatient clinics might determine that certain choices need to be discussed and decided on in the course of one visit, when ideally more time would be taken. Generally speaking, however, time should be allowed for the patient to absorb the information given and think about the choices they need to make.

This could be particularly true, for example, when someone is faced with choices soon after receiving bad news. Oncologists have claimed that once a patient has been given a cancer diagnosis little of what is said in the remainder of the consultation is heard, let alone taken in.[28] Therefore to ensure that consent can be given to any treatment proposed, it seems particularly important to first deal with the initial information about disease status and only later move on to a discussion about treatment choices. Specialist nurses have an important role to play in such situations, and their experience will enable them to judge how to pace the information given and how to assess what the patient has heard and understood.

7.11   The right to refuse or accept

It could be argued that many health care professionals perceive consent as relatively unproblematic just so long as people make the choices they expect or advise them to make. If people agree with what we say, particularly when we consider ourselves to be experts in some regard, we rarely question their readiness to do so. However, it should be allowed that an autonomous patient might choose *not* to follow medical or nursing advice, hence Gillon's requirement that when discussing consent, we acknowledge a right to accept *or* refuse a proposed course of action.

Once again Gillon's way of thinking seems nicely in step with the law, which not only allows a competent patient to refuse medical treatment proposed to them, but allows them to do so for what might appear to be eccentric reasons or indeed no reason at all. This can be much more difficult for a caring health care professional to accept.

Clearly, some treatment refusals will be the product of misinformation, ignorance or cognitive impairment, and in these cases the professional is minded to correct or compensate for the deficits, if possible. So, for example, if a nurse discovers that a patient is refusing a particular drug because they mistakenly believe it will cause them to put on weight, it is entirely appropriate to correct that misapprehension. However, other patients will withhold their consent on the basis of opinions or beliefs which are not subject to correction by the health care professional. So, for example, some people might attach themselves willingly and strongly to cultural or spiritual/religious beliefs which mean that certain health care options are unacceptable to them. A devout Catholic might refuse an offer of antenatal screening for Down's syndrome because she knows that her beliefs exclude the possibility of terminating the pregnancy which will be offered in response to a positive result.

In the case of the person with religious views, the situation is complicated by the fact that we sometimes have a very narrow conception of the types of choices autonomous people make, and the types of belief that they can acceptably attach themselves to. In fact it could be even more complicated than this with us demonstrating a tendency to respect views based on science but not those based on religion. It would sometimes seem as if we have little difficulty in allowing certain religions to determine the choices people make for themselves, yet in other cases we find the religious beliefs and consequent choices more difficult to accept. For example, a health care professional might allow that a devout Catholic would choose to risk a life-threatening tenth pregnancy rather than use contraceptives, whereas the same person might find it more difficult to accept a Jehovah's Witness rejection of a life-saving blood transfusion. It could be argued that the difference here is not between the choices being made, both of which could have devastating effects, but in our attitude to the two bodies of faith, one of which is considered mainstream and 'acceptable', the other less so.[29]

In fact it could be argued that the perceived difference between these cases is the result of mere prejudice, given the equivalence of the consequences. Therefore, one obstacle to respecting the autonomy of others and their right to accept or refuse medical treatment might be the fact that we operate in an ideological context which is quick to define ideas outside the mainstream as 'other' and thereby unlikely products of rational choice. In doing this we then call into question the capacity of decision-makers and thereby provide ourselves with a platform from which to challenge their autonomy.

The law deals with this tendency by excluding reasons from the equation, concentrating instead on capacity to choose. If I can show that I have capacity, I can make a choice that others find strange on the basis of beliefs they find incomprehensible. However, philosophers might find it hard to argue that reasons don't count, so another value has be employed to protect those who make choices we find difficult to accept. Hence the need to combine a commitment to respect for autonomy and the valuing of consent with a commitment to the virtue of tolerance, that is a willingness to accept that people will make choices that we find unacceptable.

For as long as competent peoples' choices do not entail an unacceptable degree of harm to others, we are obliged to accept what they choose and the reasons they give for doing so precisely because they are competent and autonomous, rather than on the basis of what and how they choose.

The dilemmas nurses might face as a result of this issue are real, particularly when they see the demand that they should respect a patient's autonomy conflicting with their beneficently motivated duty of care towards them. One of the great challenges one might face as a health care professional is a competent patient's request that you assist them in some way that you consider to be clearly against their best interest (remembering that this evaluation should go beyond the purely medical).

Fortunately, in this situation the health care professional can again make reference to the law in the knowledge that it is in step with ordinary moral thinking. Your professional duty of care towards a patient means you cannot be *required* to do things to them which are clearly against their best interests. This is because when a third party is required to intervene, consent cannot trump best interest.

However, if a patient tells you *not* to do something you cannot use the claim that it would be in their best interest to impose that treatment upon them – unless their autonomy and capacity are very clearly in question – without falling foul of the accusation of paternalism or worse. When caring for a competent patient, the health care professional's claim that something would be in their best interest cannot trump the patient's refusal to consent.

7.12   The consent process: Translating theory into practice

To translate a theoretical commitment to respect for autonomy into a practical reality requires that a nurse acquires specific skills and accepts a responsibility to practise them. Given the contact the nurse has with patients and the situations within which they meet and interact, the nurse will be required at different times to assess capacity, voluntariness and autonomy, enhance it where it is lacking, respect it where it is present, and find ways of promoting the patient's best interests and well-being where it is not present.

   The nurse will be a significant provider of information, and will often be best placed to judge the extent to which the patient has understood, digested and deliberated upon it. The nurse is often a key figure in the consenting process and her attitude can help to determine whether it becomes an unsatisfactory form-filling exercise or a meaningful communicative process. In her education and on-going professional development the modern nurse is minded to prepare for the substantial responsibilities that acquiring consent in a clinical or research setting can entail, but she should also be aware of the everyday importance of acquiring consent in order to protect a patient's identity and dignity. A skills checklist might look something like the following:

- *Good communication skills*
  One of the prerequisites to acquiring a morally and legally valid consent is to communicate effectively with the patient and, if needs be, their family. Only by doing so will you understand them as an individual, and learn enough about the context from which they have come to the health care setting. Communication is a two-sided exercise. On the one hand, the nurse needs to establish how the individual is coping with being in the health care setting, and what they hope to gain from their contact with health care professionals – this involves asking and listening. On the other hand, information needs to be effectively and appropriately communicated to the patient and other parties involved in the decision-making process such as the doctor– this involves listening and then re-telling.
- *Cultural literacy*
  Given the earlier claims about the extent to which a person's autonomy might be compromised or simply overlooked as a result of their cultural context, there are clearly important reasons for nurses to understand the cultural context within which they operate and the beliefs and practices of the different groups they live and work alongside. Cultural differences must be respected; however, tolerance and understanding does not necessarily commit one to permitting all choices because they are defended as culturally significant.[30] So, for example, the apparent lack of objection of a female minor to undergo circumcision and the clear wish of her parents that she should do so, would not be sufficient reason for a UK-based health care professional to offer this procedure. Tolerance is not required when a practice entails inflicting significant harm on another person, particularly when they are powerless to object.

- *Clinical knowledge-base*

  Modern medicine prides itself on being evidence-based, and an interesting shift in recent years has been the opening up-of access to the evidence upon which clinical decisions are made. The well-informed patient may in fact be more up to date about a condition from which they suffer than some of those treating them. However, the information highway is also littered with irresponsible information and advice which some patients might nonetheless rely on. The nursing profession has played a significant part in improving the information provided directly to patients in the clinical setting and now faces the challenge of providing an element of quality control in terms of information patients find for themselves.

- *Patient experience*

  Today's nurses do not have to personally meet a person living with a particular diagnosis in order to hear something of what it is like and the impact it has. Disease is no longer defined simply by medical or nursing textbooks, we can now access the first-person accounts of thousands of patients at the click of a mouse.[31] All health care practitioners have a responsibility to engage with these patient narratives as a way of taking some simple first steps to understanding what might be the shaping experiences of a particular patient.

- *Support and advocacy*

  The nurse has an important supportive role in helping those who find it difficult to engage in the consenting process and might ultimately be unable to do so. This might entail acting as the patients' advocate or supporting the person who has been appointed in this role. It could entail facilitating the patient in getting their own views heard, sometimes in situations where the patient is in conflict with both their family members and other professionals. To perform this role effectively the nurse will need to develop and enhance her own professional autonomy, and thereby increase her power to represent the patient's view to her medical colleagues. Thus her individual responsibility to a patient may feed into a bigger professional and political issue.

When supporting a patient in this way the nurse needs to be non-judgemental and willing to convey views that may be counter to her own and decisions that she may consider unwise and maybe even harmful.

One of the difficult balances to strike in such situations is that between being non-directive, which is seen as a good thing, and unsupportive, which is not. One of the most difficult questions a health care professional can face in a situation where a patient has a difficult decision to make is, 'what would you do, nurse?' There is no easy way to say how one should respond. On the one hand, to say what you, the nurse, would do is not strictly relevant and may even be counterproductive, but on the other hand, it is an appeal to your expertise and knowledge to which you would feel some need to respond.[32] One might suggest that the way forward in this situation is to return to the notion of best interests and say to the patient 'given what you have told me about what is important to you, what you hope to achieve and what you wish to avoid and given what I know about the relative costs and benefits of options A and B, I think you are probably well advised to think about taking Option A.'

7.13   Conclusion

The nursing profession has a valuable contribution to make in ensuring that patients understand the significance of the consent they are asked for, and the obstacles that might lie in the way of their giving it. Individual nurses can help patients to exercise their autonomy, and provide them with the information they need to make choices consistent with their interests and goals. They can support their patients in what is often an alien and intimidating environment, and where necessary can act as their advocates. The nursing profession should continue to challenge those aspects of the health care delivery system which work against the patient body being able to participate meaningfully in the decision-making processes which affect their care, and they should increasingly ensure that their crucial role in the consenting process is acknowledged and that they receive the education and on-going training required to do it justice.

7.14   Notes and references

1. Reference to page numbers of Jean McHale's section.
2. R. Gillon, *Philosophical Medical Ethics* (Chichester, John Wiley and Sons, 1985; reprinted 1996), p. 115.
3. Mental Capacity Act 2005 available in full at http://www.legislation.gov.uk/ukpga/2005/9/contents
4. T. Beauchamp & J. Childress, *Principles of Biomedical Ethics*, 5th edn (Oxford, Oxford University Press, 2011).
5. *Ibid*, p. 113.
6. J. Feinberg, The idea of a free man. In R.F. Dearden (ed.), *Education and the Development of Reason* (London, Routledge and Kegan Paul, 1972), p. 30.
7. R.F. Dearden, Autonomy and education. In R.F. Dearden (ed.), *Education and the Development of Reason* (London, Routledge and Kegan Paul, 1972), p. 453.
8. J. Rawls, *A Theory of Justice* (Cambridge, MA, Harvard University Press, 1971), p. 516.
9. J.L. Lucas, *Principles of Politics* (Oxford, Oxford University Press, 1966), p. 101.
10. G. Dworkin, *The Theory and Practice of Autonomy* (Cambridge MA, Cambridge University Press, 1988).
11. Dworkin, *op. cit.*, p. 20.
12. See C. Farsides, Autonomy and its implications for palliative care: a Northern European perspective, *Palliative Medicine* **12**(3) (1998), pp. 147–51.
13. C. Farsides, Autonomy and responsibility in midwifery. In S. Budd & U. Sharma (eds), *The Healing Bond* (London, Routledge, 1994).
14. For an excellent introduction to paternalism, see Gerald Dworkin, 'Paternalism', *The Stanford Encyclopedia of Philosophy (Summer 2010 Edition)*, Edward N. Zalta (ed.), http://plato.stanford.edu/archives/sum2010/entries/paternalism
15. J. Jackson *Truth Trust and Medicine* (London, Routledge, 2001) esp. chapter 9, pp. 130–46.
16. See Chapter 7A on omitting information.

17. J. Tobias & R. Souhami, Fully informed consent can be needlessly cruel, *BMJ (Clinical Research Ed.)*, **307** (1993), pp. 1199–201. Reproduced in L. Doyal & J.S. Tobias, *Informed Consent in Medical Research* (London: BMJ Books, 2001).
18. See R. Buckman, *How to Break Bad News* (London, Pan Books, 1994), esp. Chapter 4.
19. See T. Cullinan, Other societies have different concepts of autonomy. Letter to the *BMJ* republished. republished in L. Doyal & J.S. Tobias (eds), *Informed Consent in Medical Research* (London, BMJ Books, 2001).
20. R. Rena, *Testing Women, Testing the Fetus: The Social Impact of Amniocentesis in America* (Taylor & Francis Group, 1999).
21. S. Wolf, Erasing difference: race ethnicity and gender in bioethics. In A. Donchin & LM. Purdy (eds), *Embodying Bioethics: Recent Feminist Advances* (Maryland, Rowman and Littlefield, 1999).
22. J. Harris, *The Value of Life* (London, Routledge, 1985).
23. P. Alderson, In the genes or in the stars? Children's competence to consent. *Journal of Medical Ethics*, **18** (1992), pp. 119–24.
24. A.E. Buchanan & D.W. Brock, *Deciding for Others: The Ethics of Surrogate Decision Making* (Cambridge, Cambridge University Press, 1989).
25. J. Coggon, M. Brazier, P. Murphy, D. Price & M. Quigley, Best interests and potential organ donors. *British Medical Journal*, **336** (2008), pp. 1346–7.
26. Available in full at http://www.legislation.gov.uk/ukpga/2004/30/contents.
27. For further discussion of this issue, see B. Farsides, Respecting wishes and avoiding conflict: understanding the ethical basis for organ donation and retrieval, *British Journal of Anaesthesia*, **108** (Suppl. 1) (2012 Jan), pp. i73–9.
28. P.E. Schofield, P.N. Butow, J.F. Thompson, M.H.N. Tattersall, L.J. Beeney & S.M. Dunn, Psychological responses of patients receiving a diagnosis of cancer, *Annals of Oncology*, **14**(1) (2003), pp. 48–56.
29. For an interesting discussion of this issue, see Des Autels *et al.*, *Praying for a Cure When Medical and Religious Practice Conflict* (Lanham, MD, Rowman and Littlefield Publishers Inc., 1999).
30. See R. Macklin, *Against Relativism: Cultural Diversity and the Search for Ethical Universals in Medicine* (Oxford, Oxford University Press, 1999), Chapters 1–5; also David Heyd (ed.) *Toleration An Elusive Virtue* (Bognor Regis, Princeton, 1996).
31. See, for example, http://www.healthtalkonline.org and http://www.patientslikeme.com.
32. C. Williams, P. Alderson & B. Farsides, Is non-directiveness possible within the context of antenatal screening and testing? *Social Science & Medicine*, **54** (2002), pp. 339–47.

8 Responsibility, Liability and Scarce Resources

A The Legal Perspective

Tracey Elliott

Lecturer in Health Care Law, School of Law, University of Leicester, Leicester

8.1 Introduction

When the NHS was created in 1948, the service was based upon three core principles: that it meet the needs of everyone; that it be free at the point of delivery and that provision of medical treatment would be based on clinical need, not on ability to pay for it.[1] Although when the NHS was being established it was believed that providing the population with free health care would ultimately lead to a decrease in governmental spending on health care services, as the general health of the population improved,[2] it soon became clear that this expectation was both optimistic and unrealistic.[3] Increases in life expectancy, medical and pharmaceutical developments (which mean that many previously untreatable conditions may now be medically managed or cured and the scope for preventive medicine has been greatly expanded) and the rise of patients' expecta-

Nursing Law and Ethics, Fourth Edition. Edited by John Tingle and Alan Cribb.
© 2014 by John Wiley & Sons, Ltd. Published 2014 by John Wiley & Sons, Ltd.

tions as to what medicine can achieve, have all contributed to health care demand outstripping supply.[4] Successive governments have pledged their commitment to the NHS, but the problem of how fairly to allocate finite medical resources remains and is a matter of 'hot' political controversy, generating much philosophical discussion.[5] In 1999 the National Institute for Health and Clinical Excellence (NICE) was set up 'to ensure that everyone has equal access to medical treatments and high quality care from the NHS'.[6] NICE has played a key role in the rationing of treatment within the NHS, through the making of 'health technology appraisals', undertaking evidence-based assessments of the health benefits and costs of technologies, and making recommendations to the NHS, which primary care trusts (PCTs) are (at the time of writing in 2012) required to implement within three months.[7] Under the Health and Social Care Act 2012, NICE is established as a corporate body and renamed the National Institute for Health and Care Excellence, to reflect the fact that its remit has been expanded to include the development of quality standards in relation to social care in England.[8] The Act will abolish PCTs and strategic health authorities (sections. 33 and 34), whose work will be taken over from April 2013 by local commissioning care groups (CCGs) and an NHS Commissioning Board.[9] The full impact of the reforms remains to be seen, but the role of NICE in relation to health care rationing is likely to diminish when the provisions of the Health and Social Care Act 2012 with regard to the commissioning and pricing of health care services come fully into force.[10] The Government's expressed aim is to introduce a 'value-based' approach to the pricing of drugs by 2014.[11]

The courts have considered applications for judicial review of the legality of recommendations made by NICE and decisions made by NHS trusts on a number of occasions in recent years.[12] A detailed consideration of this body of law is beyond the scope of this chapter because the resource decisions involved are made by committees or panels specifically set up to consider such questions, and the making of these decisions does not therefore form part of the normal responsibilities of nursing staff. To summarise the position, the courts are generally reluctant to interfere with decisions about how to allocate scarce resources between patients, unless some specific flaw can be identified in the decision-making process – for example, if relevant factors have not been taken into account when the decision was being made,[13] or the decision may be regarded as an irrational one.[14] The courts are prepared to subject the decision-making process in relation to decisions to refuse treatment to intense scrutiny, but will not express opinions about the effectiveness of medical treatment or the merits of a particular medical judgement.[15] It is lawful for an NHS body to have a policy to decline to fund a treatment save in exceptional circumstances, provided that such a policy is applied in a fair and rational manner and it is possible to envisage such circumstances. For example, in *R (on the application of Ross)* v. *West Sussex PCT* (2008),[16] the claimant was a cancer sufferer who had undergone a number of unsuccessful treatments, including thalidomide. The PCT had refused to fund the only remaining available treatment, a drug which had not been assessed by NICE, on the basis that it was their policy only to fund exceptional cases, and his case was not exceptional because a cohort of patients with the same condition being treated with thalidomide would have suffered similar side-effects. The

Administrative Court held that this was not truly a policy for exceptional cases and was therefore unlawful because it effectively disqualified a patient if his case could be likened to that of another patient. In order to qualify, Mr Ross had to show that he was, in effect, unique, rather than merely exceptional, and this was, in practice, impossible.

The purpose of this chapter is not to focus upon legal challenges in relation to NHS refusals to fund medical treatment, but to examine legal issues which may arise where nurses are working in circumstances of economic constraint. Important issues in this context include whether and to what extent the courts dealing with a negligence claim will make allowances for inexperience, and a lack of resources, and the options available to a nurse who feels that they are being required to carry out work or assume professional responsibilities beyond their competence. Before I consider such issues, however, the standard of care that the law requires of nurses must first be considered.

8.2   Negligence: The standard of care

Nurses owe their patients a duty of care.[17] This raises the question of when a duty of care arises. Usually, this will be uncontentious. In the case of hospital treatment, a duty of care will arise when a patient is admitted to the hospital.[18] Where a hospital has an Accident & Emergency (A&E) department, a duty of care is owed to people who present themselves at the department for treatment, even before they are actually treated or admitted to a hospital ward.[19] In recent years, the A&E departments of many smaller hospitals have been closed, and hospitals which do not have such departments will display notices stating that they do not accept A&E patients and referring people to the nearest hospital that does. It appears that, as a matter of law, such a hospital may refuse to accept an A&E patient for treatment and to advise them to go straight to the nearest A&E department. In this instance it is likely that the hospital would be held not to have assumed a duty of care in respect of the patient.[20] If, however, the hospital were to choose to admit the patient, then a duty of care would arise.

Liability in negligence is likely to arise if a nurse breaches their duty of care to a patient, causing injury. A breach of duty will occur if a nurse fails to meet the relevant standard of care. What then, is the standard of care? English law requires that a nurse exercises the ordinary skill of their specialty: a nurse 'is not guilty of negligence if he [or she] has acted in accordance with a practice accepted as proper by a responsible body of medical men skilled in that particular art'.[21] This is an established and well-known legal principle known as the *Bolam* test. The standard set by the *Bolam* test is an objective one. The test was, however, criticised as being too deferential to the medical profession because the standard of care was being determined by doctors. A medical practitioner defending a clinical negligence action could escape liability provided that he could call upon expert evidence which could be regarded as truthful and representing a 'responsible body of medical men', to say that his practice was 'accepted as proper'.[22] In the case of *Bolitho* v. *City and Hackney Health Authority* (1998),[23] the House of Lords adopted a less deferential approach towards the *Bolam* test. Following *Bolitho*, if

a judge considering expert evidence as to whether the practice of a medical practitioner acted in accordance with responsible professional practice concludes
that '. . . in a rare case,[24] it can be demonstrated that the professional opinion is
not capable of withstanding logical analysis, the judge is entitled to hold that the
body of opinion is not reasonable or responsible'[25] and to reject it. As part of this
determination, 'the judge before accepting a body of opinion as being responsible, reasonable or respectable, will need to be satisfied that, in forming their
views, the experts have directed their minds to the question of comparative risks
and benefits and have reached a defensible conclusion on the matter'.[26] It appears
that there have been relatively few cases in which courts have rejected expert
evidence on the basis that it is not reasonable or responsible.[27]

Given that the standard of care is objective, the question then arises as to the
extent to whether matters such as inexperience, tiredness or lack of resources may
be taken into account if a nurse fails to meet the standard of care. The impact (or
lack of it) of these matters upon the standard of care will now be considered.

8.3   Inexperience and the standard of care

The training of both doctors and nurses inevitably involves some element of
'learning on the job', as was recognised by Lord Justice Mustill in the case of
Wilsher v. *Essex Area Health Authority* (1987):

> Public hospital medicine has always been organised so that young doctors and
> nurses learn on the job. If the hospitals abstained from using inexperienced
> people, they could not staff their wards and theatres, and the junior staff could
> never learn.[28]

If a newly qualified nurse or doctor makes an error because of their inexperience, is any allowance made for their inexperience? May an inexperienced nurse
argue that the standard of care which she is expected to meet is lower than that
of an experienced nurse? The answer is that the standard of care required is not
reduced to take account of a nurse's inexperience.[29] In *Nettleship* v. *Weston* (1971)
the Court of Appeal rejected an argument that the standard expected of a learner
driver should be lower than that of a more experienced driver:

> . . . in my judgment, in cases such as the present it is preferable that there
> should be a reasonably certain and reasonably ascertainable standard of care
> . . . the standard of care required by the law is the standard of the competent
> and experienced driver.[30]

The issue was considered in relation to the provision of medical care in the
case of *Wilsher* v. *Essex Area Health Authority* (1987),[31] in which a junior doctor
treating a premature baby in a special care baby unit mistakenly inserted a catheter, which was required to monitor the baby's arterial blood oxygen levels, into
a vein rather than an artery. The majority of the Court of Appeal took the view
that the standard of care was not adjusted to take account of the junior doctor's
inexperience. Lord Justice Mustill took the view that the duty of care should be
related not to the experience of the individual doctor, but to the post which he
occupied:

... the standard is not just that of the averagely competent and well-informed junior houseman (or whatever the position of the doctor) but of a person who fills a post in a unit offering a highly specialised service.[32]

According to this approach, it appears that the standard of care might vary according to the post occupied by the health care practitioner. Glidewell LJ, on the other hand, did not specifically link the standard of care to the post occupied by the doctor, but agreed with Mustill LJ that the standard of care was not to be reduced to take account of inexperience:

In my view the law requires the trainee or learner to be judged by the same standard as his more experienced colleagues. If it did not, inexperience would frequently be urged as a defence to an action for professional negligence.[33]

Wilsher was subsequently followed in *Djemal* v. *Bexley Health Authority* (1994),[34] where the treating doctor was a senior house officer with about four months' experience on the job. The trial judge ruled that the standard of care to be applied was 'that of a reasonably competent senior houseman acting as a casualty officer without reference to the length of experience'.[35] In *Bova* v. *Spring* (1994),[36] Sedley J made it clear that the minimum standard of care to be expected of a trainee general practitioner was no lower than that to be expected of an experienced one: '[H]is professional duty of care did not require him to be omniscient or right – only to be as knowledgeable and as careful for his patient's welfare as a competent general practitioner ought to be'. The use of the term 'post' by Lord Mustill in *Wilsher* is perhaps not very helpful, since it would be unfortunate if different standards of care applied to a particular medical task, depending on whether it was being performed by a nurse, a junior doctor or a consultant.[37] It is suggested that the standard of care ought to be judged according to the service that is being provided by the doctor or nurse. A nurse who undertakes a particular task must perform that task with reasonable skill and care.[38]

The law's refusal to take account of inexperience when determining the standard of care may at first blush seem harsh, but it should be noted that an inexperienced nurse who recognises that they are inexperienced and seeks the advice and help of their superiors will usually not be held to be liable.[39] For example, in *Wilsher*, the junior doctor was held not to be liable in negligence because he had asked a registrar to check his work. The registrar, on the other hand, was held to be liable.[40] However, a nurse or doctor who undertakes treatment for which they lack the necessary care or skill would be negligent.[41] This does mean that it is important that a nurse is aware of the limits of their competence and can recognise where a task is 'over their head' and call for assistance. For example, in the Canadian case of *Dillon* v. *LeRoux* (1994),[42] a family doctor with no emergency-room training was working as an emergency-room doctor when a patient was admitted complaining of symptoms which included sharp chest pain, tingling in the hands and feet, difficulty breathing and feeling sweaty and clammy. The doctor initially diagnosed acid reflux, when in fact the patient had suffered a heart attack. It was held that the doctor was negligent in failing to call the on-call internist to assist him with his diagnosis. A more senior nurse or doctor is likely to be found to be in breach of their duty to a patient if they fail properly to supervise more inexperienced colleagues.[43] For example, in *Drake* v. *Pontefract Health Authority*[44] (1998) a consultant psychiatrist was held to have been negligent in allowing a house officer to assess and treat a suicidal patient without proper supervision. A trust or health authority may also be in breach of their duty of care to a patient if they do not made adequate provision for the supervision of junior doctors and nurses. In *Jones* v. *Manchester Corporation* (1952),[45] an inexperienced junior doctor negligently administered an anaesthetic to a patient, causing his death. The hospital board was held to be not merely vicariously liable for the fault of their employee, but to be directly responsible in negligence:

> . . . mistakes of this kind should not occur. The Board should so run their hospital that they do not occur. They should not leave patients in experienced hands without proper supervision.[46]

8.4   Emergencies, overwork and the standard of care

Sometimes medical treatment will be provided in less than ideal conditions, particularly in situations of emergency, when hospitals may be faced with treating large numbers of casualties who require very urgent medical attention. In *Wilsher*, Mustill LJ recognised that:

> . . . I accept that full allowance must be made for the fact that certain aspects of treatment may have to be carried out in . . . 'battle conditions' An emergency may overburden the available resources, and, if an individual is forced by circumstances to do too many things at once, the fact that he does one of them incorrectly should not lightly be taken as negligence.[47]

For example, in the Canadian case of *Rodych* v. *Krasney* (1971),[48] a very drunken car accident victim was taken to a doctor's house at night. The injured victim refused to enter the doctor's house, so the doctor examined him in his vehicle, where the only available light was a torch and a nearby streetlight. The doctor observed minor injuries but failed to spot the much more serious chest injuries that had been sustained in the accident. It was held that the doctor was not negligent in failing to diagnose the full extent of the injuries in the circumstances prevailing at the time. In such cases the court will take into account the emergency circumstances when considering whether the practitioner is in breach of their duty of care. In an emergency, mistakes may be made that would not have been made in a calmer situation. If a nurse in such circumstances makes a mistake that a reasonably competent nurse would have made, then they will not have acted negligently. However, a nurse 'may still be found to be negligent if, notwithstanding the emergency, his acts are found to be unreasonable'.[49]

What if a nurse makes a mistake because they are tired, overworked, or stressed out? Will the courts approach such cases as if the nurse is acting in an 'emergency situation'? It appears not. The courts may well be sympathetic,[50] but if the nurse is unable to reach the objective standard of care, they will be found to be negligent.[51] For example, in *McCormack* v. *Redpath Brown & Co* (1961),[52] a usually careful and competent casualty officer who failed to diagnose a depressed skull fracture was held to be negligent in spite of the fact that he was overworked at the time.

8.5   Lack of resources

Given that no allowance for matters such as inexperience or overwork is made when a court is deciding whether negligence is established, the question then arises as to whether and to what extent a court may consider the scarcity of resources when determining the appropriate standard of care. In *Knight* v. *Home Office* (1990),[53] Pill J considered that it would not be 'a complete defence for a government department . . . to say that no funds are available for additional safety measures',[54] but recognised that a consideration of the available resources was relevant to his determination that the standard of care provided for a mentally ill prisoner detained in a prison hospital did not have to be as high as that provided in a psychiatric hospital:

> In making the decision as to the standard to be demanded the court must, however, bear in mind as one factor that resources available for the public service are limited and that the allocation of resources is a matter for Parliament . . . Even in a medical situation outside prison, the standard of care required will vary with the context. The facilities available to deal with an emergency in a general practitioner's surgery cannot be expected to be as ample as those available in the casualty department of a general hospital, for example.[55]

However, in *Brooks* v. *Home Office* (1999),[56] Garland J refused to accept that the appropriate standard of care in relation to the provision of antenatal care in Holloway was less than that that could be expected outside prison.

The courts are generally unwilling to become embroiled in difficult decisions as to how finite resources should be allocated. This was recognised by Simon J in *Ball* v. *Wirral Health Authority* (2003):

> In the field of medicine where resources are limited and the demands on those resources are many, it may be necessary to make difficult decisions as to how resources are to be allocated. In general, English public and private law leaves such decisions to those who have the legal responsibility for making such decisions. The fact that an area of medicine may be under-funded (for example, neonatal care in the 1970's) or that a particular hospital may not have the facilities that another hospital has, may give rise to a concern among the general public and experts in the field; but it does not necessarily provide the basis of a claim in negligence by a patient who may suffer from the effects of the under-funding or the lack of facilities . . . [57]

In *Hardaker* v. *Newcastle Health Authority* (2001),[58] a diver suffering from decompression illness (DCI) suffered serious permanent disability as a result of a delay in getting him to a decompression chamber because the local hospital's decompression chamber was closed at weekends. Mr Justice Stanley Burnton accepted that, although the Health Authority owed Mr Hardaker a duty of care, 'Their duty was however qualified by the resources available to them'.[59] Given that cases of DCI were relatively rare, the Health Authority could not be held to be negligent for failing to keep the decompression chamber open at all times because 'such an allegation involves an assessment of the priority of allocation of resources which a Court cannot perform.'[60]

A hospital will be vicariously liable for the negligent acts of its staff.[61] Those responsible for the operation of a hospital will also generally owe 'a non-delegable duty to its patients to ensure that they are treated with skill and care regardless of the employment status of the person who is treating them'.[62] In *Robertson v. Nottingham Health Authority* (1997), Brooke LJ described this as being a 'non-delegable duty to establish a proper system of care just as much as it has a duty to engage competent staff and a duty to provide proper and safe equipment and safe premises hospital staff, facilities and organisation provided are appropriate to provide a safe and satisfactory medical service for the patient'.[63] However, in *Farraj v. King's Healthcare NHS Trust* (2010),[64] Dyson LJ took the view that the precise scope of this principle was still being developed,[65] and that the extent to which a hospital owed a non-delegable duty to ensure that its patients are treated with due skill and care would depend on the facts of the particular case and whether it was 'fair just and reasonable that a hospital should owe such a duty of care to its patients' in the circumstances.[66] The rationale for imposing direct liability upon the hospital has been described as follows:

> . . . the hospital undertakes the care, supervision and control of its patients who are in special need of care. Patients are a vulnerable class of persons who place themselves in the care and under the control of a hospital and, as a result, the hospital assumes a particular responsibility for their well-being and safety.[67]

A hospital may therefore be found to be directly liable in negligence for failures in the system that has been set up to provide treatment and care to patients. In *Bull v. Devon Area Health Authority* [1993],[68] there had been a delay of over an hour between the deliveries of twin babies, as a result of which the second twin suffered asphyxia, which caused disabilities. At that time, the hospital operated on two sites, with two hospitals about a mile apart, and it was argued that, given these circumstances and the manpower resources available, the delay was inevitable and excusable and the health authority was not negligent. It was held that the health authority were liable in negligence: in the circumstances the system had broken down and the standard of care had fallen below that reasonably to be expected.[69]

It was suggested on behalf of the health authority that the hospital 'could not be expected to do more than their best, allocating their limited resources as favourably as possible', but Mustill LJ indicated that he was dubious about this argument:

> I have some reservations about this contention, which are not allayed by the submission that hospital medicine is a public service. So it is, but there are other public services in respect of which it is not necessarily an answer to allegations of unsafety that there were insufficient resources to enable the administrators to do everything which they would like to do. I do not for a

moment suggest that public medicine is precisely analogous to other public services, but there is perhaps a danger in assuming that it is completely sui generis, and that it is necessarily a complete answer to say that even if the system in any hospital was unsatisfactory, it was no more unsatisfactory than those in force elsewhere.[70]

Because the hospital had failed to meet an acceptable minimum standard of care, the Court of Appeal did not need to resolve these wider issues, although Lord Mustill recognised that they involved 'important issues of social policy, which the courts may one day have to address'. It does, however, appear that if a hospital is claiming that, because of limited resources, they were not negligent because they were doing the best that they could in the circumstances, they will have to produce some evidence to support this case.[71]

While a hospital trust or health authority[72] may, in an appropriate case, be directly liable in negligence for their failure to provide a system reasonably sufficient for the foreseeable requirements of their patients, the full extent of their 'non-delegable duty' and the extent to which the courts are prepared to take into account issues relating to the allocation of funding when considering whether a claim in negligence is established, remain to be fully worked out by the courts.

8.6   Case study 1

Alex is the nurse in charge of a small hospital situated in a market town. The hospital's emergency A&E unit was closed six months ago and the nearest emergency A&E facility is now ten miles away. A large sign is displayed at the entrance to the hospital, informing the public of these facts and advising anyone requiring emergency treatment to attend at the nearest emergency A&E unit. At about 1 am on a foggy and icy winter's night, Marion and Geoff arrive at the hospital by car. Marion states that she found Geoff sitting by the side of the road next to a mangled bicycle a short distance from the hospital, and that it appeared that he had been hit by a car, which had then driven off without stopping. Marion is a trained volunteer first-aider in her spare time and administered first aid to Geoff at the scene before driving him to hospital. Geoff is conscious, although a little shocked, and has sustained a head injury. He has extensive bruising to his torso and may have fractured some ribs in the accident. Alex decides to keep Geoff at the hospital and offer what treatment she can to him until an ambulance can arrive to take him to the nearest emergency A&E department.[73]

As a matter of law, Marion was not under any duty to go to Geoff's assistance: English law does not impose a 'duty to rescue' in such circumstances. However, by stopping and administering first aid to Geoff, Marion has assumed a duty of care in relation to him. The standard of care of a first-aider in such circumstances is that of an 'ordinary skilled first-aider'.[74] So far as Alex is concerned, because the hospital does not have an A&E department and is displaying notices to that effect, she could have refused to admit Geoff and advised them to travel as a matter of urgency to the nearest hospital with an A&E department. If Geoff's condition deteriorated as a result of the delay involved, it appears that neither

Alex nor the hospital would be liable in negligence because they had not assumed a duty of care in relation to Geoff.[20] However, once Alex decides to keep Geoff at the hospital and to provide interim treatment until an ambulance arrives, she will be under a duty of care towards him. So far as the standard of care is concerned, the emergency nature of the situation will be taken into account in assessing the applicable standard of care.

8.7   Scarce resources: Public disclosures and confidentiality

Nurses are under a professional duty to put the interests of people in their care first and to take steps to protect them if they consider that they may be at risk.[75] The Nursing and Midwifery Council (NMC) has made it clear that this duty extends not merely to a nurse's actual patients, but also to people that they encounter or become aware of during the course of their work.[76] The NMC's Code of Professional Conduct, *The Code: Standards of Conduct, Performance and Ethics for Nurses and Midwives* (2008),[77] requires nurses to:

- 'act without delay if you believe that you, a colleague or anyone else may be putting someone at risk' (clause 32)
- 'inform someone in authority if you experience problems that prevent you working within this code or other nationally agreed standards' (clause 33), and
- 'report your concerns in writing if problems in the environment of care are putting people at risk' (clause 34).

   If a nurse believes that patients are being put at risk because reasonable standards of care are not being achieved and wishes to draw wider attention to this, they should be aware that, by publicising failures of the system, they may breach principles of patient confidentiality.

   The NMC Code makes it clear that nurses must 'respect people's right to confidentiality' (clause 5), and 'ensure people are informed about how and why information is shared by those who will be providing the care' (clause 6). However, the Code not merely permits, but requires nurses 'to disclose information if you believe someone may be at risk of harm, in line with the law of the country in which you are practising' (clause 7). The NMC 2009 Advice Sheet on confidentiality provides some further guidance as to the circumstances in which nurses may disclose patient information without consent. Although disclosure is generally 'only lawful and ethical if the individual has given consent to the information being passed on', in 'exceptional circumstances' it is accepted that the public interest may 'justify overruling the right of an individual to confidentiality in order to secure a broader social concern'.[78] In addition, the NMC advice sheet on confidentiality states that: 'Under common law, staff are permitted to disclose personal information in order to prevent and support detection, investigation and punishment of serious crime and/or to prevent abuse or serious harm to others'. Further guidance on confidentiality and the circumstances in which the disclosure of confidential information by health care professionals may be justified in the public interest may be found in the Department of

Health's NHS Code of Practice on *Confidentiality*,[79] their supplementary guidance on *Public Interest Disclosures*,[80] and the GMC's 2009 extensive ethical guidance on *Confidentiality*.[81]

Since the professional guidance makes it clear that any disclosures of confidential information without the consent of the patient must be within the law, it is necessary to consider what the legal position is. In *Attorney-General* v. *Guardian Newspapers (No.2)* (1990),[82] Lord Goff stated that a duty of confidence arises:

> . . . when confidential information comes to the knowledge of a person (the confidant) in circumstances where he has notice, or is held to have agreed, that the information is confidential, with the effect that it would be just in all the circumstances that he should be precluded from disclosing the information to others.[83]

At common law, medical information will generally be treated as being confidential information and health care professionals will owe a duty of confidence to their patients. In *Hunter* v. *Mann* (1974),[84] Boreham J accepted that a doctor, 'in common with other professional men', was under a duty not voluntarily to disclose, without the consent of his patient, information gained in his professional capacity, save in exceptional circumstances.[85] In addition, Article 8(1) of the European Convention on Human Rights (ECHR) protects a patient's 'right to respect for his private and family life'. The European Court of Human Rights has held that respect for patient confidentiality in respect of medical data is of fundamental importance so far as a patient's Article 8 rights are concerned.[86] The duty to respect patient confidentiality continues after the patient has died.[87]

However, the duty of confidentiality is not absolute. This was recognised in *Attorney-General* v. *Guardian Newspapers (No.2)*[83] by Lord Goff, who stated:

> . . . although the basis of the law's protection of confidence is that there is a public interest that confidences should be preserved and protected by the law, nevertheless that public interest may be outweighed by some other countervailing public interest which favours disclosure.[88]

In the case of medical information, there is a strong public interest in maintaining confidentiality: if patients feared that intimate details in relation to their health might be more widely disclosed, people might be deterred from seeking medical advice or treatment.[89] This public interest may only be overriden if there is a stronger public interest in disclosure.[90] In *X Health Authority* v. *Y* (1988),[91] the High Court granted an injunction to restrain the publication by a newspaper of information identifying two doctors with AIDS who were practising in the United Kingdom. It was held that the public interest in free and informed press debate on the question of whether a doctor with AIDS should continue to practise was outweighed by the public interest in preserving confidence, because there was a risk that, if confidence was breached, patients might be reluctant to come forward for counselling or treatment.

By contrast, in *W* v. *Egdell* (1990),[92] the court held that a breach of confidence was justified in the public interest. The patient, W, had shot and killed five people and injured two more, and had been detained in a secure hospital, having pleaded guilty to manslaughter on the grounds of diminished responsibility. His solicitors commissioned a report from Dr Egdell, an independent consultant psychiatrist, with a view to this report being used at a forthcoming tribunal hearing, either to obtain W's discharge from hospital, or his transfer to a regional secure unit. The report disclosed that W had a long-standing and continuing interest in home-made bombs, and made it clear that Dr Egdell did not accept the view that W was no longer a danger to the public. In the light of this negative report, W's solicitors withdrew the tribunal application. However, when Dr Egdell discovered that the report was not to be used, he disclosed a copy of his report to the medical director of W's secure hospital. The hospital then sent a copy of the report to the Home Secretary, who in turn forwarded a copy to the tribunal. The Court of Appeal held that, where a patient in W's position commissioned an independent psychiatric report, the doctor making the report was undoubtedly under a duty of confidence, but that that duty was not absolute. In the circumstances, disclosure to the relevant authorities was lawful because there was a strong public interest in reducing the risk that W posed to public safety:

> Where a man has committed multiple killings under the disability of serious mental illness, decisions which may lead directly or indirectly to his release from hospital should not be made unless a responsible authority is properly able to make an informed judgment that the risk of repetition is so small as to be acceptable. A consultant psychiatrist who becomes aware, even in the course of a confidential relationship, of information which leads him, in the exercise of what the court considers a sound professional judgment, to fear that such decisions may be made on the basis of inadequate information and with a real risk of consequent danger to the public is entitled to take such steps as are reasonable in all the circumstances to communicate the grounds of his concern to the responsible authorities.[93]

Similarly, although a patient's right to confidentiality is protected by Article 8 ECHR, this right is qualified by Article 8(2):

> There shall be no interference by a public authority with the exercise of this right except such as is in accordance with law and is necessary in a democratic society in the interests of national security, public safety or the economic well-being of the country, for the prevention of disorder or crime, for the protection of health or morals, or for the protection of the rights and freedoms of others.

Any interference with a patient's Article 8 rights must be justified as being in accordance with law, pursuing one of the legitimate aims that are identified in Article 8(2), and must be 'necessary', which requires that the interference 'corresponds to a pressing social need' and is 'proportionate to the legitimate aim pursued'.[94]

Clearly, the balancing exercise involved in determining whether a disclosure of confidential information may be justified in the public interest may be very difficult. To assist staff making these decisions, more detailed guidance may be found in the Department of Health's *Confidentiality: Code of Practice*, Annex B, and the 2010 *Supplementary Guidance: Public Interest Disclosures*. The *Supplementary Guidance* states that:

In some cases, it is clear that a proportionate disclosure is required to:

- Prevent serious harm being caused to one or more other individual(s), such as child abuse, or a serious assault;
- Report a doctor or nurse with Hepatitis B who carries out exposure–prone procedures without taking proper precautions to protect patient safety; and/or
- Prevent, detect or prosecute what is clearly a serious crime like murder or rape.[95]

However, in other less serious cases, it is advised that further guidance should be sought before disclosure is made because it is less clear that a public interest defence is applicable.[96]

8.8   Whistleblowing and modern technology

Social networking sites are a popular way of communicating with friends and acquaintances: the NMC has estimated that around 355,000 registered nurses and midwives are on Facebook.[97] A nurse considering 'whistleblowing' may be tempted to post information on a social networking site. The issues discussed above in relation to confidentiality will have to be carefully considered, but it should also be noted that in July 2011 the NMC updated its guidance on the use of social networking sites by nurses, midwives and students. This guidance makes it clear that such sites should not be used to discuss work-related issues online, including complaints about colleagues, and that such discussions are likely to be inappropriate even if individuals discussed are anonymised. With the popularity of 'smart phones', which have in-built cameras, there may also be the temptation to photograph issues of concern and to post such photographs on a social networking site. This temptation is best avoided: the guidance states that mobile phone cameras should not be used in the workplace and that pictures of patients and service users should never be placed on social networking sites, even if they request you to do so. In relation to the use of social networking sites to raise and escalate concerns, the guidance clearly states that these sites should not be used for whistleblowing purposes. Instead, nurses should follow the NMC's specific guidance on *Raising and Escalating Concerns*.[98]

8.9   Whistleblowing and the Public Interest Disclosure Act 1998

As I have indicated, the NMC requires nurses, midwives and students to report concerns which they may have about any aspect of their workplace which may put the safety of people in their care, or the public at risk. This applies to a wide range of situations, including the following:

- danger or risk to health and safety, e.g. health and safety violations
- issues regarding staff conduct, e.g. unprofessional attitudes or behaviour and concerns related to equality and diversity issues
- issues regarding care delivery involving nurses, midwives or other staff members
- issues related to the environment of care, e.g. resources, products, people, staffing or organisation-wide concerns
- issues related to the health of a colleague, which may affect their ability to practise safely
- misuse or unavailability of clinical equipment, including lack of adequate training
- financial malpractice, including criminal acts and fraud.[99]

However, a nurse considering reporting concerns which relate to any of these issues may fear that they making such a report might have negative consequences for their future employment and might lead to disciplinary proceedings, or even dismissal. The fear about 'speaking out' may be particularly great where a nurse is concerned about the conduct of a consultant or institutional bad practice.[100] The 2010 NHS Staff Survey indicated that, while 82 per cent of staff participating in the survey felt encouraged to report errors, near-misses and incidents, 11 per cent still feared that the reporting of errors might lead to them being punished or blamed.[101] The *Report of the Robert Francis Inquiry into the Mid Staffordshire NHS Foundation Trust* (2010)[102] highlights the problems that can arise where poor practice and low standards of care within a hospital are combined with poor complaint procedures and management, with staff being afraid to complain because of reprisals, complaints not being properly followed up and the internal reporting of issues relating to staffing being discouraged.

The relevant legislation in relation to whistleblowing is the Public Interest Disclosure Act 1998 (PIDA), which inserts a new Part IV into the Employment Rights Act 1996. It provides legal protection from victimisation or dismissal to all workers in England and Wales who disclose concerns in the public interest and in good faith, provided that the procedure set out in the Act is followed. Volunteer workers are not protected by PIDA, although the Department of Health has stated that it regards it a good practice for NHS organisations to extend their whistleblowing practices to include volunteers.[103] The protection provided by PIDA may extend to detriment suffered after the employment contract has been terminated.[104]

First, certain disclosures are regarded as being 'qualifying disclosures', in other words, as qualifying for protection under the 1996 Act. These are disclosures of information which, in the reasonable belief of the worker making the disclosure, tends to show one or more of the following:

(a) that a criminal offence has been committed, is being committed or is likely to be committed

(b) that a person has failed, is failing or is likely to fail to comply with any legal obligation to which he is subject

(c) that a miscarriage of justice has occurred, is occurring or is likely to occur

(d) that the health or safety of any individual has been, is being or is likely to be endangered

(e) that the environment has been, is being or is likely to be damaged, or

(f) that information tending to show any matter falling within any one of (a) to (e) above has been, is being or is likely to be deliberately concealed.[105]

A number of other conditions must be satisfied for the disclosure to be protected. The disclosure must be made in good faith, either to the worker's employer, or, where the employee reasonably believes that a person other than his/her employer has sole or main responsibility for the matter, then disclosure may be made to that other person.[106] Qualifying disclosures are also protected if they are made in the course of obtaining legal advice,[107] or if the employer is a body any of whose members are appointed under any enactment made by a minister of the Crown, the disclosure may be made in good faith to a Minister of the Crown.[108] This last provision would apply to NHS employees and would permit them, for example, to make a qualifying disclosure in good faith to the Secretary of State for Health. Protected disclosures may also be made to a 'prescribed person' under section 43F of the Employment Rights Act. The list of prescribed persons is contained in Schedule 1 of the Public Interest Disclosure (Prescribed Persons) Order 1999,[109] and currently includes: the Care Quality Commission (CQC); the General Social Care Council; the Care Council for Wales; the Independent Regulator of NHS Foundation Trusts; the Health and Safety Executive; and numerous other regulatory bodies. A disclosure to a prescribed person is protected if it is made in good faith and the disclosing employee reasonably believes that: (a) the relevant failure is within the responsibility of the prescribed person, and that (b) the information disclosed and any allegation contained within it are substantially true.[110]

Disclosure in other cases is protected if the conditions set out in section 43G of the Employment Rights Act are satisfied:

- The worker must make the disclosure in good faith[111]; and
- The worker must reasonably believe that the information disclosed and any allegation contained in it are substantially true; and
- At the time that the disclosure is made:
  (i) the worker reasonably believes that he will be subjected to a detriment by his employer if he/she makes a disclosure to his/her employer or to a 'prescribed person',
  (ii) in a case where there is no relevant 'prescribed person', the worker reasonably believes that it is likely that evidence relating to the relevant failure will be concealed or destroyed if disclosure is made to the employer, or
  (iii) The worker has previously made a disclosure of substantially the same information to the employer or a prescribed person; and
- In all the circumstances of the case it is reasonable to make the disclosure.

Factors which are to be taken into account in determining whether it is reasonable for the worker to make the disclosure include, in particular, the identity of the person to whom the disclosure is made; the seriousness of the failure and whether it is likely to recur; whether the disclosure is made in breach of a duty of confidence; any previous disclosures made to the employer or to a prescribed person, and whether the worker has complied with any internal procedures in relation to the making of disclosures.[112]

Where a worker encounters an exceptionally serious failure, a public disclosure may be made as a matter of urgency without the need for the worker to have previously reported the matter to his/her employer or to a prescribed person, or to show that they fear that they will be victimised if they make a disclosure.[113] Disclosure of a failure of an exceptionally serious nature will be protected if the disclosure is made in good faith and in the reasonable belief that the information disclosed and any allegation contained in it are substantially true, the disclosure is not made for personal gain, and it is, in all of the circumstances of the case, reasonable for the disclosure to be made.[114] In deciding whether it is reasonable for the disclosure to be made, regard is had to the identity of the person to whom the disclosure is made,[115] so it is unlikely that a nurse would be justified in rushing straight to the press to make a disclosure without first contacting a relevant regulatory or professional body, or, for example, raising the matter with his or her Member of Parliament, or, in a case where it is reasonably believed that a crime has been committed, with the police.

If a worker makes a disclosure that is protected by PIDA and is subjected to victimisation by their employer, they may bring a claim against their employer in the Employment Tribunal. The employer will be liable if the disclosure is a material factor in a decision made by them (or by their employees) to subject the worker to a detrimental act.[116] The Court of Appeal has recently indicated that, where a whistleblower has suffered a detriment without being at fault in any way, 'tribunals will need to look with a critical – indeed sceptical – eye to see whether the innocent explanation given by the employer for the adverse treatment is indeed the genuine explanation'.[117] If the whistleblower's claim is successful, there is no cap on the awards that an Employment Tribunal can make – the award will be based on what is just and equitable in all the circumstances.

If an employer seeks to prevent an employee from making a disclosure that is protected by PIDA, by placing a 'gagging' clause in the contract of employment, such a clause is void and ineffective.[118] However, concern has been expressed in the media that 'gagging' clauses are still being used in compromise agreements being made between NHS bodies and whistleblowers, and that workers may feel pressurised into accepting such clauses because of the length of time that employment litigation may take, and fears that they may be left with a large legal bill because the Employment Tribunal does not normally award successful claimants their costs.[119]

Every NHS trust is required to have in place policies and procedures that comply with PIDA,[120] and a guide, *Speak up for a Health NHS* (2010), has been published by the Social Partnership Forum to help NHS bodies to follow best practice in relation to whistleblowers.[121] The NMC has produced additional guidance, *Raising and Escalating Concerns* (2010),[122] which suggests a four-stage process be followed when concerns are being raised. It advises that concerns should initially be raised with a line manager, or, if that is not possible, with the person designated by their employer's policy on raising concerns. Thereafter, if the concern is not adequately addressed and/or there is immediate risk to others, it is suggested that the issue is raised at a higher level within their organisation and then, if necessary, with a health care regulatory organisation, although nurses are advised always to seek advice before taking this final step.[123] The NHS Constitution and Handbook were updated in 2012 to include: an expectation that staff raise concerns at the earliest opportunity; a pledge that NHS organisations support staff by ensuring that concerns are fully investigated and that they have an independent person to speak to in relation to their concerns, and to clarify the existing legal right under PIDA for staff to raise concerns about safety, malpractice, or other 'qualifying disclosures', without suffering detriment.[124] The CQC has produced guidance on whistleblowing and how to raise concerns with the CQC, for those who work for providers of health, social and dental care registered with the CQC.[125]

8.10   Whistleblowing and Article 10 ECHR

An employer who victimises or dismisses a whistleblowing employee may also breach their right to freedom of expression under Article 10(1) ECHR. A recent illustration of this may be found in the case of *Heinisch* v. *Germany* (2011).[126] In that case, the whistleblower, Ms Heinisch (H) was employed by a company that specialised in health care for the elderly, working as a geriatric nurse in a nursing home. The Medical Review Board had found that there were serious shortcomings in the daily care provided at the home, which were caused by a shortage of staff. Regular complaints were also made to the management by H and her colleagues that they were overburdened because of the staff shortages and therefore had difficulty in carrying out their duties to an acceptable level, but these did not lead to an improvement in the situation. H fell ill on a number of occasions: one medical certificate stated that she was ill because of overworking. Eventually, H instructed a lawyer, who wrote to the management of the nursing home asking them to state how they intended to avoid criminal liability and ensure that sufficient care was taken of the home's residents. When these concerns were rejected, H lodged a criminal complaint against the company through her lawyer, but this complaint was subsequently discontinued by the public prosecutor's office. Having been given notice of termination of her employment on account of her repeated illness, H contacted her trade union, calling for the withdrawal of her dismissal, and the union issued a leaflet stating that the H had been dismissed on account of her illness, called for the withdrawal of the dismissal, and described the dismissal as a 'political disciplinary measure taken in order to gag those employed'. H sent one copy of this leaflet to the nursing home, where it was distributed. It was only at this stage that the employer because aware of H's criminal complaint, and H was dismissed without notice on suspicion of having instigated the production and dissemination of the leaflet. H brought proceedings before the national courts, which held on appeal that H's dismissal was lawful as her criminal complaint had provided a compelling reason for dismissal without notice. H then instituted a claim in the European Court of Human Rights (ECtHR), arguing that her dismissal and the refusal of the national courts to order her reinstatement infringed her Article 10 right to freedom of expression.

The ECtHR felt that the information disclosed by H was 'undeniably of public interest', given the context of H's employment at an institution responsible for the care of elderly and potentially vulnerable individuals:

> In societies with an ever growing part of their elderly population being subject to institutional care, and taking into account the particular vulnerability of the parties concerned, who often may not be in a position to draw attention to shortcomings in the care rendered in their own initiative, the dissemination of information about the quality or deficiencies of such care is of vital importance with a view to preventing abuse. This is even more evident where institutional care is provided by a state-owned company, where the confidence of the public in an adequate provision of vital care services by the State is at stake.[127]

The Court felt it was reasonable to conclude that any further internal complaints would not have been effective to remedy the matters complained of, and concluded that H's external reporting by means of a criminal complaint was justified. They also accepted that she had acted in good faith in making the complaint. In the circumstances, the Court felt that the public interest in having information about deficiencies in the provision of institutional care for the elderly by a state-owned company was so important in a democratic society that it outweighed the company's interest in protecting its business reputation and interests, and that H's dismissal without notice was disproportionately severe, having regard to the risk that such a sanction might have a serious chilling effect, not only on the company's other employees, but also on other employees in the nursing service sector, discouraging them from reporting any shortcomings in institutional care.[128]

It appears from this case that a court, when assessing whether action taken by an employer against a whistleblower is disproportionate and breaches Article 10, will consider the following factors:

- the public interest in the information disclosed by the whistleblower
- whether there were alternative methods which the whistleblower could have taken to remedy the wrong complained of
- whether the whistleblower acted in good faith
- the authenticity of the information disclosed
- the damage suffered by the employer, and
- the penalty imposed on the whistleblower by the employer.

8.11   Case study 2

Jo is a night-duty charge nurse on a geriatric acute ward. She believes that the standard of care of her patients has declined considerably in recent weeks due to two events: (1) the permanent withdrawal of one night nurse, and (2) the replacement of experienced nurses with much less experienced agency staff. She becomes particularly concerned when a patient dies in circumstances which she believes were largely due to insufficient experienced staff being available.

Under the NMC Code, *Standards of Conduct, Performance and Ethics for Nurses and Midwives*, Jo is required to act without delay if she believes that patients are being put at risk and to report concerns about problems in relation to the care environment in writing. A failure on her part to do this should amount to misconduct on her part. Jo clearly has such concerns and ought therefore to report them promptly. If her employer has a complaints procedure, she would be well advised to follow that procedure. Otherwise, she would be advised to follow the NMC's procedure in relation to raising and escalating concerns and raise the matter initially with her line manager. In addition, she may also wish to contact the Royal College of Nursing (RCN) to raise her concerns. She should also seek advice either from the NMC, her union or PCaW. If her concerns are still brushed aside, she may ultimately wish to raise the matter with the Care Quality Commission or other health care regulatory organisation, but she should take advice before taking this step.

In raising her concerns, she should be aware of NMC guidance in relation to confidentiality and should follow her employer's written information-sharing protocols in relation to the disclosure of patient information to others within the health care system. She should not use patient identifiable information, unless that is absolutely necessary. A proportionate disclosure of confidential information to third parties for the protection of the health of patients is likely to be lawful. If Jo is victimised or subjected to disciplinary proceedings as a result of raising her concerns, then she may wish to avail herself of the protection provided by PIDA. Her disclosure will be regarded as a qualifying disclosure under section 43B of the Employment Rights Act, and she will be protected under section 43C if it is made in good faith to her employer. If she suffers a detriment as a result of making a qualifying disclosure, then she may bring a claim against her employer in the Employment Tribunal. She may also have a claim for breach of her Article 10 right to freedom of expression.

8.12   Conclusion

This chapter has considered a wide variety of legal issues which may arise in a cash-strapped health service. Staff working within the NHS are constantly under pressure to provide an acceptable standard of service and to meet service targets within a system where difficult decisions in relation to the allocation of finite resources are constantly having to be made. Cost-cutting measures may mean that inexperienced nurses are placed in a position where they feel that they are being asked to undertake tasks that are beyond their competence. Staff shortages may mean that even experienced staff are overburdened with tasks, or have to work when they are overtired or ill. In such circumstances, as we have seen, although the courts may be sympathetic to the nurses' plight, the standard of care is not reduced to take account of these factors.

On the other hand, the scarcity of NHS resources places additional responsibilities and pressures upon nursing staff. Where financial restraints affect the quality of care provided to patients, putting them at risk, the nurse is required by the NMC Code to report the matter. However, in voicing their concerns, nurses may be required to consider difficult issues relating to patient confidentiality and may need real courage to comply with their professional responsibilities in the face of inaction by their employer and fears that whistleblowing may lead to disciplinary action or even dismissal. PIDA offers important legal protection to the nurse who is victimised for acting in good faith to highlight failures in the standard of care being provided to patients, but staff who are concerned about the cost and stress involved in pursuing a claim before an employment tribunal may feel under pressure to compromise their claims. The problem of how to allocate finite resources within the NHS may not be for individual nurses to resolve, but the negative impact that economic pressures may have upon patient care may nevertheless have significant legal ramifications for nursing staff.

8.13   Notes and references

1. http://www.nhs.uk/NHSEngland/thenhs/about/Pages/nhscoreprinciples.aspx
2. D. Hunter, *Desperately Seeking Solutions: Rationing Health Care* (London, Longman, 1997), p. 20.
3. See *e.g. Report of the Committee of Inquiry into the Costs of the National Health Service* (Cmnd. 9663) (1956) para. 95.
4. For discussion of these issues see: C. Newdick, *Who Should We Treat?* 2nd edn (Oxford, OUP, 2005), at pp. 5–8; E. Jackson, *Medical Law: Text, Cases and Materials* (Oxford, OUP, 2010), pp. 34–6.
5. See *e.g.* I. Kennedy, The technological imperative and its application in health care. In *Treat Me Right: Essays in Medical Law and Ethics* (Oxford, Clarendon Press, 1988), pp. 287–99; N. Daniels, Health-care needs and distributive justice, *Philosophy and Public Affairs*, **10** (1981), pp. 146–79; J. Harris, Qualifying the value of life, *Journal of Medical Ethics*, **13** (1987), pp. 117–23; B. New & J. Le Grand, *Rationing in the NHS: Principles and Pragmatism* (London, King's Fund, 1996).
6. http://www.nice.org.uk/aboutnice/whoweare/who_we_are.jsp. NICE was established as a Special Health Authority: National Institute for Clinical Excellence (Establishment and Constitution) Order 1999 (SI 1999/220).
7. http://www.nice.org.uk/media/B52/A7/TAMethodsGuideUpdatedJune2008. pdf. NICE uses the QALY (Quality Adjusted Life Year) measurement to assess the clinical and cost effectiveness of health technologies: http://www.nice.org.uk/newsroom/features/measuringeffectivenessandcosteffectivenesstheqaly.jsp. Generally a drug will not be considered to be cost-effective if its cost is more than £30,000 per QALY.
8. Health and Social Care Act 2012, sections 232–234. The relevant provisions are expected to come fully into force in 2013. The RCN has produced a briefing document upon the Act, *What does the Health and Social Care Act 2012 mean?* which may be found at: http://www.rcn.org.uk/__data/assets/pdf_file/0008/461798/HSCA_FINAL.pdf
9. Health and Social Care Act 2012, sections13–28.
10. Health and Social Care Act 2012, Chapter 4, makes provision for pricing within the NHS and provides for the establishment of a national tariff to determine the price

payable by commissioners for NHS services. *C.f.* M. Brazier & E. Cave, *Medicine, Patients and the Law*, 5th edn (London, Penguin Books, 2011), para.2.17.

11. The purpose of a value-based approach toward the price of medicines would be to ensure that the price paid by the NHS for a drug reflected the value of that drug in improving the length and quality of patients' lives: A. Maynard & K. Bloor, The future role of NICE, *BMJ*, **341** (2010), c6286; DH, *A new value-based approach to the pricing of branded medicines: Government Response to Consultation*, (2011) http://www.dh.gov.uk/prod_consum_dh/groups/dh_digitalassets/documents/digitalasset/dh_128404.pdf

12. See *e.g. Eisai Ltd v. NICE* [2008] EWCA Civ 346; *R (on the application of Fraser) v. NICE* [2009] EWHC 452 (Admin); *Servier v. NICE* [2010] EWCA Civ 346; *R v. Cambridge DHA ex parte B* [1995] 1 WLR 898; *R v. North Derbyshire HA, ex parte Fisher* [1997] 8 Med LR 327; *R v. North West Lancashire HA, ex parte A, D & G* [2000] 1 W.L.R. 977; *R (Rogers) v. Swindon NHS Primary Care Trust* [2006] 1 WLR 2649; *R (on the application of Otley) v. Barking and Dagenham NHS Primary Care Trust* [2007] EWHC 1927; *R (on the application of Murphy) v. Salford Primary Care Trust* [2008] EWHC 1908 (Admin); *R (on the application of Ross)* [2008] EWHC 2252 (Admin); *R (on the Application of Booker) v. NHS Oldham and Direct Line Insurance Plc* [2010] EWHC 2593 (Admin); *AC v. Berkshire West Primary Care Trust* [2010] EWHC 1162 (Admin); *R (on the Application of Condiff) v. North Staffordshire Primary Care Trust* [2011] EWHC 872 (Admin).

13. *R v. North Derbyshire HA, ex parte Fisher* [1997] 8 Med LR 327. See also: *R v. Cambridge Health Authority, ex parte B* [1995] 1 WLR 898; *AC v. Berkshire West Primary Care Trust* [2010] EWHC 1162 (Admin).

14. See, for example, *R (Rogers) v. Swindon NHS Primary Care Trust* [2006] 1 WLR 2649; *R (on the application of Ross)* [2008] EWHC 2252 (Admin).

15. *R (Rogers) v. Swindon NHS Primary Care Trust* [2006] 1 WLR 2649; *R (on the application of Otley) v. Barking and Dagenham NHS Primary Care Trust* [2007] EWHC 1927; *R (on the application of Murphy) v. Salford Primary Care Trust* [2008] EWHC 1908 (Admin).

16. [2008] EWHC 2252 (Admin).

17. *Gold v. Essex CC* [1942] 2 KB 293; *Barnett v. Chelsea and Kensington Hospital Management Committee* [1969] 1 QB 428.

18. *Jones v. Manchester Corporation* [1952] QB 852, Denning LJ, 867; *Barnett v. Chelsea and Kensington Hospital Management Committee* [1969] 1 QB 428, Nield J, 435–6.

19. *Barnett v. Chelsea and Kensington Hospital Management Committee* [1969] 1 QB 428, Nield J.

20. See M. Brazier & E. Cave, *Medicine, Patients and the Law*, 5th edn (London, Penguin Books, 2011). para.7.2.

21. *Bolam v. Friern Hospital Management Committee* [1957] WLR 582, McNair J., p.587. This test was subsequently approved by the House of Lords: *Whitehouse v. Jordan* [1981] 1 WLR 246; *Maynard v. West Midlands RHA* [1984] 1 WLR 634.

22. See e.g. M. Jones, The *Bolam* test and the responsible expert, *Tort Law Review*, (1999), p. 226; *Maynard v. West Midlands RHA* [1984] 1 WLR 634, Lord Scarman, at p. 639.

23. [1998] AC 232. *C.f. Hucks v. Cole* [1993] 4 Med LR 393 (decided in 1968).

24. 1998] AC 232, Lord Browne-Wilkinson at 243. *C.f.* R. Mulheron, Trumping *Bolam*: a critical analysis of *Bolitho*'s 'gloss', *Cambridge Law Journal*, **69** (2010) p.609, where it is suggested that the *Bolitho* test has altered the outcome of clinical negligence cases more commonly than the label 'rare case' would suggest.

25. *Bolitho v. City and Hackney HA* [1998] AC 232, Lord Browne-Wilkinson, 243. For more detailed analysis of the decision in Bolitho, see *e.g.*: M. Brazier & J. Miola, Bye-bye bolam: A medical litigation revolution? *Medical Law Review*, **8** [2005] p. 85; A. Maclean,

Beyond Bolam and Bolitho, *Medical Law International*, **5** [2002] p. 205; R. Heywood, The logic of Bolitho, *Professional Negligence*, **6** [2006] p. 225; Mulheron, *supra* note 24.

26. *Bolitho, supra* note 25, Lord Browne-Wilkinson, at p. 241. See e.g. *Marriott* v. *West Midlands RHA* [1999] Lloyds Rep Med 23; *French* v. *Thames Valley Strategic HA* [2005] EWHC 459 (QB), Beatson J, [112]; *Brown* v. *Scarborough and North East Yorkshire Healthcare NHS Trust* [2009] EWHC 3103 (QB); *Campbell* v. *Borders Health Board* [2011] CSOH 73 (affirmed [2012] CSIH 49).

27. See Maclean, *supra* note 25; Mulheron, *supra* note 24.

28. [1987] 1 QB 730, at p.750.

29. [1971] 2 QB 691.

30. *Ibid.*, at p.709.

31. [1987] 1 QB 730. The case was appealed to the House of Lords on the issue of causation: [1988] AC 1074.

32. [1987] 1 QB 730, at p. 751. See also: *Jones* v. *Manchester Corporation* [1952] 2 QB 852, at p. 871.

33. [1987] 1 QB 730, at p.754. *C.f.* the minority approach of Sir Nicholas Browne-Wilkinson VC, who considered that 'a doctor who has properly accepted a post in a hospital in order to gain necessary experience should only be held liable for acts or omissions which a careful doctor with his qualifications and experience would not have done or omitted', because he felt that otherwise, 'the young houseman or the doctor seeking to obtain specialist skill in a special unit would be held liable for shortcomings in the treatment without any personal fault on his part at all' (at p. 777).

34. (1994) (QB) Unreported, Lexis Transcript.

35. *Ibid.* Sir Haydn Tudor Evans (sitting as a High Court Judge), at p. 3. *C.f. Cattley* v. *St. John's Ambulance Brigade* (1988) (QB) Unreported, Lexis Transcript 87 NJ 1140/1986 C 133, a case involving alleged negligence on the part of a St John's Ambulance first-aider, where it was held that the standard of care in that case was that of an 'ordinary skilled first-aider exercising and professing to have that special skill of a first-aider'.

36. [1994] 5 Med LR 120.

37. M. Jones, *Medical Negligence*, 4th edn (London, Sweet & Maxwell, 2008), paras 3-099-101.

38. *Ibid.* 3–100.

39. *Wilsher* v. *Essex AHA* [1987] 1 QB 730, Glidewell LJ, at p. 774, Sir Nicholas Browne-Wilkinson VC, at pp.778–9. *C.f. Junior* v. *McNichol* (1959) *The Times*, February 11: House surgeon acting on instructions of consultant surgeon not liable.

40. *Ibid.*, Mustill LJ, at p.758, Glidewell LJ, at p. 774.

41. *Ibid.*, Sir Nicholas Brown-Wilkinson VC, at p. 777; *Payne* v. *St Helier Group HMC* [1952] CLY 2992; *Poole* v. *Morgan* [1987] 3 WWR 217. However, it should be remembered that, for an action in negligence to succeed, the claimant would have to prove that the negligence had caused: see e.g. *Wilsher* v. *Essex AHA* [1988] AC 1074 (HL).

42. [1994] 6 WWR 280 (British Columbia Court of Appeal).

43. It is part of the role of a ward sister/manager to 'set care standards; observe, support and supervise ward staff in nursing practice': RCN, *Breaking Down Barriers, Driving Up Standards: The role of the ward sister and the charge nurse* (2009), p.14.

44. [1998] Lloyds Rep Med. 425.

45. [1952] QB 852.

46. *Ibid.*, Denning LJ, at pp. 871–2. The Board was adjudged to be responsible for paying 80 per cent of the damages.

47. [1987] 1 QB 730, at p.749.

48. [1971] 4 WWR 358.

49. *Cattley* v. *St John's Ambulance Brigade* [1988] LexisNexis Transcript, transcript No. 87 NJ 1140/1986 C 133, HHJ Prosser QC, p. 7. In relation to the standard of care in an emergency, the learned judge said: 'Anyone confronted with an emergency situation is not to be held to the standard of conduct normally applied to one who is not in that situation. This does not mean that any different standard is to be applied in the emergency. The conduct required is still that of a reasonable person under the circumstances as they would appear to one who was using proper care, and the emergency is to be considered only as one of the circumstances.'

50. See e.g. *Barnett* v. *Chelsea and Kensington Hospital Management Committee* [1969] 1 QB 428, Neild J, at p.437.

51. Jones, *supra* note 37, para. 3–104.

52. (1961) *The Times*, 24 March. *C.f. Deacon* v. *McVicar and Leicester Royal Infirmary* (1984) LexisNexis transcript: Plaintiff had had a Shirodkar suture inserted because she had an incompetent cervix. During labour doctors failed to remove this suture because they were busy, as a result the plaintiff suffered a torn cervix. The hospital was found to be negligent as the plaintiff had not been treated with proper professional care and skill. *C.f. Nickolls* v. *Ministry of Health* (1955) *The Times*, 4 February (CA): surgeon who continued to operate while ill would be liable for continuing to perform surgery while unfit to do so.

53. [1990] 3 All ER 237.

54. *Ibid.*, 243.

55. *Ibid.*, 243.

56. [1999] 48 BMLR 109.

57. [2003] Lloyds Rep Med 165, at [32].

58. [2001] Lloyds Rep Med 512.

59. *Ibid.*, at [54].

60. *Ibid. C.f. Bull* v. *Devon AHA* [1993] 4 Med LR 117.

61. *Cassidy* v. *Ministry of Health* [1951] 2 KB 343; *Roe* v. *Ministry of Health* [1954] 2 QB 66.

62. *Farraj* v. *King's Healthcare NHS Trust* [2010] 1 WLR 2139, Dyson LJ, at [88].

63. *Robertson* v. *Nottingham Health Authority* [1997] 8 Med LR 1, Brooke LJ, at p. 13. See also: *Wilsher* [1987] QB 747, Sir Nicholas Browne-Wilkinson V-C, at p. 778 and Glidewell LJ, at p. 775; *Child A* v. *Ministry of Defence* [2005] QB 183, at [32]. In the *Child A* case it was held that the MOD did not owe a non-delegable duty to the wife and child of a British Army officer to ensure that due care and skill was taken by those carrying out treatment in a German hospital. In *Farraj*, the CA held that the NHS hospital did not owe the claimant a non-delegable duty of care in respect of tests which had been contracted out to an independent laboratory.

64. [2010] 1 WLR 2139.

65. *Ibid.*, [77].

66. *Ibid.*, See *Caparo Industries* v. *Dickman* [1990] 2 AC 605, 618. In *Farraj* Dyson LJ stated (at [79]) that the general observations of Brooke LJ quoted above were *obiter* since the point decided in *Robertson* was that the Health Authority was liable for a patient being injured because of a negligent breakdown in the system for communicating relevant information to the clinicians responsible for the patient's care.

67. *Farraj* v. *King's Healthcare NHS Trust* [2010] 1 WLR 2139, Dyson LJ, [88], following Mason J in *Kondis* v. *State Transport Authority* (1986) 154 CLR 672, at p.686.

68. [1993] 4 Med LR 117.

69. See e.g. *Loraine* v. *Wirral University Teaching Hospital NHS Foundation Trust* [2008] EWHC 1565 (QB) for a recent example of a hospital trust being held to be directly liable. In that case the hospital communications system was held to be flawed and to expose patients to unacceptable risk because it relied upon the patient to identify

potential complications, with the patient's hospital records only being retrieved if that appeared to be necessary from the patient's account. *C.f. Garcia* v. *East Lancashire Hospital NHS Trust* [2006] EWHC 2314 (QB) where delay was held not to be negligent.

70. [1989] 4 Med LR 117, 141–2.
71. *Richards* v. *Swansea NHS Trust* [2007] EWHC 487 (QB), Field J, at [31]; Jones, *supra* note 37, 4–123.
72. It appears that direct liability may extend to other bodies or even, in an appropriate case, to the Secretary of State: see *Re HIV Haemophiliac Litigation* (1990) BMLR 171, in which the Court of Appeal decided that there was an arguable case in negligence against the Secretary of State for failing to warns of the risks of HIV contamination.
73. The case studies in this chapter are adapted and updated versions of case studies written by Robert Lee and included in the third edition of this work.
74. *Cattley* v. *St. John's Ambulance Brigade, supra*, note 49.
75. NMC, *Raising and Escalating Concerns: Guidance for Nurses and Midwives* (2010), p. 1.
76. *Ibid.*
77. See www.nmc-uk.org
78. http://www.nmc-uk.org/Nurses-and-midwives/Advice-by-topic/A/Advice/Confidentiality/
79. (2003) http://www.dh.gov.uk, Annex B.
80. (2010) http://www.dh.gov.uk
81. (2009) http://www.gmc-uk.org
82. [1990] 1 AC 109.
83. *Ibid.*, at p. 281.
84. [1974] QB 767.
85. *Ibid.*, at p. 772. See also: *W* v. *Egdell* [1990] Ch 359, Bingham LJ, at p. 419.
86. *Z* v. *Finland* (1998) 25 EHRR 371; *MS* v. *Sweden* (1999) 28 EHRR 313; *Szuluk* v. *United Kingdom* (2010) 50 EHRR 10.
87. *Bluck* v. *Information Commissioner* (2007) 98 BMLR 1; *Lewis* v. *Secretary of State for Health* [2008] EWHC 2196 (QB); *C.f.* GMC, *Confidentiality* (2009), paras. 70-72.
88. *Ibid.*, at p. 282.
89. See e.g. *Z* v. *Finland* (1998) 25 EHRR 371, 393.
90. *W* v. *Egdell* [1990] Ch 359.
91. [1988] RPC 379. See also: *H (a Healthcare Worker)* v. *Associated Newspapers Ltd* [2002] EWCA Civ 195.
92. (1990) Ch 359.
93. *Ibid.*, Bingham LJ, 424. *C.f. Stone* v. *South East Coast SHA* [2006] EWHC 1668 (Admin).
94. *Szuluk* v. *United Kingdom* (2010) 50 EHRR 10, [45]. *C.f. Re General Dental Council's Application* [2011] EWHC 3011 (Admin).
95. (2010) http://www.dh.gov.uk, para. 25.
96. *Ibid.*, para. 26.
97. http://www.nmc-uk.org/Nurses-and-midwives/Advice-by-topic/A/Advice/Social-networking-sites/
98. (2010)http://www.nmc-uk.org/Documents/RaisingandEscalatingConcerns/Raising-and-escalating-concerns-guidance-A5.pdf
99. *Ibid.*, p. 5.
100. See e.g. The Ritchie Report, *An Inquiry into quality and practice within the National Health Service arising from the actions of Rodney Ledward* (2000), paras 12.2.3, 12.5, 18.1.1, 18.3.3, 18.3.6, http://www.dh.gov.uk/en/Publicationsandstatistics/Publications/PublicationsPolicyAndGuidance/DH_4093337

101. Published March 2011, see: http://www.cqc.org.uk. These findings are reported in *The NHS Constitution and Whistleblowing, Consultation Report: September 2011*, p. 11: http://www.dh.gov/publications.
102. http://www.dh.gov.uk/en/Publicationsandstatistics/Publications/Publications PolicyAndGuidance/DH_113018
103. *Ibid*.
104. *Woodward* v. *Abbey National Plc (No.1)* [2006] EWCA Civ 822, [2006] ICR 1436, reversing *Fadipe* v. *Reed Nursing Personnel* [2005] ICR 1760, on this point.
105. Employment Rights Act 1996 (ERA), section 43B(1).
106. ERA, section 43C.
107. ERA, section 43D.
108. ERA, section 43E.
109. SI 1999/1549. This list has periodically been added to by Order, see e.g. the Public Interest Disclosure (Prescribed Persons)(Amendment) Order 2009, SI 2009/2457; the Public Interest Disclosure (Prescribed Persons)(Amendment) Order 2010, SI 2010/7 (in force: 1.10.2012).
110. ERA, section 43F.
111. A complaint not made in good faith, e.g. because it is made as part of a 'campaign against other staff', will not be a protected disclosure. See e.g. *Ezsias* v. *North Glamorgan NHS Trust* [2010] UKEAT/0399/09/CEA.
112. ERA, section 43G(3). For an example of a successful claim made under section 43G, see *Kay* v. *Northumberland NHS Trust* (2001), reported on the Public Concern at Work (PCAW) website: http://www.pcaw.co.uk/law/casesummaries.htm
113. ERA, section 43H.
114. *Ibid*.
115. ERA, section 43H(2).
116. *NHS Manchester* v. *Fecitt* [2011] EWCA Civ 1190: wrongs committed by employees during the course of their employment are imputed to the employer.
117. *Ibid*. Elias LJ, [51].
118. ERA section 43J; Health Service Circular, HSC 2004/001.
119. See e.g. the 'Medicine Balls' column in *Private Eye*, written by Dr Phil Hammond: 'Shoot the Messenger', (2011) volume 1292; 'NHS Gagging Wars (cont)', (2011) volume 1303; H. Puttick, 'Gagging clause silences NHS whistle-blowers' (2012) *Sunday Herald* 26 August, http://www.heraldscotland.com/news/health/gagging-clause-silences-nhs-whistle-blowers.18669895
120. Health Service Circular HSC 1999/198.
121. http://www.pcaw.co.uk/policy/policy_pdfs/SpeakupNHS.pdf
122. http://www.nmc-uk.org/Nurses-and-midwives/Raising-and-escalating-concerns/
123. *Ibid*., at p. 15. The NMC suggests that advice be sought from either the NMC, a professional body, trade union or Public Concern at Work (PCaW). PCaW operate a free, confidential whistleblowing telephone advice service: 020 7404 6609; http://www.pcaw.co.uk/index.htm and the Royal College of Nursing (RCN) operates a whistleblowing hotline: 0345 772 6300, http://www.rcn.org.uk/support/raising_concerns_raising_standards. See also the GMC guidance, *Raising and acting on concerns about patient safety* (2012), http://www.gmc-uk.org/static/documents/content/Raising_and_acting_on_concerns_about_patient_safety_FINAL.pdf
124. http://www.dh.gov.uk/health/2012/03/nhs-constitution-updated/. See: The NHS Constitution for England (2012 edition), section 3a, p.11, http://www.dh.gov.uk/prod_consum_dh/groups/dh_digitalassets/@dh/@en/documents/digitalasset/dh_132958.pdf; *The handbook to the NHS Constitution for England* (2012 edition),

pp. 90, 100–1, 112–5, 143, http://www.dh.gov.uk/prod_consum_dh/groups/dh_digitalassets/@dh/@en/documents/digitalasset/dh_132959.pdf

125. CQC, *Whistleblowing: Guidance for workers of registered care providers* (2012), http://www.cqc.org.uk/sites/default/files/media/documents/rp_poc_100494_20120410_v3_00_whistleblowing_guidance_for_employees_of_registered_providers_afte_pcaw_comments_with_changes_tracked_for_publication.pdf

126. [2011] IRLR 922.

127. *Ibid.*, [71].

128. The ECtHR awarded 10,000 euros for non-pecuniary damage.

B   An Ethical Perspective – How to Do the Right Thing

David Seedhouse

CEO of VIDe Ltd, and Visiting Professor, University of Cumbria

8.14   Introduction

Health care resources are scarce. This is an unfortunate fact of life. In those cases where there are not enough to go round, difficult choices must be made. Sometimes nurses must make these choices. This may mean that they cannot help everyone they would like to. It may mean that they will not be able to offer as much to each patient as they would ideally wish to, but this is not a perfect world. In order not to waste resources, and in order to be as fair as possible across the health service, all nurses must be aware that rationing is sometimes necessary.

Nurses must recognise these facts; nurses must do the right thing. This, at least, is the official position: it is held (and fostered) by governments preoccupied by the need to keep health care costs in check,[1] by several health economists,[2] some of whom devote considerable energy to the production of technical 'rationing formulae', and it is increasingly (though often grudgingly) accepted by many nurses. Slowly but surely the 'official line' has also come to be believed by many of the general public, who listen to the various experts and – not unreasonably – conclude that if those in the know see the need to ration, then there must indeed be such a need.

But is the official position true? Certainly, not everyone accepts it. For instance, it has been argued that the basic duty of any government must be to defend its people against threats to life and safety, and that since in normal circumstances health care does this much better than any other sort of public provision (and is infinitely more useful than an idle army), governments must – as a matter of obligation to their subjects – switch military funding to health services.[3] It is also claimed that in the USA, where spending on health care consistently consumes around 14 per cent of the gross domestic product, there are already more than enough health services to go round; the problem is that not everyone who needs them can get access (millions of Americans do not have health insurance and cannot afford to pay privately to get the help they need).[4]

It is further argued, against the official view, that the belief that the development of new medicines and technologies must fuel growing patient demand ad infinitum is based on a myth.[5] It is argued that just as a doubling of public toilets or public bus services would not automatically double the desire (or need) of the public to make use of them, so too there is a finite amount of kidney disease, a limit to the number of people who can benefit from coronary by-pass surgery, and so on. Perhaps if more buses were supplied very cheaply, or even at no cost to the user at all, their use would increase, but even so there will always be a natural limit on the number of people who would like to travel from A to B at any one time.

It is not easy to judge which one of these positions – the 'official line' or that of the 'rebel camp' – is correct. Clearly, both are at least partly true. For instance, where there are more potential recipients than donated organs, there is an undeniable scarcity of this particular resource. On the other hand, it is equally incontrovertible that if money were to be taken from some expensive 'high-tech' or over-provided medical services, and spent instead on the provision of better and more comprehensive preventive services' many 'health needs now not met because of scarcity could be provided for.

What is clearest of all, however, is that there are considerable philosophical and practical uncertainties underlying the 'resources debate', most of which are unlikely to be resolved in the foreseeable future. The nature of 'health care cost' and 'health care benefit' is not agreed in theory.[6] Nor is it yet physically possible to collate even the simple financial costs of many modern health services.[7] And even if credible classifications and calculations were to be developed, even if someone were to invent a comprehensive 'health service slide rule', the accuracy and appropriateness of these taxonomies and methods of calculating would inevitably be challenged. It would, for instance, remain the case that different individuals would value even identical services (and identical results) in different ways. For one person a few more days of life, even in great pain, might be of immense value – while for another there would be no point at all.

8.15   Nursing in scarcity

What can nurses do when faced with such intangibles? These days almost all nurses work in environments where managers, and others, are openly concerned about efficiency, avoiding waste and reducing cost wherever possible. What is the nurse, concerned about how best to use scarce resources, to do? How can she be fair? How can she deal with perceived injustice? How can she make any difference at all?

Whether or not any individual can make a difference within massive, complex systems depends on two factors. First, and obviously, what she can do depends on whether or not she is in a position of any power and influence. Second, and less obviously, what she can do depends upon the clarity with which she has formulated her goals. Philosophy (or clear thinking) can do nothing about the first factor, but it can help (albeit only a little) with the second. With practice a nurse can improve her understanding of both general situations and her own circumstances, she can learn to define the meaning of key terms (such as 'resource', 'rationing' and 'fairness'), and she can become better able to identify her role (and the limits of her role).

It is not possible in this chapter to provide a philosophical education. In order to learn philosophy there is no substitute for a carefully formulated programme of study undertaken over several years. However, it is possible to show how a philosophically informed nurse might at least begin to react to resource allocation problems, and in so doing to offer insight into one method of coping with seemingly impossible situations.

8.16   A number – or a free person?

Nursing is a hierarchical and often authoritarian profession. All groups of nurses have a 'pecking-order', and those nurses who do not toe the line can, in some circumstances, suffer severe reprimand. This is a deep-seated aspect of nursing culture. It is an equally long-established tradition that most nurses are of a lower rank than doctors. These circumstances are changing somewhat nowadays, with the advent of nurse managers and as nursing is increasingly thought of as a profession. However, for very many nurses it remains the case that they are able to exert only a very limited influence on health service policy. So, when it comes to 'doing the right thing', most nurses apparently have very little choice; the 'right thing' is defined by 'the system' in which they are a 'cog' or a 'number', and their only option is to implement it. The 'right thing', in other words, is handed down to them (this might be called 'doing the right thing 1'). Of course, there is an alternative form of 'doing the right thing', which can be defined as a nurse taking the course of action that she has, after careful deliberation, deemed to be the best – whether or not this is the action recommended by the system. The 'right thing', in this form, is a matter of conscience and intelligent reflection (and might be called 'doing the right thing 2'). How might the nurse 'do the right thing' in the two case studies offered by Tracey Elliott in Part A of this chapter?

8.16.1   Case study 1

Consider again the first case study of the nurse, A, on night duty in charge of a small hospital where M brings G, the victim of a hit-and-run accident, despite the sign at the gate advising that there is no A&E unit there (Section 8.6).

As far as 'doing the right thing 1' is concerned, Tracey Elliott has already given part of a possible answer that 'in purely legal terms, A would be free to refuse treatment to G and urge M and G to present themselves at the nearest A&E department'. Officially, the hospital does not provide A&E services, so there is no legal obligation on the nurse to do anything. Furthermore, if this hospital is cost-conscious, and if the management have made it clear that emergency cases are not to be treated, then to 'do the right thing 1' the nurse must turn the potential patient away – and must do so whatever her feelings about it, and whatever help she might have been able to give. Since she would have 'done the right thing', there would be no sanction 'the authorities' could take against the nurse.

However, in this case (as in all cases) the nurse might instead consider 'doing the right thing 2' – that is, she might not simply follow the regulation course, but might first take the trouble to analyse the situation for herself, and then act according to the result of her own reasoning. Of course, if she decides that she must advise G and M that she cannot help them, and that they must attend the nearest A&E hospital, then the practical outcome will be the same. However, the nurse herself will have thought more thoroughly than if she had merely obeyed the rules, and may well feel more confident (and more in charge) as a result. But how is she to carry out this analysis? How might she structure her thinking if she decides to 'do the right thing 2'? A does have the option to help the injured person, but if she does so, she might well place herself at greater personal risk than if she were simply to turn M and G away. As stated in Section 8.6, 'once A opts to render care and assistance to G, then a duty of care arises and the question then relates to the applicable standard of care. It is clear that liability may result from negligent treatment or advice rendered by A or any failure of communication in providing G with emergency treatment.' So what should A do?

Certainly, 'doing the right thing 2' is the more complicated – and potentially more fraught – option. What factors should the nurse take into account? How might she begin to think clearly about this case? If she does decide to deliberate on the situation, she must do so quickly, and under considerable emotional pressure – neither of which is conducive to clear reasoning. Given this, the nurse might find it helpful to organise her thinking under three distinct headings: context, outcomes and obligations.

8.16.1.1   Context

First, A must assess the risk. 'Risk', of course, is a general term that might be interpreted in several ways. The nurse might, for instance, think about the risk to the injured party (if he is not instantly helped, how will he be affected?); the risk to her conscience (what if she begins to help and the patient dies – or what if she does not help and the patient dies?); the risk to her future career, and so on. She must also, prior to any further deliberation, decide whether any intervention she could make would do any good. If it would not, and if it is clearly better that G attends a working clinic, then obviously that is where he should go. If, on the other hand, she decides she could give some help, she must also work out how effective she would be and how certain she is of her judgement about her effectiveness. Also, if there are other patients whom she might be helping instead of G, she must consider whether she should assist them before she turns her attention to G.

The context, in this case as in most cases that nurses have to deal with, is one of uncertainty. A simply does not know for sure what the outcome of any of her options will be. Because of this, it is very important that she reflects, in the abstract, on her priorities.

8.16.1.2   Outcomes

Is she, for example, most concerned with the reputation of the hospital? Is she concerned for the safety of her other patients, who may be endangered if she devotes herself solely to the care of G? Or is her priority the injured person directly in front of her? She may not, in a short space of time, be able to think through all the ramifications, but it will help her considerably if she feels she understands which of these possible goals are, in principle, the most important.

8.16.1.3   Obligations

Does she have any obligations or duties that override the context? Must she, for instance, as a 'caring professional', do all she can to help G, who is clearly suffering? This is for her to decide. However, as she thinks about this, she must be aware that not only must she justify her decision to herself but she may also have to justify it to others. So if she decides she is obliged to intervene wherever she sees suffering, she must also be able to say whether this is a general obligation and is always incumbent on her, or whether there are factors (such as context and outcome) that may sometimes cancel out such a duty.

8.16.2   Case study 2

Consider now the second case study (set out in Section 8.11) of J, the night-duty charge nurse believing that the standard of care had dropped prior to a patient's dying in distressing circumstances. In this case, even more than the first, there are evidently two distinct 'right things' to do. 'Doing the right thing 1' in this case is either to do nothing because the context is so overwhelming (the nurse may know that similar staffing difficulties are being experienced across the country – how can her situation be made an exception?), or to pursue the matter through the 'official channels', as explained in Section 8.11. However, since all the 'official channels' are themselves part of the system that allows (or is forced to allow) such a situation to arise, it is extremely unlikely that this course of action will bring about an improvement in the situation on the nurse's ward. 'Doing the right thing 1' would almost certainly mean that little would change.

   However, if the nurse were to 'do the right thing 2', it might be a different matter. Although she might in the end reach the same conclusions as generated by 'doing the right thing 1', the nurse must first try to think as an individual uninfluenced by the system. What, she might ask, ought to be done in these circumstances? The questions she must address are similar to those considered by A in Case study 1, and again might usefully be divided into the three categories. What are the risks in this context? Will 'whistleblowing' be effective? How important is the nurse's career? (There are well-known examples of nurses destroying their careers in the pursuit of causes they believe to be just.) Are the nurse's obligations to her patients paramount, or does she have wider duties (to her colleagues or to those future patients she might not be able to care for, if she is suspended from work or sacked)? In principle, what outcomes does she value most highly? Is her own happiness paramount? Or is it crucial that the patients on her ward get the best possible service? If the latter, does it matter that if she succeeds in getting what she wants for her ward, resources may be moved from other hard-pressed parts of the hospital – so decreasing the quality of service to other patients? If she finally decides that the context is simply unacceptable, and that something must be done to improve it, then 'doing the right thing 1' may very well cease to be an option.

8.17   Principled solutions?

Some nurses may find it helpful to try to apply 'ethical principles' to resource allocation dilemmas. This approach has been widely recommended in recent years, and most texts on 'nursing ethics' contain sizeable sections on 'basic', 'ethical' or 'philosophical' principles.[8] A quartet of principles are regularly advocated, and it is likely that most nurses will at least have heard of them. They are: 'nonmaleficence' (do no harm), 'beneficence' (do good), 'respect autonomy' (respect the patient's choice) and 'justice' (see Chapter 2).[9] The attraction of this group of principles is that they seem to offer an uncomplicated structure within which to organise one's thoughts. Moreover, it seems possible to seize on just one of these principles in order to 'solve' a dilemma. If, for instance, a nurse feels that a doctor is not taking the wishes of a patient seriously, she might describe this as 'unethical' behaviour purely because the doctor is not 'respecting autonomy' (so ignoring or overriding any alternative justifications the medic might have). Most nurses will have personal experience of cases in which this has happened – and might well consider it fair criticism – but it is very important not to confuse the assertion of single principles (however justifiable) with 'ethical analysis'. The latter is a much more complicated procedure which – if it is to be done at all properly – must involve reflection upon a range of 'ethical principles' together with the other considerations (context, outcomes, obligations) already mentioned in this section.

This is not to say that the use of the principles is unhelpful. The point is that any thoughtful ethical analysis is bound to place considerable intellectual demands on the health care analyst. In Case study 2, it might appear that the hub of the matter is a straightforward clash between the ideal of 'efficiency' and the principles of 'justice'. It might, in other words, seem to nurse J that her patients are being unjustly treated, and that their interests are regarded as secondary to those of the hospital as a whole (which must be run as 'efficiently' as possible). However, if J is seriously to argue this case, then it is not enough for her merely to cry 'unjust!', since 'justice' can be understood in more than one way, and can even be interpreted in ways that contradict each other.

For example, there are those who think that the key to understanding 'justice' is to treat people first and foremost in accord with what they deserve; others disagree, arguing that the basic criterion of justice is need; and there is a further group who believe that justice can come about only when people's rights are upheld.[10] What is more, sophisticated analysts tend to blend and adapt these different understandings in subtle ways, depending on the matter under scrutiny. Any contemplative analysis of the merits (or justice) of the management of the acutely ill patient must consider and explain what justice means in this case (whether the patients have the same right to treatment as other patients in the hospital, and so no special priority; whether they have needs of such gravity that they are entitled to treatment before those with lesser needs; whether this set of patients merits privileged attention and so deserves priority treatment for some reason). Philosophers are used to such discussions, and often spend much time trying to disentangle the various issues, only to see them knot together again the moment they move their attention elsewhere. Such detailed reflection requires a fair amount of expertise – and countless hours – neither of which is usually available to the nurse. And this can place the nurse who sees that these are complex matters, and who recognises that they can be properly dealt with only by careful analysis, at a considerable disadvantage. If she tries to protest in an intelligent way, it is very easy to defeat her. Her opponent can say: 'We don't have the time for this sort of reflection'; or, 'What you are suggesting requires an analysis of everything we do, and this is not a practical proposition' (which of course means that everything can continue unchanged – inertia is not only a natural tendency but also a powerful weapon in the hands of those who are happy with the status quo). Her opponent might also ask: 'What do you mean by justice?', knowing full well that any credible answer must take more time and effort than almost any nurse can give (and knowing that even if the nurse does attempt an answer it will be very easy to say later: 'Please spell out your inter- pretation of need/rights/equity,' or whatever other terms she has not fully explained).

In such circumstances the nurse has three strategies open to her. She might spend many hours developing her case (she might even enlist the help of a trained philosopher); she might take a simpler course and analyse her work problems using the 'context, outcomes and obligations' framework (in the knowledge that this is by no means all there is to ethical analysis); or she might take her opponent on, on his own terms. Whenever he says, 'Could you expand on that?' or 'What do you mean?', the nurse might ask in turn, 'What do you mean by efficiency?', 'How do you justify removing resources from this ward and increasing them on that?' or 'What are your principles for resource allocation within this hospital, and on what grounds do you justify these?'

8.18   Conclusion

This part of the chapter has raised questions, but only sketched out answers to them. The rest is for the individual nurse to decide, and there are many books and papers available to which she might turn for more detailed guidance. What is most important is that each nurse realises the complexity of any resource problem she is facing and, if she so decides that she is able to tackle it in a sys- tematic manner. If she genuinely tries to do this, and if she feels she has arrived at a defensible decision, then there is probably little more she can do. She cannot change the world, and whatever she does, she is hardly likely to unsettle govern- ments focused so intently on financial balance sheets.

Nevertheless, there will always – if only occasionally – be times when the nurse can do something to change things for the better. If, for example, she decides not only to treat G (in Case study 1) but to publicise the fact in local newspapers (so both promoting the hospital as a compassionate organisation and letting it be known that were funds available an accident and emergency service could be provided or reinstated) then she might have an impact. Moreover, if the nurse were to contact the relatives of the patient who died 'in distressing circumstances' (in Case study 2) and enlist their support she might campaign intelligently and effectively for more resources. On both strategies she would face very significant risks – indeed, she could expect censure from the system were her involvement to become known – but she would at least stand a chance of making a desirable difference. She would, in other words, be working for justice as a combination of meeting needs and deserts and upholding rights – through positively discriminating in favour of those patients closest to her.

In general, a great deal rests on the following question, and how it is answered in the coming years: whether nurses in general continue mostly or only 'to do the right thing 1' or whether the profession increasingly aims 'to do the right thing 2' (and commits its own resources to ensuring this). If the former, then it is hard to see how nurses will be able to justify their claim to professional status, but if the latter, and the majority of nurses become able and willing to think through the question 'How best might I act in this situation?' (rather than asking 'What am I supposed to do here?'), then nurses, as a group, might perform an enormous service: they might open up the health service to internal debate, to genuine conversation (without fear of sanction and reprisal) about how best to deliver public health services – not least when there are not enough of them to go round. And it is certain that it is only by continually considering whether to 'do the right thing 1' or to 'do the right thing 2' that nurses will exercise their 'moral muscles' sufficiently to effect resource allocation injustices for the better, since never to consider 'doing the right thing 2' eventually and inevitably destroys the capacity for moral reasoning.[11,12]

8.19   Notes and references

1. See *Health Care Analysis*, **1** (1) (1993), passim.
2. A. Williams, Cost-effectiveness analysis: is it ethical? *Journal of Medical Ethics*, **18** (1992), pp. 7–11.
3. J. Harris, Unprincipled QALYs: a response to Cubbon, *Journal of Medical Ethics*, **17** (1991), pp. 185–8.
4. C. Hackler, Health care reform in the United States, *Health Care Analysis*, **1** (1) (1993), pp. 5–13.
5. A. Smith, Qualms about QALYs, *The Lancet*, **329** (8542) (1987), pp. 1134–6.
6. D.F. Seedhouse, *Fortress N.H.S: A Philosophical Review of the National Health Service* (Chichester, John Wiley and Sons, 1994).
7. A. Culyer, The morality of efficiency in health care: some uncomfortable implications, *Health Economics*, **1** (1) (1992), pp. 7–18.
8. I. Thompson, K.M. Melia & K.M. Boyd, *Nursing Ethics* (Edinburgh, Churchill Livingstone, 1988).
9. R.P. Gillon, *Philosophical Medical Ethics* (Chichester, John Wiley and Sons, 1986).
10. D. Miller, *Principles of Social Justice* (Cambridge MA, Harvard University Press, 2001).
11. D.F. Seedhouse, *Practical Nursing Philosophy: The Universal Ethical Code* (Chichester, John Wiley and Sons, 2000).

12. D.F. Seedhouse, *Health: The Foundations for Achievement*, 2nd edn (Chichester, John Wiley and Sons, 2001).

8.20   Further reading

Seedhouse, D.F. (2007) *Ethics: The Heart of Healthcare*, John Wiley and Sons, Chichester.
Seedhouse, D.F. (2005) *Values Based Health Care: The Fundamentals of Ethical Decision-Making*, John Wiley and Sons, Chichester.

9 Mental Health Nursing

A The Legal Perspective

Leon McRae

Lecturer in Law, Birmingham Law School, University of Birmingham, Birmingham

The potential for tension between responding effectively to perceived clinical need and promoting patient autonomy is a familiar theme in this book.[1] In mental health care, difficulty resolving this tension has resulted in over 50 years of legislative cut-and-paste. In late 2008, however, following a decade of discussion, the Mental Health Act 2007 (hereinafter 'MHA 2007') introduced substantial amendments to the Mental Health Act 1983 (MHA) and, to a lesser extent, the Mental Capacity Act 2005 (MCA). For many commentators, the 2008 amendments represented the Government's promise of protecting the public, at all costs, from the small minority of patients who act violently. A broader definition of mental disorder; the abandonment of the justification for compulsory treatment based on treatability; and the introduction of Community Treatment Orders are illustrations of this. The MHA (as amended) does, nevertheless, introduce patient safeguards in respect of administration of electro-convulsive therapy and medication beyond three months, to name but two. Further amendments to the MHA were the direct response of the enactment of the MCA and decisions of the

Nursing Law and Ethics, Fourth Edition. Edited by John Tingle and Alan Cribb.
© 2014 by John Wiley & Sons, Ltd. Published 2014 by John Wiley & Sons, Ltd.

European Court of Human Rights in relation to the Human Rights Act 1998. Together, the MHA and MCA provide statutory frameworks under which people with mental disabilities can be deprived of their liberty and treated in the absence of consent.

An ancillary development under the MHA is the recent redeployment of professional roles in respect of detention and treatment decision-making. The MHA effectively replaces the 'approved social worker' (ASW) with the 'approved mental health professional' (AMHP). Prior to 2008, the ASW was 'an officer of a local social services authority' having primary responsibility for matters including making applications for compulsory admission to hospital and advising responsible medical officers (RMO) (a psychiatrist with overall control of the patient's care) of alternatives. Under the MHA, the role of RMO was replaced by the 'responsible clinician' (RC), and the scope of the AMHP and RC broadened to include participation by nurses, psychologists and occupational therapists. Both roles remain competency-based: to be eligible for approval as an approved clinician (AC), schedule 2 of the Mental Health (Approved Clinician) Directions 2008 states that the professional must possess the necessary competencies. These include understanding the legal responsibilities under the MHA – such as assessment, treatment and multi-disciplinary team working – and the ability to apply the MCA (where applicable). The responsibilities of the RC include the power to renew detention for treatment (sections 3 or 37), grant leave of absence (section 17), the power to discharge in certain circumstances (section 23) and deem a patient suitable for Community Treatment Orders (section 17A(1)).

Professional expansion is not, however, without possible problems. While training for AMHP's builds upon well-established training programmes devised for ASWs, some commentators have expressed concern that additional monetary costs may result in specific training needs of nurses not being met.[2] The Explanatory Notes accompanying the 2008 Directions merely state that 'psychiatrists and psychologists of consultant status' are expected to be among the *first* to be approved. While it is not yet clear the extent to which nurses will be approved, it is tacit that added professional accountability and the necessity to keep abreast of further policy and practice changes are increasingly becoming part of the therapeutic milieu. For nurses working within hospital-based multi-disciplinary teams or care homes, this Chapter offers an insight into some of the more onerous, or contentious, issues of current mental disability service provision. Owing to the complexity of the issues involved, an exhaustive account is not provided; rather, interested readers are referred to additional sources.[3] This Chapter will instead focus on circumstances in which compulsory treatment may be lawfully provided under the MHA; when people lacking capacity may be treated under the MCA, and the impact of the *Bournewood* litigation on lawful deprivation of liberty; the nurse's holding power under the MHA; management of violent and aggressive patients in hospital (with especial reference to seclusion); psychiatric treatment in the community (Community Treatment Orders); and the process of discharge from hospital under the First-tier Tribunal (Mental Health) process.

9.1   Treatment under the Mental Health Act 1983

Treatment may lawfully be given to any patient detained under the MHA not subject to emergency section. If the patient is refusing, or lacks the capacity, to consent to treatment proposed by the nurse, additional safeguards apply under the MHA and the MCA. In some cases, the MHA deems certain treatments to be so invasive that special oversight is required (see further below). Additional patient protection is promoted by the more generic principles of the Mental Health Act Code of Practice 2008.[4] Chapter 1 of the Code of Practice comprises 'a set of guiding principles which should be considered when making decisions about a course of action under [the Act]'.[5] The guiding principles include imposing the least minimal restriction on a patient's right to consent; consideration of the patient's 'views, wishes and feelings' before implementing the proposed treatment; participation by patients, family members and carers in treatment decision-making; and the requirement to act 'in the most effective, efficient and equitable way' to meet the needs of the patient. While the Code does not impose 'a legal duty' on nurses and other professionals to ensure the principles are adhered to, in the event of legal challenge the court will 'scrutinise the reasons for the departure to ensure there is sufficiently convincing justification in the circumstances'.[6]

The Code of Practice explicitly states that lawful departure from its principles means having complied with the Human Rights Act 1998 (HRA, incorporating the European Convention of Human Rights 1950 (ECHR)).[7] This means 'taking into consideration' the case law of the European Courts of Human Rights (section 2) on the question of breach of articles such as 2 (right to life), 3 (no one shall be subjected to torture or to inhuman or degrading treatment or punishment) and 8 (right to private life). However, in reality, while the courts have often referred to their inherent jurisdiction to question the logic of compulsory treatment in light of the HRA, they have been reluctant to call into question medical treatment decisions.[8] In *R(B)* v. *Ashworth Hospital Authority* [2005], for instance, Baroness Hale opined:

> Psychiatry is not an exact science . . . Once the state has taken away a person's liberty and detained him in hospital with a view to medical treatment, the state should be able (some would say obliged) to provide him with the treatment which he needs. It would be absurd if a patient could be detained in hospital but had to be denied the treatment which his doctor thought he needed for an indefinite period while some largely irrelevant classification was rectified.[9]

With changes to the RMO role now encouraging wider professional participation in medical decision-making, it is increasingly likely that nurses will have to make complex decisions about whether or not to administer compulsory psychiatric treatment without consent under the MHA. Even if she is not directly responsible for this responsibility, she is likely to be involved in the administration of various treatments, and for this reason the Mental Health Act Commission (MHAC, now the Care Quality Commission) has stressed the importance of the nurse's role.[10] Clearly, before administrating any treatment, the nurse will wish to be satisfied that the patient is detained under the MHA.

9.1.1   First stage: is the patient detained?

Detention under the MHA must be proceeded by two medical recommendations that the patient should be sectioned; this will be demonstrated by completion of the relevant forms.[11] The relevant forms broadly require a psychiatrist to state the reasons for admission and to declare why informal admission is not appropriate (see further below). If it turns out that the forms are insufficiently completed, and this is not apparent to the nurse, she will face no liability if she subsequently conveys the patient to hospital.[12] Nevertheless, the nurse will wish to ensure she is aware of the section applicable to the respective patient, and the treatment implications of this. The relevant sections to which the admission forms relate are located in Parts II (civil provisions) and III (criminal provisions) of the MHA, and include the following:

- section 2 (for assessment)
- section 3 (for treatment)
- section 35 (remand of a criminal accused person to hospital for the completion of reports on his mental condition)
- section 36 (remand of a criminally accused person to hospital for treatment)
- section 37 (hospital order for treatment, with potential discharge restrictions applying to the detaining authority under section 41)
- section 46 (an order relating to a member of the armed forces)
- section 47 (admission of a prisoner for treatment, with potential discharge restrictions applied under section 49)
- section 48 (admission of a civil or remand prisoner, with potential discharge restrictions applied under section 49).

The majority of patients will be detained under Part II of the Act (sections 2 and 3 above).[13] If the two medical recommendations were completed at the same time, the nurse will be looking for form A3 (admission for assessment) or form A7 (admission for treatment).[14] If the assessments were conducted separately, the relevant forms are A4 and A8.[15]

9.1.1.1   Legal reform

The more commonplace technical requirements of the MHA risk obscuring significant legislative changes that have been implemented with the enactment of the MHA 2007. In the last edition of this book, the Mental Health Bill 2006 had proposed sweeping reform to the admission requirements of the Act in respect of the classification of different mental disorders and their amenability to treatment. Underlying the proposals were three agendums: (1) reducing stigma, protecting against discrimination, and promoting social inclusion; (2) management of risk to the public and to sufferers themselves; and (3) protection of human rights.[16] It remains a requirement of section 6 of the HRA that detaining authorities act in compliance with Convention rights, and for a number of years the consolidation of a rights-based discourse in European jurisprudence has ensured debate about ethical legal reform.[17]

For many, the introduction of the MHA 2007 was evidence of the Government's preoccupation with public protection and a desire to increase control over the lives of those with mental disorder. A key catalyst was the finding by several homicide inquiries during the 1990s of serious shortcomings in supervision, provision of treatment and aftercare arrangements of people previously treated in psychiatric services.[18] Upon the conviction of Michael Stone, following the peculiarly brutal murders of members of the Russell family, concerns that medical practitioners were unwilling to engage with patients suffering from 'psychopathy' were scrutinised.[19] Two reasons for medical apathy were particularly in view. First, patients with psychopathy (or the more common anti-social personality disorder (ASPD)[20]) are generally averse to receiving treatment which they do not believe they need.[21] Psychiatrists may respond by favouring the admission of patients who may be more motivated to engage.[22] Second, prior to 2008, long-term admission (most notably, under section 3) required medical reports to classify individuals as suffering from mental illness, psychopathic disorder, mental impairment or severe mental impairment before recommending detention for up to six months. In the case of psychopathy (and mental impairment), treatment had to be certified as likely to alleviate or prevent deterioration in health (the oft-termed 'treatability test'). Stone was discharged from hospital after his carers assessed him to be a 'classic psychopath' whose condition was deemed unresponsive to treatment.[23] The Government subsequently opined:[24]

> The 1983 Act . . . fails to address the challenge posed by a minority of people with mental disorder who pose a significant risk to others as a result of their disorder . . . We . . . need to move away from the narrow concept of treatability which applies to certain categories of mental disorder in the 1983 Act. New legislation must be clearly framed so as to allow all those who pose a significant risk of serious harm to others as a result of their mental disorder to be detained in a therapeutic environment where they can be offered care and treatment to manage their behaviour.[25]

The amended MHA now incorporates a simplified definition of mental disorder ('any disorder of the mind' (section 1(2)); and, in respect of long-term admissions, refers only to the 'availability of appropriate treatment' necessary for the 'health or safety of the patient' or 'the protection of others persons', where treatment in the community or as an informal patient would not suffice (section 3(4)).[26] On the one hand, it is uncontroversial that the law ought to be amended to prevent social exclusion;[27] on the other hand, the requirements of 'effectiveness', 'equity' and 'participation [by patients]' underlying the Code of Practice are untenable if public protectionism is the primary policy driver.[28] For those patients effectively indeterminately detained for public safety purposes, it will come as cold comfort that the 'appropriate treatment' standard has been ruled compliant with article 5 (deprivation of liberty) of the ECHR.[29]

9.1.2   Can treatment lawfully be given under 'section'?

Once the nurse is satisfied that the patient's admission has been lawfully conducted, she will wish to be confident that the proposed treatment is recognised
under the MHA. The meaning of 'medical treatment' under the MHA was
widened by the MHA 2007. Section 145(1) now reads:

> '[M]edical treatment' includes nursing, psychological intervention and spe-
> cialist mental health habilitation, rehabilitation and care.

The reference to 'psychological intervention' merely recognises that many
patients already benefit from cognitive-behavioural therapy, psychotherapy,
counselling or related talking therapies either in isolation or combined with other
treatments. The reference to 'includes' in this section ensures that the list of treatments that can lawfully be given is non-exhaustive. Nevertheless, some treatments are considered to be so invasive, or potentially deleterious to health, that
mental health legislation specifies that additional safeguards must be met before
treatment can go ahead. Such treatments are identified in Part IV of the MHA as
electro-convulsive therapy (ECT), implantation of hormones for the reduction of
male sex drive, medications beyond three months, and neurosurgery (also known
as psychosurgery) for mental disorder (NMD).[30] Sections 57–58A of the MHA
discuss the most invasive forms of treatment, namely hormone therapy and
NMD, while section 62 deals with treatment given in emergency situations.
These provisions will be considered shortly. Section 63 governs treatment not
requiring consent.

9.1.2.1   Treatment not requiring consent

The majority of treatments broadly identified above can be administered without
the need for the patient's prior consent. Section 63 of the MHA states:

> The consent of the patient shall not be required for any medical treatment
> given to him for the mental disorder for which he is suffering [, not being a
> form of treatment to which section 57, 58 or 58A above applies,] if the treat-
> ment is given by or under the direction of the [approved clinician in charge of
> the treatment].

As noted by the section, the range of therapeutic interventions which may
be compulsorily administered is subject to statutory safeguards (see below).
Furthermore, invoking section 63 will be useless if consent is a prerequisite
to the effectiveness of the proposed treatment. In the case of *R* v. *Ashworth Hospital Authority, ex parte B*,[31] Baroness Hale discussed this problem in the context
of ASPD:

> A patient [with personality disorder] may be offered various forms of psycho-
> therapy . . . but clearly these can only take place with his co–operation. Oth-
> erwise the treatment is counselling and guidance from the nursing staff, with
> a view to helping patients to observe appropriate boundaries in their behav-
> iour and controlling their impulsivity.[32]

NICE guidelines have identified a 'small but positive [therapeutic] effect' in offenders with ASPD who do engage with psychological therapies.[33] In contrast to other more common mental disorders, administering medications has not proven effective in this group.[34] Without more, one finds sympathy with commentators who have long questioned whether unacceptable behaviour linked to personality difficulties is really evidence of symptoms of mental disorder.[35]

In recent years, significant controversy has also been voiced about justifying compulsory *physical* interventions by reference to a patient's underlying mental disorder. Consider, in particular, interventions for Caesarean section (see Chapter 7) and force-feeding reluctant, or anorexic, patients. Jean McHale explains in section 7.2.5 about the legal and ethical problems that abound when the need for a forced Caesarean section is attributed to an underlying mental disorder.[36]

The leading authority on force-feeding is the case of *B v. Croydon Health Authority* [1995]. In this case, B suffered from borderline personality disorder;[37] during the course of a section 3 admission, she refused all food. When her RC proposed naso-gastric feeding, she contended that there was no authority under section 63 to do so. Hoffman LJ responded that the treatment was 'concurrent with the core treatment'.[38] He concluded:

> It would seem to me strange if a hospital could, without the patient's consent, give him treatment directed to alleviating . . . suicidal tendencies, but not without such consent be able to treat the consequences of a suicide attempt.[39]

Some years later, Ian Brady, who was detained in Broodmoor under Part III of the MHA, sought judicial review of his doctor's decision to force-feed him.[40] His argument was that he had competently embarked on a hunger strike as a protest over the conditions of his detention, and that his behaviour was not a consequence of personality disorder. Maurice Kay J, however, agreed with the RC's opinion that Brady's underlying personality disorder explained his behaviour, and that naso-gastric tube feeding could be justified to treat the symptom of resistance to medical authority. It did not seem to matter that a rational individual might challenge their conditions of detention in the same way.[41]

The *ex parte Brady* case demonstrates the limitations of justifying a physical intervention on the basis of unacceptable behaviour attributed to mental disorder. It also demonstrates that the law sometimes fails to promote the involvement of capable patients in treatment decision-making. The result for the (capable) patient in the case of forced naso-gastric feeding is undoubtedly unpleasant; but no special safeguards attach to its administration. In contrast, the MHA adopts a position of reserve when it comes to the administration of potentially harmful treatments under sections 57–58A.

9.1.2.2   Treatment under section 58

Additional safeguards are provided under section 58 for the administration of long-term medication and ECT. The MHA is clear that the nature of those safeguards depends upon whether or not the patient has consented at the material time, and has capacity to do so. In respect of both treatments, the patient retains the right to withdraw their consent (section 60); moreover, since the passing of the MCA, if the patient loses capacity to consent once treatment begins, he or she must be treated as if consent has been withdrawn. In respect of medication, this only poses a problem if treatment is proposed to continue beyond three months. In that case, treatment can continue only if the patient's AC, or a second opinion approved doctor (SOAD),[42] certifies that the patient is capable of consenting and is consenting (section 58(3)(a)). If the patient withdraws his or her consent, treatment may only proceed if a SOAD certifies that the patient lacks capacity or is refusing treatment which he or she believes is appropriate in the circumstances (section 58(3)(b)). Before making a determination as to whether the decision of the AC is reasonable, the SOAD will consult two other people: one person will be a nurse, and the other will not be a nurse or a doctor but someone professionally involved in the patient's treatment (section 58(4)). A nurse responsible for administering medication will, therefore, wish to record the date when treatment began. By doing so, she avoids the potential for unpleasant legal action. The nurse will also wish to make sure that the SOAD has provided the patient with reasons for the decision before administering medication. While non-disclosure of reasons is permitted if disclosure would likely cause the patient to experience serious physical or mental harm,[43] the provision of reasons should ordinarily be construed as minimising unnecessary interference with a patient's right to autonomous refusal arising from the professional's fear that the patient may lack awareness of their condition.

Unlike the administration of medication beyond three months, ECT can no longer be forcibly administered to a competent patient (section 58A(2)). A refusing patient who lacks capacity, and who is over 18 (section 58A(4)), may be treated with ECT only if a SOAD certifies that it is appropriate for treatment to be given, and the patient has not made a valid advance directive – or someone with authority has not opposed treatment. Nevertheless, the nurse will wish to ensure the SOAD has considered whether the proposed treatment – be it ECT, medication or otherwise – is in the best interests of the patient. In *R(B)* v. *Dr SS and others* [2006], best interests was defined as treatment,

(a)   which is either immediately necessary to save the patient's life; or
(b)   which (not being reversible) is immediately necessary to prevent a serious deterioration of his condition; or
(c)   which (not being irreversible or hazardous) is immediately necessary to alleviate serious suffering by the patient; or
(d)   which (not being irreversible or hazardous) is immediately necessary and represents the minimum interference necessary to prevent the patient from behaving violently or being a danger to himself or others.

In 2009 the MHAC reported a dramatic increase in second opinions since the 1990s, explaining this as evidence of good practice in following procedures under the MHA.[44] However, in the same report the MHAC criticised the willingness of ACs to administer high-dose medication.[45] Given the problematic impact that this particular form of treatment can have on a patient's health, the patient's refusal should be clearly noted in form T4.[46] If the patient is consenting, form T2 should be completed.[47] While the completion of the latter form does not give rise to statutory review by the SOAD, the Code of Practice 2008 states that the AC should ensure that 'the number of drugs authorised in each class is indicated, by the classes described in the *British National Formulary* (BNF). The maximum dosage and route of administration should be clearly indicated for each drug or category of drug'.[48] Changes in drug preference should also be recorded. Failure to do so may be deemed unlawful. In the case of form T4, the SOAD does not need to specify which drugs are being approved; only those categories engaged within the BNF. Moreover, the SOAD is not expected to certify that the dosages preferred by the AC are reasonable, unless they exceed the BNF recommended upper limits.

However, these requirements tell us nothing about the (in-)effectiveness of the SOAD appointments scheme at curtailing medical power in reality. In *R (Wilkinson)* v. *Broadmoor Hospital Authority* [2001], Simon Brown LJ hinted at a system working well.

> Whilst, of course, it is proper for the SOAD to pay regard to the views of the [AC] . . . that does not relieve him of the responsibility of forming his own judgment as to whether or not 'the treatment should be given'. And certainly, if the SOAD's certificate and evidence is to carry any real weight in cases where, as here, the treatment plan is challenged, it will be necessary to demonstrate a less deferential approach than appears to be the norm.[49]

While the court's willingness to advocate the questioning of contested medical opinion is salutary, problems with the SOAD are likely to persist. Nell Munro explains:[50]

> [T]he SOAD knows that ongoing responsibility for the patient will remain with the approved clinician. As a result the SOAD's role is not to provide an independent assessment of the patient, but merely to review the appropriateness of a pre-ordained treatment plan, whilst bearing in mind that the Code of Practice suggests that she give due weight to the opinions of those who already know the patient, and also urges the SOAD and clinician in charge to compromise on the treatment plan as far as possible.[51]

In 2004–5, SOAD's acted in 10,500 cases, and in 9.3% of cases the treatment plan was slightly changed; in 2.2% of cases it was significantly altered (11.5% in total).[52] In 2008, the MHAC reported that the percentage of changes had increased to 27%.[53] It is not clear, however, to what degree treatment plans had actually changed, and the MHAC recommended further research.[54] Indeed, in the same year, the MHAC found an increase in the relative proportion of patients deemed to lack capacity for the purposes of refusing treatment.[55] It would be timely if such research could clarify the effect, if any, that the introduction of section 58A is having on the assessment of capacity in the event of treatment refusal, particularly as it is clear that patients face great difficulty in achieving judicial review of a SOAD's decision.[56]

In practical terms, this point speaks to the importance of the nurse helping patients to achieve capacity-oriented decision-making, by communicating his or her findings on a respective patient to either the AC or, more directly, to the SOAD.[57] In the unlikely event that the nurse is concerned that their findings, or concerns, are not being listened to, this should be communicated to the Care Quality Commission.[58]

9.1.2.3   Treatment under section 57

Neurosurgery (NMD) and surgical implantation of hormones to reduce male sex drive are particularly invasive. The MHA does not allow surgery on a patient who has not given consent for the procedure, which has been verified by a medical professional other than the AC in charge of treatment, and two other people appointed by the Care Quality Commission (section 57(2)). The effect of this is that an individual who lacks capacity may never be permitted to undergo a 'section 57 treatment'. Moreover, if the AC deems that either procedure is inappropriate, it is unlawful to conduct them (section 57(3)). In practice, the question of whether it is appropriate rarely arises: in respect of NMD, referrals for second opinions have been decreasing steadily. Between 2007 and 2009, there were only two applications, both of which were granted.[59] Applications for surgical implantation of hormones are virtually non-existent; if a reduction in male sex hormone is desired, the use of hormonal medication will be preferred, and this will bring the treatment within the safeguards contained within section 58. The decrease in requests for NMD may be explained by the wider availability of talking therapies as an alternative,[60] as well as caution on the part of the AC.

9.1.2.4   Emergency treatment under section 62

The MHA states that the additional safeguards contained within sections 57–58 do not apply in cases of emergency (section 62(1)). This means that in the case of medication beyond three months and ECT, sections 58 and 58A are not engaged if either treatment is immediately necessary to save the patient's life, or if treatment ('not being irreversible') is necessary to prevent serious deterioration in the patient's condition (section 62(1A)). Section 62(3) defines 'irreversible' treatment as that which may have 'unfavourable irreversible physical or psychological consequences', and 'hazardous' treatment as that which 'entails a significant physical hazard'. The addition of 'unfavourable' in this section is of uncertain application: it is not presumed that NMD, for instance, would be proposed *unless* the clinician expected a favourable outcome. Since the outcome cannot be known prior to the operation, the better view is that NMD is *always* hazardous. The section would also seem to disapply surgical implantation of hormones to control male sex drive, which has potentially hazardous consequences, even if medication is selected as the preferred route of administration.

The MHAC has cautioned against over-reliance on section 62 to negate the protection afforded to patients for whom ECT is proposed under section 58A.[61] Where section 62 is applied for this purpose, a sympathetic reading is that medical professionals may not always know when their request for a SOAD will be acted upon. However, recourse to section 62 should not be necessary for the administration of medication which extends beyond three months. It is preferable that even if medication has only been administered once during a three month period, good practice dictates that a SOAD assessment is instigated.

9.2   Treatment falling within the Mental Capacity Act 2005

The MCA is the second significant statutory framework permitting treatment decisions to be made on behalf of people who lack capacity. This includes patients informally admitted under the MHA and people in residential or care homes. However, the MCA is distinct from the MHA in a number of important ways. First, though determination of capacity-status is pivotal to whether some treatments may be administered under the MHA (see section '9.1.2.2 Treatment under section 58' above), the MCA does authorise the administration of those treatments in the absence of consent (section 28(1)). This is because the MHA already provides such authority under Part IV on the basis of medical necessity. By comparison, treatment decisions reached under the MCA on behalf of the person lacking capacity must be in their best interests. Second, unlike the MHA, the MCA is a principles-based piece of legislation. The aim of the statutory principles is to offer greater clarity than the common law from which they are derived by supplying one source of reference for the law on providing treatment and care to those lacking capacity by setting out a clearer set of prioritised options for decision-makers.

9.2.1   Does the person lack capacity because of a mental disability?

Autonomy is central to the spirit of the MCA: treatment must only be provided where it is ascertained that the patient lacks capacity to consent, or refuse, the proposed intervention. If treatment is to be given to any person under the MCA, it must be deemed to be in the person's best interests. These central tenets are incorporated within the five overarching principles contained within section 1 of the MCA:

(2)   a person must be assumed to have capacity unless it is established that they lack capacity;

(3)   a person is not to be treated as unable to make a decision unless all practicable steps to help him do so have been taken without success;[62]

(4)   a person is not to be treated as unable to make a decision merely because he makes an unwise decision;[63]

(5)   an act done, or decision made, under this Act for or on behalf of a person who lacks capacity must be done, or made, in his best interests;

(6)   before an act is done, or the decision is made, regard must be had to whether the purpose for which it is needed can be effectively achieved in a way that is less restrictive of the person's rights and freedom of action.

Section 2 of the MCA states that a person lacks capacity in relation to a matter 'if at the material time he is unable to make a decision for himself because of an impairment of, or a disturbance in the functioning of, the mind or brain'.[64] Reference to 'at the material time' is further defined in the Code of Practice:

> An assessment of a person's capacity must be based on their ability to make a specific decision at the time it needs to be made, and not their ability to make decisions in general.[65]

Capacity must be determined on the balance of probabilities (section 2(4)), notwithstanding that the mental disability in question may be temporary or permanent (section 2(2)). The test for capacity is contained within section 3, and provides that an individual is unable to make a decision for themselves if they are unable:

(a)   to understand the information relevant to the decision
(b)   to retain that information
(c)   to use or weigh that information as part of the process of making the decision,[66] or
(d)   to communicate his decision (whether by talking, using sign language or any other means).

Two points deserve clarification here. First, a person does not lack capacity merely because their decision is deemed to be 'irrational' or 'contrary to what is expected of the majority of adults'.[67] Further, the person's 'condition' (which includes mental disorder under the definition of MHA or temporary conditions such as drunkenness) or any associated 'physical characteristics' or 'aspects of behaviour' should not influence the final determination of whether the patient lacks capacity.[68] Second, the nurse who is assisting in the assessment of capacity should pay particular attention to whether or not the person is unable to 'use or weigh' relevant information by making enquiries as to the underlying circumstances giving rise to disbelief:

> If [it] were the result of a psychotic delusion, the effect of the delusion on the belief of the information would unquestionably be relevant to the assessment of incapacity. If the lack of belief flowed for example from a view that the person providing the information was not adequately qualified, however – a house officer rather than a consultant, for example – it would not necessary bespeak incapacity. In other cases, the failure to believe may flow from a refusal to accept that the facts are as presented – a manifestly unrealistic view that P can return to his or her own home and a consequent refusal to move to a nursing home, for example. Once again, a failure to be realistic about one's prospects does not necessarily bespeak incapacity. The robustly capable may behave in this fashion without any challenge to their right to do so; it does not follow from the fact that an individual has marginal capacity or is in a position or relative vulnerability that this should change.[69]

In practice, the nurse may not be required to conduct a capacity assessment; however, in a civil or criminal action based on alleged administration of treatment in the absence of consent, he or she would be required to show, on the balance of probabilities, that their actions arose out of a reasonable belief that the person lacked capacity.[70] A check of the person's medical records will avail him or herself of such a belief before proceeding with treatment. If there is doubt as to the person's capacity at 'the material time', an assessment by the Court of Protection should be sought before administering treatment. Nevertheless, as the *Brady* case reveals (see section '9.1.2.1 Treatment not requiring consent' above), the court may also struggle to convincingly extricate a person's competent, but unsatisfactory, refusal to cede to the proposed treatment from the question of whether the person is unable to 'weigh' in the balance the relevant factors.[71]

9.2.2   The person is deemed to have capacity

The position at common law is that a patient who has capacity may refuse pro-posed treatment, even if it is potentially life-saving.[72] Where acts of care and treatment are carried out on a non-consenting person *with* capacity, sections 5 and 6 of the MCA provide the nurse with a defence against a tort of battery if reasonable steps were taken to assess capacity and the subsequent acts were carried out in the patient's perceived best interests.

9.2.3   The person is deemed to lack capacity

It is a key principle of the MCA that any act done or decision made for or on behalf of a person who lacks capacity must be done, or made, in his or her best interests (section 1(5)). In *Re A (Male Sterilisation)* [2000], Butler Sloss LJ held that best interests may derive from 'medical, emotional and all other welfare issues'.[73] In the earlier case of *Re Y (Mental Patient: Bone Marrow Donation)* [1996], Connell J noted that when deciding on a course of action it is the *patient's* best interests, not the interests of others, which are to be determined.[74] However, in practice there may be many 'ethical differences . . . within care teams concerned with the treatment of incapable patients'.[75]

In *Re S (Adult Patient: Sterilization)*,[76] Butler Sloss LJ was of the opinion that disputes between the medical team should be cured by referring the matter to court for determination of the best option. For some commentators, this more restrictive definition of best interests is just as problematic, for there are many options which might be beneficial to the patient, but only the patient can realisti-cally claim to have privileged knowledge of what those are. Much like a wide definition, then, a restrictive definition applied by the courts also evokes 'incal-culable and insoluble moral dimensions'.[77]

The MCA, in part, avoids addressing the problem of multidisciplinary deci-sion-making in medicine by referring to 'the person making the determination' (section 4(1)). Moreover, the putative restrictions placed on patient autonomy are mitigated to some extent by section 4(6), which states that the person making the decision

must consider, so far as is reasonably ascertainable,

(a)   the person's past and present wishes and feelings (and, in particular, any relevant written statement made by him when he had capacity);

(b)   the beliefs and values that would be likely to influence his decision if he had capacity; and

(c)   the other factors that he would be likely to consider if he were able to do so.

Under subsection (7), the person making the determination (in the best interests of the patient) must take into account, 'if it is practicable and appropriate to consult them', the views of

(a)   anyone named by the person as someone to be consulted on the matter in question or on matters of that kind

(b)   anyone engaged in caring for the person or interested in his welfare

(c)   any donee of a lasting power of attorney granted by the person; and

(d)   any deputy appointed for the person by the court, as to what would be in the person's interests and, in particular, as to the matters mentioned in subsection (6).

Moreover, a patient who is over 18 can circumvent the best interests test entirely – and so the effect of section 4(6)(c) above – by making an advance decision to take effect during a period of incapacity.[78] Section 24(1) states that if:

(a)   at a later time and in such circumstances as he may specify, a specified treatment is proposed to be carried out or continued by a person providing health care for him, and

(b)   at that time he lacks capacity to consent to the carrying out or continuation of the treatment

the specified treatment is not to be carried out or continued.

Advance decisions (AD) and the lasting power of attorney (LPA) are given a restrictive interpretation under the MCA. The AD applies only to treatment *refusal*, and the LPA enables treatment preferences to be specified but does *not* preclude treatment being given in the best interests of the patient. Both the AD and the LPA have no jurisdiction to ensure a certain treatment is administered in the event of incapacity (section 4(7)). An AD cannot be used to justify causing or hastening death (section 62), or to refuse basic or essential care.[79] Further, if the AD is to be valid, it must state 'precisely' what treatment is being refused.[80] And its contents are subject to recapitulation if the patient's subsequent conduct contradicts its contents.[81] Additional reasons for inapplicability of the AD are set out in section 25(4):

(a)   that treatment is not the treatment specified in the advance decision;

(b)   any circumstances specified in the advance decision are absent; or

(c)   there are reasonable grounds for believing that circumstances exist which the patient (P) did not anticipate at the time of the advance decision and which would have affected his decision had he anticipated them.

The AC will not incur liability for declaring the AD inapplicable if he or she is 'satisfied' that the AD is valid, nor conversely incur liability for withholding or withdrawing treatment if he or she 'reasonably believes' that the AD is 'valid and applicable to the treatment'.[82] Peter Bartlett explains the potential consequences for treatment providers thus:

These standards of certainty differ: satisfaction implies a higher level of certainty than reasonable belief. A margin is thus created within the system, serving to protect treatment providers from liability in cases of honest doubt. A valid and applicable advance decision is effective as if P were competent and refusing the treatment at the time the treatment is offered, however, so treatment of P if the provider is satisfied that such a valid and applicable advance decision exists would be battery and, potentially, a criminal offence. Similarly, failure to treat when there is no reasonable belief that such an advance decision exists is likely to constitute negligence . . . In the event of doubt, the matter of validity and applicability can be referred to the Court of Protection [under section 26(4)].[83]

It is important to note that the AD has no bearing upon whether treatment under Part IV of the MHA can be lawfully given.[84] Once a patient is formally detained in hospital, the nurse will consider whether the patient has capacity in light of the special safeguards of sections 57, 58 and 58A before administering treatment (as above). But, what is the position of an incompetent patient who is *informally* detained but acquiescent?

Until recently, the lacuna in law was that patients who lacked capacity but who did not protest against their informal detention or treatment had no procedural treatment safeguards under Part IV of the MHA. This position was challenged in the *Bournewood* litigation, when the pivotal question for determination was: when, and in what circumstances, is an informal patient deprived of their liberty?

9.2.3.1   The *Bournewood* litigation and the deprivation of liberty safeguards

The question of when an informal patient is effectively detained was considered in *HL* v. *United Kingdom* [2005].[85] HL was an adult with severe autism, who lacked capacity to make treatment decisions. He was admitted as an informal patient to hospital under section 131 of the MHL ('requires treatment for mental disorder'), and for five months was treatment and detention compliant. However, it later transpired that had HL attempted to leave the hospital, he would have been formally detained. A request made by HL's parents that he be released into their care was refused, and they sought judicial review. Both the Court of Appeal and House of Lords held that HL was not detained, and leave was granted to examine a question of law at the European Court of Human Rights (ECtHR). The ECtHR subsequently held that HL had been unlawfully deprived of his liberty under article 5(1) of the ECHR. The Court reasoned:

The contrast between [the] dearth of regulation and the extensive network of safeguards applicable to psychiatric committals covered by the Act . . . is, in the Court's view, significant . . . As a result of the lack of procedural regulation and limits, the Court observes that the hospital's health care professionals assumed full control of the liberty and treatment of a vulnerable incapacitated individual . . . While the Court does not question . . . that they acted in what they considered to be the applicant's best interests, the very purpose of procedural safeguards is to protect individuals against any misjudgments and professional lapses.[86]

The decision of the ECtHR came too late to modify the MCA, so the Government responded by inserting new – highly complex[87] – deprivation of liberty safeguards (DOLS) into the MHA 2007. Sections 4A and 4B of the MCA (as amended) now stipulate that detention of incapacitated persons is only lawful if authorised by the Court of Protection; by the procedures set out in schedule A1; or because deprivation is necessary to provide treatment to present serious deterioration in the person's condition, while a decision is sought from the Court.[88]

Schedule A1 provides that the 'managing authority' of the NHS hospital or care home must request a standard authorisation for the deprivation of liberty from 'the supervisory body' (a primary care trust or local authority). The Code of Practice to the DOLS provides some limited guidance as to when deprivation of liberty should be suspected; relevant considerations are:

- All the circumstances of each and every case.
- What measures are being taken in relation to the individual? When are they required? For what period do they endure? What are the effects of any restraints or restrictions on the individual? Why are they necessary? What aim do they seek to meet?
- What are the views of the relevant person, their family or carers? Do any of them object to the measures?
- How are any restraints or restrictions implemented? Do any of the constraints on the individual's personal freedom go beyond 'restraint' or 'restriction' to the extent that they constitute a deprivation of liberty?
- Are there any less restrictive options for delivering care or treatment that avoid deprivation of liberty?
- Does the cumulative effect of all the restrictions imposed on the person amount to a deprivation of liberty, even if individually they would not?[89]

The standard authorisation request must be received within 28 days of the deprivation of liberty, which will either be at the point of admission or when the relevant person loses capacity.[90] If it is not possible to seek a standard authorisation, because the need to detain is urgent, the managing authority can deprive liberty for up to seven days pending the outcome of the request.[91] If standard authorisation is granted, the supervisory body must appoint someone, who may be a carer, friend or family member, to maintain contact with the person and provide support during their deprivation of liberty (patient representative).[92] Where no such person exists, an Independent Mental Health Advocate (IMHA) will be appointed to fulfil that role.

The decision to grant a standard authorisation will be determined by the supervising body on account of whether six qualifying requirements are met:

- The relevant person is over 18 years of age (age requirement).
- The relevant person suffers from a mental disorder, as defined in the MHA (mental health requirement).
- The relevant person must lack capacity to decide upon whether to agree to detention for care or treatment (mental capacity requirement).

- Admission must be in the best interests of the relevant person; that is, [it] constitutes a proportionate response to the threat of harm to the relevant person (best interests requirement).
- The relevant person is not subject to compulsory treatment under the MHA and has not refused admission, unless overridden by a court–appointed deputy of the holder of a lasting power of attorney (eligibility requirement).
- The relevant person has made a valid and applicable advance directive under the MCA refusing treatment, or if admission conflicts with the valid decision of a court–appointed deputy or lasting power of attorney (no refusals requirements).[93]

Assessments under DOLS may be carried out by the same assessor,[94] except in the case of the best interests and mental health assessments.[95] The mental health assessor must be a doctor authorised to admit patients under the MHA,[96] who has three years' post-registration experience in diagnosing or treating mental disorder, and has undergone the prescribed training. However, the best interests' assessor – who must also carry out the age and no refusals assessment –[97] can be either an AMHP, a registered social worker, first-level nurse or occupational therapist, or a chartered psychologist, provided the professional has two years' experience and has undergone the prescribed training.[98]

Once granted, the standard authorisation lasts for a maximum of 12 months, but may be renewed. The relevant person, the managing authority and those consulted as part of the best interests assessment should be notified of the outcome.[99] The relevant person should also be notified of their right of review.[100] In general, it is expected that the managing authority will alert the supervisory body that one or more of the qualifying requirements appears to be reviewable during the ordinary course of monitoring the relevant person's case. The supervisory body should also carry out a review of the assessments if requested to do so by the relevant person or his or her personal representative.[101] An assessor will then determine whether any qualifying requirement is 'reviewable', and if necessary carry out a separate assessment. If it appears that none is reviewable, no further action is needed. If there remains disagreement, either on the reviewability of a qualifying requirement; re-assessment of one or more qualifying requirement; the duration of the standard authorisation, its purpose, or the conditions subject to which it was given,[102] the Court of Protection may vary or terminate the standard authorisation or direct the supervising authority to do so.[103] Failure of the managing authority to remit the matter in question to the Court of Protection could engage article 5(4) (right to a speedy hearing) as well as article 5(1) (right to liberty) of the ECHR. Where the issue is failure to notify the supervising body of a potential deprivation of liberty, nurses should ensure that any concerns about the capacity-status of an informal patient or person in a care home is raised with the RC, hospital manager or care home manager, pursuant to an application for standard or urgent authorisation being made by the managing authority. Indeed, it is only through good faith that some very vulnerable people will be afforded points of challenge against arbitrary decisions involving deprivation of liberty.

9.3   Miscellaneous provisions of the MHA and MCA

The remainder of this chapter discusses other significant amendments introduced by the MHA 2007 and MCA. The issues chosen have especial relevance to nursing practice, and complement those provisions already discussed. The first of these is the nurse's holding power; the second is the management of violent or aggressive patients; the third is compulsory treatment orders in the community; and, fourth, the First–tier Tribunal (Mental Health).

9.3.1   Informal inpatients and the nurse's holding power

It has already been pointed out that a patient may consent to admission (either for assessment or treatment) as an informal patient under the MHA. In respect of a patient with capacity who revokes their consent to be treated informally, the only options are discharge or formal detention (section 3(2)). Formal detention may be appropriate, for example, if the condition of the patient has deteriorated since informal admission and treatment under Part IV of the MHA is deemed necessary.[104] Occasionally, the patient may try to leave hospital before his or her legal status can be changed. To prevent this from happening, section 5(4) of the MHA provides that nurses of 'the prescribed class'[105] can hold an informal patient for up to six hours pending the arrival of a doctor, if it reasonably appears to the nurse:

(a)   that the patient is suffering from mental disorder to such a degree that it is necessary for his health or safety or for the protection of others for him to be immediately restrained from leaving the hospital; and

(b)   that it is not practicable to secure the immediate attendance of a practitioner or clinician for the purposes of furnishing a report under subsection 2 . . .

Before invoking the power, the nurse will compare the arrival time of the doctor or AC[106] with the patient's intentions of leaving hospital and the likely consequences of doing so. The Code of Practice 2008 states that every effort should be made to 'persuade the patient to wait until a doctor or approved clinician arrives to discuss the matter further'.[107] Further relevant factors include:

- any evidence of disordered thinking
- the patient's current behaviour and, in particular, any changes in their usual behaviour
- whether the patient has recently received messages from relatives or friends
- any recent disturbances on the ward
- any relevant involvement of other patients
- any history of unpredictability or impulsiveness
- any formal risk assessment which have been undertaken
- any other relevant information from other members of the multidisciplinary team.[108]

The decision of the nurse to use the holding power must be recorded on an H2 form,[109] and this must be sent to the hospital managers before the power is invoked.[110] Once the form is recorded, the patient may be detained for up to 72 hours, if on arrival the doctor or AC exercises their own respective holding power through completion of a further report (section 5(5)). But not unless a civil section has been applied, should the nurse consider administering treatment under Part IV of the MHA.

In some (limited) circumstances, the completion of a form may be impracticable, or irrelevant; for example, a patient may behave aggressively, or otherwise be perceived to constitute a risk to others, though they are not threatening to leave the hospital. In these circumstances, section 3(1) of the Criminal Law Act 1967 allows a person, who may be a nurse, to use 'such force as is reasonably required in the circumstances in the prevention of crime' for the duration of the risk. Reasonable force is also sanctioned under the common law to prevent breach of the peace, which includes fear of assault, an affray or other disturbance.[111] If, however, the patient is adjudged to be attempting to leave hospital, the H2 form should be completed as soon as possible after applying restraint.

A patient who lacks capacity may also be reasonably and proportionately restrained from leaving hospital, if doing so is in their best interests (section 6 of the MCA). The legality of restraint (but not the extent to which it is applied) turns on whether the nurse reasonably believes the patient to lack capacity, and whether it is applied to prevent harm to the patient that is both likely and possibly severe.

In 2005, the MHAC commented that the use of section 5(2) restraint had declined, and that this 'should *probably* be welcomed, since the drop in its use could be reflective not in any lessening of coercion in mental health services, but by the greater use of de facto detention'.[112] It is clear that, if the patient in hospital lacked capacity from the outset, they will have been formally detained, or the eligibility criteria of DOLS will have been applied (the latter not applying to patients formally detained). However, for informally detained patients who do not lack capacity, the threat of coercive detention still looms large.

Hoge *et al.*, for instance, found that 38.6 per cent of patients sampled ($n = 34$) believed they would face formal detention if they did not agree to informal detention; and, moreover, 'multiple influence attempts were recorded'.[113] While the potential impact of family, friends and carers on admission 'decisions' should not be ignored, coercion by medical professionals, in particular, has the potential to damage therapeutic relationships or cause patients to avoid seeking psychiatric treatment or care in the first place.

9.3.2   The management of violent or aggressive patients

It has already been noted that informally detained patients who pose a risk to themselves or others may be forcibly restrained by the nurse pursuant to being considered for formal detention. In the case of a formally detained patient presenting as violent and aggressive, compulsory medication may be administered under Part IV of the MHA, if necessary by force, whether or not the behaviour is caused by the underlying disorder or its symptoms.[114]

The MHA Code of Practice warns that 'disturbed behaviour' can be the result of many factors unrelated to the underlying disorder, including boredom, too much stimulation, overcrowding, difficulties in communication, emotional distress, patient mix, provocation and alcohol or drugs.[115] This common sense analysis suggests that policies of early recognition, prevention and de-escalation techniques are to be preferred over more invasive procedures such as medication, restraint or seclusion (see 9.3.2.1 below). Yet, for disorders like ASPD this may be impracticable, as such patients may demonstrate a 'willingness to use untamed aggression to back up the need for control or independence'.[116] While compulsory medication such as antipsychotics is an option for this patient group, their administration is more likely to occur 'for the sake of the psychiatrists, nurses and other staff who care for [these] very troubled patients'.[117] This (further) blurring of the distinction between treating the disorder and its symptoms should raise legal objections. Furthermore, ethically speaking, it is a paradox that nurses who do not wish to use medication to 'restrain' problematic patients are more likely to resort to *management*, rather than treatment, strategies. For dangerous, violent and problematic patients, this may include the controversial use of seclusion.

9.3.2.1 Seclusion

The MHA Code of Practice defines seclusion as 'the supervised confinement of a patient in a room, which may be locked'.[118] The MHA makes no reference to seclusion, though it *could* be construed as an element of 'care' within the meaning of section 145, but arguably not treatment. 'Its sole aim,' the Code of Practice states, 'is to contain severely disturbed behaviour which is likely to cause harm to others',[119] where de-escalation techniques have proven insufficient for the time being.[120] Consequently, it should be reserved as a measure of last resort, for the shortest possible time, not as a punishment or a threat or because of a shortage of staff, and not as a means of managing self-harming behaviour.[121] If seclusion is being considered for informally detained patients, this should be taken as evidence of the need to consider formal detention.[122]

The decision to seclude a patient can be made by a doctor, the AC or the professional in charge of the ward.[123] A multidisciplinary team should review its necessity 'as soon as practicable' after seclusion begins[124]; and if the need for continued seclusion is affirmed, it must be continually reviewed every two hours by *two* nurses (or other suitably skilled professionals, one of whom will have been involved in the initial decision) and every four hours by a doctor or AC.[125] According to the Code of Practice:

A suitably skilled professional should be readily available within sight and sound of the seclusion room at all times through the period of the patient's seclusion.[126]

The aim of this observation is to monitor the condition and behaviour of the patient and to identify the time which seclusion can be ended. The level of observation should be decided on an individual basis. A documented report must be made at least every 15 minutes.[127]

Moreover, the room used for seclusion should:

- provide privacy from other patients
- be safe and secure
- be adequately furnished, heated, lit and ventilated
- be quiet but not soundproofed and should have some means of calling for attention (operation of which should be explained to the patient).[128]

There have been repeated calls to ban the practice of seclusion, and the non–binding status of the Code of Practice has been challenged by patients in recent years. In the seminal case of *R (on the application of Munjaz)* v. *Mersey Care NHS Trust*,[129] the policy of Ashworth high-secure hospital to provide one medical review following three days' seclusion was challenged as being contrary to the Code of Practice. The court held that the Code of Practice has the status of guidance only, which, while not binding, should be followed, unless there are good reasons not to do so. The court argued that the fact that Ashworth was a high-security hospital justified departure from the Code of Practice because 'patients are there because they cannot be dealt with by mental health services elsewhere in a way that will protect others from harm'.[130] Lord Bingham added: 'The procedure adopted by the Trust does not permit arbitrary or random decision making. The rules are accessible, foreseeable and predictable.'[131]

The MHAC has paid particular attention to unethical seclusion practices in recent years. In 2008, it pointed out that 'euphemisms' are commonly applied to the practice of seclusion, which effectively deprives patients of the safeguards of the Code of Practice.[132] High-secure forensic care was singled out, with evidence provided of poor sanitation and the lack of toilet facilities in seclusion rooms (raising the possibility of a breach of article 3 of the ECHR (prohibition of degrading treatment)).[133] Most recently, the Care Quality Commission (CQC) has commented on the use of protracted seclusion, absent prior de-escalation attempts and evidence of disturbed behaviour prior to its use, as envisaged by the Code of Practice. In one case, the CQC complained:

> [T]he commission is extremely concerned that the threshold for seclusion did not appear to be met, nor was it used for the shortest time, nor as a last resort . . . Human rights issues are possibly engaged based on the poor recording and rationale for initial and ongoing seclusion.[134]

In *Munjaz*, counsel for the applicant submitted that the trust's seclusion policy was disproportionate to one of the justifications (protection of health or morals) for restricting the right to private life guaranteed by Article 8. However, Lord Bingham, having already declared that the trust's policy did not breach Article 3, stated that 'properly used the seclusion will not be disproportionate because it will match the *necessity* giving rise to it'.[135] The fact that seclusion *can* be and *is* improperly used suggests that the necessity 'giving rise to it' is in some cases professional expediency. It is therefore vital that the nurse employs seclusion only for good reason, and then, as far as practicable, in line with the letter of the Code of Practice.

9.3.3   Community treatment orders

The discussion so far has focused on treatment and the provision of care of those detained formally or informally within a hospital or care facility. This emphasis is undoubtedly correct: the numbers of patients admitted formally to hospital-based care,[136] and the coercive thrust of disability-centred health legislation, necessitate an understanding of the application and limits of medical power. Nevertheless, the last 50 years or so have seen a marked contraction of hospital-based care in favour of community care,[137] including detention of the elderly in (private) care homes under the MCA. Many people with capacity in the community do not require formal admission to hospital, and the disapplication of Part IV of the MHA invites consent into the process of care and treatment.

Prior to the amendments introduced to the MHA by the MHA 2007, only patients formally detained under section 3 who were on section 17 leave from hospital could be treated compulsorily in the community. For these patients, the issue was whether a doctor could briefly invoke section 3 with a view to imposing long-term leave of absence (six months initially with the power to renew), or readmit the patient on leave of absence to hospital in order to renewal the section 3 (bearing in mind that the legal justification for invoking section 3 was that treatment could not be provided 'unless he is *detained*' (emphasis supplied)). In the case of *R v. Hallstrom, ex parte W; R v. Gardner, ex parte L*,[138] the court ruled that this use of sectioning was contrary to the intention of Parliament,[139] and that it precluded serious consideration being given to whether informal treatment was appropriate.[140] This situation is now likely to be mitigated by the introduction of Supervised Community Treatment (also known as Community Treatment Orders (CTOs)) contained in the MHA 2007 for its introduction means that the RC is now obliged to impose a CTO if section 17 leave will extend beyond seven days (sections 17(2) and (2A)).

The purpose of the CTO is to enable the patient's continued treatment following discharge from hospital, where hospital detention is no longer deemed necessary. The CTO remains one of a number of legal mechanisms authorising compulsory outpatient treatment, which include section 17 leave and guardianship.[141] However, what is immediately significant about the CTO is its increasing use. As of 31 March 2011 there were 4291 people on a CTO – an increase of 29.1 per cent on the previous year.[142] With such exponential use, their potential benefits and risks are yet to be fully understood, as John Dawson explains:

> Requiring contact to be maintained with a community service may prevent relapse in [the patient's] illness, or reduce the severity of its consequences. It may also reduce the stress imposed by a person's illness on their family and friends, reduce their potential to cause harm, prevent their arrest, or avoid their being processed through the criminal justice system with the result that they may be imprisoned or directed into forensic mental health care . . . On the other hand, CTOs may be used too readily, or for too long, or may be imposed on inappropriate categories of patient, or their use may become a form of defensive medical practice designed to deflect public concern about

the closure of psychiatric hospitals or . . . their existence may prevent greater professional efforts being made to engage patients voluntarily.[143]

The criteria for implementing a CTO are contained within section 17A of the MHA. This section states that, following agreement by an AMHP, the RC of an unrestricted patient detained in hospital – that is, not subject to discharge restrictions imposed by the Secretary of State for Justice – may 'order in writing' that the patient become a 'community patient'. Only patients detained under section 3; those on section 17 leave; those subject to a hospital order (for mentally disordered offenders) or transfer direction (transferred from prison to a secure hospital) can become a community patient. As with section 17 leave and detention for treatment (section 3), the CTO lasts for a period of six months (unless terminated by the RC or a First-tier Tribunal (Mental Health). The CTO can be renewed for a further six months (and then a year), if the relevant criteria of section 17A(5) continue to be met:

(a)   the patient is suffering from mental disorder of a nature or degree which makes it appropriate for him to receive medical treatment;
(b)   it is necessary for his health or safety or for the protection of other persons that he should receive such treatment;
(c)   subject to his being liable to be recalled . . . such treatment can be provided without his continuing to be detained in hospital;
(d)   it is necessary that the responsible clinician should be able to exercise the power . . . to recall the patient to hospital; and
(e)   appropriate medical treatment is available for him.

The MHA Code of Practice states that before placing a patient on a CTO, the RC will have assessed the patient and be of the opinion that his or her condition would deteriorate after discharge from hospital.[144] This risk of deterioration will be assessed by reference to the patient's history and 'any other relevant factors' when making this assessment.[145] It is expected that relevant factors will include the patient's current mental state and the patient's insight and attitude towards treatment.[146] These should be determined by consultation with the patient's carers and the patient, though formal consent is not a prerequisite to invoking the CTO.[147]

Whether or not the patient can be lawfully treated while on a CTO turns on the issue of capacity and, in the case of administration of medication beyond three months and ECT, SOAD certification (Part 4A).[148] If the patient *lacks* capacity, the patient may be treated in the absence of consent, but not through force,[149] and not with ECT. If the patient has made a valid and applicable advance directive, or someone is authorised to refuse on the patient's behalf, it is binding. Patients *with* capacity can only be treated with their consent, even in an emergency, unless they are recalled to hospital (in which case Part IV of the MHA applies).[150] Readmission to hospital of the non-consenting patient for the purposes of compulsory administration of medication (under section 63) may be irresistible in such instances, and this is likely to increase the risk of coercive 'negotiation' between the medical practitioner and patient, particularly if prior consultation with the patient was inadequate.

Recall may also result if unrealistic 'optional conditions' are attached to the CTO. The nature of the optional conditions will depend on the patient's circumstances, but they may cover where and when the patient is to receive treatment; residency requirements; and stipulation that the patient avoid 'known risk factors or high-risk situations' linked to their mental disorder.[151] Breach of these conditions may lead to the conclusion that the patient can no longer be 'safely treated for mental disorder in the community'.[152] Once recalled to hospital, the patient may be detained (for up to 72 hours) for reassessment and either detained under section 3 or, if the relevant provisions of the MHA are met, reissued with a CTO. If the patient is reissued with a CTO, the RC should inform the patient and those consulted of the decision and conditions which are being applied.[153]

The Code of Practice provides that conditions should 'be kept to a minimum number consistent with achieving their purpose' and evidence 'a clear rationale' linked to the criteria of for issuing the CTO.[154] In the absence of a clear rationale, the RC may be obliged to modify or remove certain conditions (without need to consult the AMHP); indeed, failure to do so may give rise to Convention challenge on the grounds that the conditions are disproportionate. More generally, section 132A of the MHA stipulates that it is a responsibility of hospital managers to inform any patient (re-)issued with the CTO 'as soon as practicable' of the provisions of the MHA engaged in their case. He or she must also inform the patient of their right to apply to the First-tier Tribunal (Mental Health) for review of the optional conditions and the need for compulsory outpatient treatment.[155]

9.3.4   Leaving hospital: the First-tier Tribunal (Mental Health)

A community or hospital patient falling within Part II of the MHA can be discharged by their RC, the hospital manager or by a First-tier Tribunal (Mental Health). A patient conveyed to hospital under Part III, following the commission of a criminal offence, can only be discharged with the consent of the Secretary of State for Justice. However, all patients deprived of their liberty, whether in the community or in hospital, are entitled to a Tribunal hearing for review of the lawfulness of continued detention.[156] Moreover, if they do not exercise this right, they should periodically be referred by hospital managers for a hearing on the expiry of six months from the period of admission and thereafter every three years (section 68).

The Tribunal is an inquisitorial rather than adversarial process, and therefore the hospital manager is required to file reports covering basic information about the patient, a medical report prepared by the RC and a social circumstances report – usually prepared by a social worker – within three weeks of the hearing or seven days, if the patient is detained under section 2.[157] In addition, if the hearing concerns an inpatient, his or her current nursing plan must be appended to the report,[158] and a nursing report filed covering the following matters:

(i)   the patient's understanding of and willingness to accept the current treatment for mental disorder provided or offered

(ii)   the level of observation to which the patient is subject

(iii)   any occasions on which the patient has been secluded or restrained, including the reasons why seclusion or restraint was considered to be necessary

(iv)   any occasions on which the patient has been absent without leave whilst liable to be detained, or occasion when he has failed to return when required, after being granted leave of absence

(v)   any incidents where the patient has harmed himself or others, or has threatened other persons with violence.[159]

Having been provided with the necessary documents, the role of the Tribunal members (legal, medical member and tribunal) is to determine whether the medical authorities have demonstrated the existence of a 'true mental disorder' justifying continued deprivation of liberty, as required by Article 5(1)(e) of the European Convention of Human Rights (see *Winterwerp* v. *The Netherlands*[160]). Under section 72(1)(b) of the MHA, the patient is entitled to discharge if the Tribunal is *not* satisfied:

(i)   that the patient is then suffering from mental disorder of a nature or degree which makes it appropriate for him to be liable to be detained in hospital for medical treatment; or

(ii)   that it is necessary for the health or safety of the patient or for the protection of other persons that he should receive such treatment; or

   (iia)   that appropriate medical treatment is available for him; or [the following *is* met]

(iii)   in the case of an application by the nearest relative following the barring of a discharge order, that the patient if released would be likely to act in a manner dangerous to himself or to other persons.[161]

The Care Quality Commission (CQC) reports that there were 12,122 Tribunal hearings in 2009, up from 7295 in the previous year.[162] An additional 50 per cent of applications did not result in a hearing; approximately 70 per cent of these were the result of the patient being discharged, with the remainder having been withdrawn by the patient[163] – most likely because the patient was changed from formal to informal status or they were issued with a CTO.

In its final report, the MHAC expressed its concern about the practice of changing a patient's status from a section 3 to a CTO, as this causes the appeal against detention to lapse but the application for section 3 admission 'shall not cease to have effect' (see section 17(D)(1)).[164] Following legal challenge,[165] it now appears that the section 3 detention lapses if the patient is discharged from the CTO following appeal. While the patient could be issued with a new section 3, a mental health professional would presumably think carefully before ignoring a Tribunal decision. Two legitimate reasons for doing so are that information relevant to the hearing was not known at the time,[166] or the detaining authorities believe the Tribunal to have erred on a point of law. Where the decision appears to be wrong, the usual approach will be to apply to the Tribunal for a stay of their decision pending appeal to the Upper Tier Tribunal.[167]

However, it is unusual for a Tribunal decision to be countermanded. In 2009, only 5 per cent out of 3500 CTO appeal hearings (29 per cent of total applications) resulted in discharge; for detained patients, the discharge rate was 14 per cent.[168] One reason for these low figures is the nature of fact-finding undertaken by the medical member of the Tribunal. He or she is required to both examine the patient *and* 'examine any records relating to the detention or treatment of the patient'.[169] While this is supposed to introduce inquisitorial objectivity into the process, there is evidence that the medical member will tend towards the RC's views of the patient's suitability for discharge.[170] Since the concepts 'nature' and 'degree' in section 72(1)(b)(i) of the MHA are medical constructs, the legal and tribunal members are likely to defer to the views of the medical member.[171] The probable result is a decision that is in conflict with the patient's own self-understanding of their condition. Nevertheless, provided the medical member does not 'form a concluded opinion until the conclusion of the hearing' and the other members are 'free to disagree' with the medical member's opinion on the evidence and submissions, then the decision cannot be impugned as contrary to Article 6 (right to a fair and public hearing) of the ECHR.[172]

Another reason for the low discharge rate may be that doctors reserve the right not to disclose medical and social documents if to do so is 'likely to cause serious harm to the physical or mental health or condition of the data subject or any other person'.[173] In the case of *Roberts* v. *Nottinghamshire Healthcare NHS Trust*,[174] Cranston J believed that harm to health should be widely construed to include: '[S]elf-harm or harm to others. The issue demands a factual inquiry, taking all the matters into account such as the personality of the applicant, his past history, the care regime to which he is subject and so on . . .'[175] Note, however, that the Tribunal Procedure (First-tier Tribunal) (Health, Education and Social Care Chamber) Rules 2008 have now implemented a more demanding non-disclosure test. Under rule 14(2), the Tribunal should order disclosure unless 'disclosure would be likely to cause that person or some other person serious harm' and 'having regard to the interests of justice, that it is proportionate to give such a direction'[176] – and provided the medical records do not contain sensitive information from third-parties.[177] While these provisions may improve patients' chances of mounting their best case, others may be discouraged from applying at all if their medical records are initially withheld. Therefore, medical practitioners should think carefully before relying on provisions justifying non-disclosure of medical reports in respect of patients detained under the MHA.

The review of detention of patients not detained under the MHA is governed by schedule A1 of the MCA. Schedule A1 requires the managing authority to review the necessity for the deprivation of liberty by reference to qualifying requirements contained within the DOLS (see section '9.2.3.1 The Bournewood litigation and the deprivation of liberty safeguards' above). This process is triggered once a request is made by the detained person, their representative (who will have been appointed by a supervisory body) or an Independent Mental Capacity Advocate. If during review it is found that one of the qualifying requirements contained within DOLS is *not* met, the patient should either be discharged or formally detained under the MHA.

However, as this chapter has highlighted, such is the potential for encroachment upon patient's autonomy once the compulsory powers of the MHA are evoked, and such is the growing emphasis on shared decision-making in disability-based legislation, this latter manoeuvre should ideally be one of last resort.

9.4   Notes and references

1. See, for example, Chapters 7A, 10A.
2. N. Glover-Thomas & J. Laing, Mental health professionals. In L. Gostin, P. Bartlett, P. Fennell, J. McHale & R. Mackay (eds), *Principles of Mental Health Law and Policy* (Oxford, Oxford University Press, 2010), p. 309. [Hereinafter Principles of Mental Health Law and Policy].
3. *Ibid.*, P. Bartlett & R. Sandland, *Mental Health Law: Policy and Practice*, 3rd edn (Oxford, Oxford University Press, 2007), with the 4th edn due in September 2013; P. Fennell, *Mental Health: The New Law* (Jordans, 2007).
4. Department of Health, *MHA Code of Practice Mental Health Act 1983* (TSO 2008). (A separate Code applies in Wales: see Welsh Assembly Government, *Mental Health Act 1983 Code of Practice for Wales*.)
5. *Ibid.*, at para. 1.1.
6. *Ibid.*, at para. iv. In practice, judicial evaluations of the legality of non–consensual treatment have in the past shown marked deference for psychiatric decision-making. See, for instance, *R (on the application of PS)* v. *G (RMO) and W (SOAD)* [2003] EWHC 2335, para. 39; *R (JB)* v. *Haddock and others* [2006] EWCA Civ 961, paras 32–3.
7. *Ibid.*, at para. 1.7.
8. See, for example, *R v. RMO, Broadmoor Hospital and Others, ex parte Wilkinson* [2002] EWHC 429, paras 22, 26.
9. *R (B)* v. *Ashworth Hospital Authority* [2005] UKHL 20, paras 30–31. Reference to 'obliged' comes from the case of *Kolanis* v. *United Kingdom* (2006) 42 EHRR 12, in which it was submitted that psychiatry is 'entitled and obliged' to provide medical care (though this obligation was not engaged on the facts) (para. 29). Nell Munro comments that the normative aim of treating mental disorder, namely, 'to maximize the health and safety both of the patient *and the community*' (emphasis supplied), results in the judiciary avoiding unnecessarily restraining professionals in their ability to treat effectively. See 'Treatment in hospital', in *Principles of Mental Health Law and Policy*, note 2 above, pp. 475–6.
10. *5th Biennial Report 1991–1993* (London, TSO, 1993), at para. 7.15.
11. As it is only a psychiatrist who can diagnose a mental disorder, his or her recommendation remains the 'cornerstone of the admission procedure'. See P. Bean, *Mental Disorder and Legal Control* (Cambridge University Press, 1986), p. 35.
12. Section 6(3) of the MHA states: 'Any application for the admission of a patient under [this] Part of this Act which appears to be duly made and to be founded on the necessary medical recommendations may be acted upon without further proof of the signature or qualifications of the person by whom the application or any such medical recommendation is made or given or any matter of fact or opinion stated in it.' Moreover, the admission remains lawful unless overruled by the court. See *R v. Managers of South Western Hospital, ex parte M* [1993] QB 683.
13. As of 31 March 2011 there were 30,092 admissions to NHS and independent hospitals between 2010/11, of which around 2138 were under Part III. See The Health and Social Care Information, Centre Health and Social Care Information Centre, *In-patients formally detained in hospitals under the Mental Health Act, 1983 and patients subject to supervised community treatment, annual figures, England 2010–11*, October 2011 (Department of Health, NHS Information Centre, 2011), pp. 4, 12.

14. Schedule 1 of the Mental Health (Hospital, Guardianship and Treatment) (England) Regulations 2008, SI 2008/1184.

15. *Ibid*.

16. Joint Pre-Parliamentary Scrutiny Committee House of Lords. House of Commons, *Report on the Draft Mental Health Bill, Session 2004–2005*, HL Paper 79–1, HC 95–1. Sessions 2004–2005, 2005, paras 18–22.

17. Notably, *X* v. *United Kingdom* (1981) 4 EHRR 188.

18. See, for example, J.H. Ritchie, D. Dick & R. Lingham, *The Report of the Inquiry into the Care and Treatment of Christopher Clunis* (London, HMSO, 1994).

19. Previously defined in law as 'a persistent disorder or disability of mind . . . which results in abnormally aggressive or seriously irresponsible conduct' (section 1(2)). The definition of psychopathy in medicine remains; identified traits are grouped within interpersonal factors (superficial charm, grandiosity, pathological lying, manipulation); affective factors (callousness, lack of remorse, shallowness, failure to accept responsibility); impulsive lifestyle (impulsivity, attention seeking, irresponsibility); and antisocial conduct (general rule-breaking). See C.S. Neumann, R.D. Hare & J.P. Newman, The super-ordinate nature of the Psychopathy Checklist – revisited, *Journal of Personality Disorders*, **21** (2007), pp. 102–17.

20. Widely defined as a 'gross and persistent attitude of irresponsibility and disregard for social norms, rules and obligations' from late adolescence, World Health Organization, *The ICD-10 Classification of Mental and Behavioural Disorders: Clinical Descriptions and Clinical Guidelines* (Geneva, WHO, 2002), p. 204.

21. W.H. Reid & C. Gacono, Treatment of antisocial personality, psychopathy, and other characterological antisocial syndromes, *Behavioural Sciences and the Law*, **18** (2000), pp. 647–62.

22. Evidence of this in respect of civil admission-making is inconclusive. In respect of admissions to secure hospitals, see A. Grounds, L. Gelsthorpe, M. Howes, D. Melzer *et al.*, Access to medium secure psychiatric care in England and Wales. 2: a qualitative study of admission decision-making, *Journal of Forensic Psychiatry and Psychology*, **15** (1) (2004), pp. 32–49.

23. South East Coast Strategic Health Authority, *Report of the Independent Inquiry into the Care and Treatment of Michael Stone* (2006), http://www.kent.gov.uk/publications/council-and-democacy/michael-stone.htm

24. Cm 5016-1, at para. 1.15.

25. Of course, the 'treatability test' posed no barrier to detention if medical professionals were willing to engage with the patient. Moreover, in the face of an uncertain prognosis, the courts had previously ruled that detention for treatment was lawful if the patient had a mental disorder. See *R* v. *Cannon Park MHRT, ex parte A* [1994] WLR 630.

26. The appropriate treatment test now also applies to admissions under sections 36, 48 and 51 of the MHA (as amended by section 4(3) of the MHA 2007). Section 7(3) inserts a new subsection (4) into section 145, which would on its face appear to re-implement a form of 'treatability' test: 'Any reference in this Act to medical treatment . . . shall be construed as a reference to medical treatment the purpose of which is to alleviate, or prevent a worsening of, the disorder or one or more of its symptoms or manifestations'. It is important to note, however, that treatment need only have the 'purpose' of alleviating or preventing a worsening of the manifestations of the disorder, which includes present – or, presumably, future – risky behaviours; the justification for detention rests on the matters already referred to.

27. Department of Health, *Personality Disorder: No Longer a Diagnosis of Exclusion. Policy Implementation Guidance for the Department of Services for People with Personality Disorder* (London, Department of Health, 2003).

28. See note 4 above, paras 1.5–1.6.
29. The European Court on Human Rights stated that there was nothing *prima facie* unlawful in detaining a patient whose condition might not be amenable to treatment; it is sufficient for the purposes of Article 5 that the patient requires control and supervision for the benefit of the public. See *Hutchinson Reid* v. *United Kingdom* [2003] 37 EHRR 211, at para 51.
30. Defined by section 57(2) as 'any surgical operation for destroying brain tissue or for destroying the functioning of brain tissue'.
31. [2005] UKHL 20. This case concerned a personality-disordered offender who was challenging the right of doctors to compulsorily treat him for any mental disorder arising during detention under the MHA.
32. At para. 10.
33. *Antisocial Personality Disorder: The NICE Guideline on Treatment, Management and Prevention* (National Collaborating Centre for Mental Health. The British Psychological Society and the Royal College of Psychiatrists, 2010), p. 191.
34. N. Khalifa, C. Duggan, J. Stoffers, N. Huband *et al.*, Pharmacological interventions for antisocial personality disorder, *Cochrane Database of Systematic Reviews*, (8) (2010), CD007667, p. 2.
35. For example, '. . . mental disorder is inferred from [his] anti-social behaviour while the anti-social behaviour is explained by mental disorder' B. Wootton, *Crime and Criminal Law* (Stevens, 1981), p. 90.
36. It now seems that the introduction of the MCA (sections 5 and 6) is likely to preclude forced Caesarean sections on competent women. This conclusion is supported by the decision in *St George's Healthcare NHS Trust* v. *S* [1998] 3 All ER 673, per Lord Justice Judge, at p. 773. For further discussion, see R. Jones, *Mental Health Act Manual*, 11th edn (London, Sweet and Maxwell, 2008), p. 329.
37. Defined as 'a pervasive pattern of instability of interpersonal relationships, self-image and affects and marked impulsiveness that begins in early adulthood, is present in a variety of contexts, and is manifested in frantic efforts to avoid real or imagined abandonment, including self-mutilation or self-harm'. See American Psychiatric Association, *Diagnostic and Statistical Manual of Mental Disorders: DSM-IV-TR, text revision* (Washington, DC, American Psychiatric Press, 2000), p. 629.
38. *B* v. *Croydon Health Authority* [1995] 1 All ER 683, at 298.
39. Ibid, at 688.
40. *R* v. *Collins and another, ex parte Brady* [2001] 58 BMLR 173.
41. In contrast, where treatment is proposed outside the psychiatric hospital, the court has upheld the right of those with personality disorder to refuse food, provided the person has the capacity to do so (for to do otherwise would constitute a tort of battery). See *Secretary of State for the Home Department* v. *Robb* [1995] 1 All ER 677 (HC); and in the case of an individual in the community, see A. David *et al.*, Mentally disordered or lacking capacity? Lessons for managing serious deliberate self-harm? *BMJ (Clinical Research Ed.)*, **341** (2010).
42. A SOAD is appointed by the Secretary of State for Health; his or her role is monitored by the Care Quality Commission.
43. *R (Wooder)* v. *Feggetter and another* [2002] EWCA Civ 554, at para. 34.
44. *Coercion and Consent: Mental Health Act Commission 13th Biennial Report 2007–2009* (London, TSO, 2010), at para. 3.35. In its 2008 edition, it stated: 'We suspect a combination of increasingly unwell patients and increasing awareness of the consent issues by clinicians, the latter including a growing appreciation by clinicians of the Second Opinion services (whether as a protection for their patient or as a protection for themselves)'. See MHAC, *Risks, Rights and Recovery 12th Biennial Report 2005–2007* (London, TSO, 2008), at para. 6.

45. Ibid, at para. 3.37.
46. Section 27(2) of the Mental Health (Hospital, Guardianship and Treatment) (England) Regulations 2008, SI 2008/1184.
47. *Ibid.*, section 27(3)(b).
48. *MHA Code of Practice 2008*, note 4 above, at para. 16.14.
49. *R (Wilkinson)* v. *Broadmoor Hospital Authority* [2001] EWCA Civ 1545, at para. 33.
50. Treatment in hospital, in *Principles of Mental Health Law and Policy*, note 2 above, p. 495.
51. See the *MHA Code of Practice 2008*, note 4 above, paras 24.64–67.
52. MHAC, *In Place of Fear, 11th Biennial Report 2003–2005* (London, TSO, 2005), at fig. 63.
53. MHAC, *13th Biennial Report 2005–2007*, note 46 above, at para. 3.36.
54. *Ibid.*, paras 3.35–3.36.
55. *Ibid.*, at para. 3.53.
56. It has been said that, 'Unless a patient can show a real prospect of establishing that a SOAD has not addressed any substantive point which he should have addressed, or that there is some material error underlying the reasons that he gave, the court will not grant permission for judicial review'. See *R (Wooder)* v. *Feggetter and another* [2002] EWCA Civ 554, at para. 35.
57. *Contra*, '[I]t is not clear why the SOAD's opinion should be preferred, beyond the obvious reason that if this were not the case it would not be necessary to request a second opinion at all. Nor is it clear why the patient's best interests are better served by the SOAD's opinion than by that of her approved clinician.' See N. Munro, Treatment in hospital, in *Principles of Mental Health Law and Policy*, note 2 above, p. 495.
58. An alternative may be to utilise the Public Disclosure Act 1998. This Act seeks to protect individuals who disclose information in the public interest and to enable the individual to claim legal redress in the event of victimisation following certain forms of disclosure.
59. See MHAC, *13th Biennial Report 2007–2009*, note 46 above, at para. 3.62.
60. *Ibid.*, at para. 6.88.
61. It reported that in 23 per cent of cases it was administered immediately prior to the arrival of the SOAD. See *13th Biennial Report 2007–2009*, note 46 above, at para. 3.57.
62. Practicable steps include 'simple language, sign language, visual representations, computer support or any other means'. See the *MCA Code of Practice 2008* (London, TSO, 2008), at para. 4.17.
63. In *Re T (Adult: Refusal of Treatment)* [1992], Lord Donaldson stated that it does not matter that 'the reasons for making the choice are rational, irrational, unknown or even non-existent', at 187.
64. Examples provided by the *MCA Code of Practice 2008* include: mental illness, dementia, significant learning disabilities, concussion following head injury, and symptoms of alcohol or drug abuse. See note 64 above, at para. 14.12. The section only applies to persons over 16 years of age (see section 2(5)); below that age, the common law test of sufficient understanding and maturity prevails. See *Gillick* v. *West Norfolk and Wisbech Area Health Authority* [1986] AC 112.
65. *MCA Code of Practice*, note 64 above, at para. 4.4.
66. In common law, the additional requirement of needing to 'believe' the relevant information. See *Re C (adult: refusal of medical treatment)* (1994) 1 WLR 290, at 295; approved in *Re MB (Medical Treatment)* [1997] 2 FLR 426.
67. *Per* Lord Donaldson in *Re T (adult: refusal of medical treatment)* [1993] Fam 93, at 796.
68. *MCA Code of Practice*, note 64 above, at paras 4.8–4.9.

69. P. Bartlett, *Blackstone's Guide to the Mental Capacity Act* 2005, 2nd edn (Oxford, Oxford University Press, 2008), pp. 51–2.

70. Section 5(1)(b) of the MCA. This approach follows the common law, in which it had been said that 'The only situation in which it is lawful for the doctors to intervene is if it is believed that the patient lacks the capacity to decide'. See *Re MB (Medical Treatment)* (1997) 38 BMLR 175 (CA), *per* Butler Sloss LJ. Nevertheless, the remedy is likely to be notional damages (for example, £100 were awarded for a technical assault in *Re B (Adult: Refusal of Medical Treatment)* [2002] 2 All ER 449 (competent patient given ventilation against her wishes)).

71. For discussion, see P. Fennell, Detained psychiatric patient: forcible feeding and the right to die, *Medical Law Review*, **8** [2000], pp. 251–6.

72. *Re MB (An Adult: Medical Treatment)* [1997] 2 FCR 541. This rationale was widely followed in subsequent cases; see, for example, *Re S (Sterilisation; Patient's Best Interests)* [2000] 2 FLR 389.

73. *Re A (Male Sterilisation)* [2000] 1 FLR 549, at 555. For a more recent example, see *Trust A v. H (An Adult Patient)* [2006] 9 CCLR 474, at paras 25–26.

74. *Re Y (Mental Patient: Bone Marrow Donation)* [1996] 2 FLR 787.

75. P. Fennell, Inscribing paternalism in the law: consent to treatment and mental disorder, *Journal of Law and Society*, **17** (29) (1990), p. 43.

76. [2001] Fam 15.

77. S. Holm & A. Edgar, Best interest: a philosophical critique, *Health Care Analysis*, **16** (2008), pp. 197–207.

78. The advance decision will take priority over any other mechanisms identified in section 4(7): see section 26(1). This also means it will also cause the nurse's defence to battery in the event of non-consensual treatment under section 5 to fail.

79. The *MCA Code of Practice 2008* states: 'An advance decision cannot refuse actions that are needed to keep a person comfortable . . . Examples include warmth, shelter, actions to keep a person clean and the offer of food and water by mouth.' See note 64 above, para. 9.28.

80. *Ibid.*, at para. 9.11.

81. *HE v. A Hospital NHS Trust, AE* [2003] EWHC 1017.

82. Section 26(2)–(3).

83. See note 71 above, pp. 82–3.

84. Schedule 1A, section 4(2) of the MCA.

85. *HL v. United Kingdom* [2005] 40 EHRR 32.

86. *Ibid.*, paras 120–21.

87. Peter Bartlett argues: '[I]t is astonishing and distressing these amendments take approximately the same space in the statute book as the whole previous MCA, excluding its schedules. The drafting is at times hideous and needlessly complicated. This is highly unfortunate. The MCA as passed in 2005 is the sort of legislation that a reasonable lay person charged with making decisions can reasonably understand; not so the amendments.' See note 71 above, p. 97.

88. For those patients with capacity who are informally detained, the (latent) threat of formal detention in the event of treatment non-compliance may act as a potent form of unregulated coercion.

89. Department of Health, *Mental Capacity Act 2005: Deprivation of Liberty Safeguards* (Code of Practice) (London, TSO, 2008), at para. 2.6.

90. MCA, schedule A1, at para. 24. Authorisation lasts for one year: see schedule A1, paras 42(2), 51(2).

91. *Ibid.*, at para. 78(2).

92. *Ibid.*, paras 139–140.

93. *Ibid.*, paras 12–20.
94. *Ibid.*, at para. 129(1).
95. *Ibid.*, at para. 129(5).
96. Mental Capacity (Deprivation of Liberty: Standard Authorisations, Assessments and Ordinary Residence) Regulations 2008 (SI 2008/1858), regulation 4.
97. *Ibid.*, regulation 5(2).
98. *Ibid.*, regulations 6–9.
99. MCA, schedule A1, paras 57–58.
100. *Ibid.*, at para. 59.
101. *Ibid.*, at para. 102.
102. *Ibid.*, section 21A(2).
103. *Ibid.*, section 21A(3).
104. Notwithstanding, before administering treatment 'the patient's consent should still be sought before treatment is given, wherever practicable' by the nurse. See *MHA Code of Practice 2008*, note 4 above, at para 23.37.
105. The 'prescribed class' is defined by regulation 2(1) of the Mental Health (Nurses) (England) Order 2008 as specialist mental health or learning disability nurses registered under the Nursing and Midwifery Order 2001.
106. Section 5(4) is an emergency measure; therefore, the doctor or approved clinician with power to detain should 'not wait six hours before attending simply because that is the maximum time allowed'. See *MHA Code of Practice 2008*, note 4 above, at para. 12.32.
107. *Ibid.*, at para. 12.27.
108. *Ibid.*, at para. 12.28.
109. See Schedule 1 of the Mental Health (Hospital, Guardianship and Treatment) (England) Regulations 2008, SI 2008/1184.
110. *MHA Code of Practice 2008*, note 4 above, at para. 12.24.
111. *Albert* v. *Lavin* [1982] AC 546 (HL).
112. *11th Biennial Report 2003–2005*, note 54 above, at para. 4.26.
113. S. Hoge, C.W. Lidz, M. Eisenberg, W. Gardner *et al.*, Perceptions of coercion in the admission of voluntary and involuntary psychiatric patients, *International Journal of Law and Psychiatry*, **20** (2) (1997), pp. 167–81.
114. *Re KB (adult) (mental patient: Medical treatment)* (1994) 19 BMLR 144, per Ewbank J, at 146.
115. See note 4 above, at para. 15.5.
116. L.S. Benjamin, *Interpersonal Diagnosis and Treatment of Personality Disorders*, 2nd edn (New York, Guilford, 1996), p. 197.
117. *Hansard*, HL Deb, Ser 5, Vol 426, col 1064–65, 1982 (1 February), per Lord Elton.
118. See note 4 above, at para. 15.43.
119. *Ibid.*, at para. 15.43.
120. *Ibid.*, at para. 15.8.
121. *Ibid.*, at para. 15.45.
122. *Ibid.*, at para. 15.46.
123. *Ibid.*, at para. 15.49.
124. *Ibid.*, at para. 15.50.
125. *Ibid.*, at para. 15.51.
126. *Ibid.*, at para. 15.55.
127. *Ibid.*, at para. 15.56.
128. *Ibid.*, at para. 15.60.
129. [2005] UKHL 58.
130. Per Lord Hope, at 70.

131. *Ibid.*, at 34.
132. *12th Biennial Report 2005–2007*, note 46 above, at para. 2.132.
133. *Ibid.*, at para 2.133.
134. *Monitoring the Use of the Mental Health Act in 2009/10*, p. 74.
135. See note 131 above, at 33 (emphasis supplied).
136. For example, on 31 March 2011 there were 16,642 patients detained in NHS and independent hospitals. See note 13 above, p. 4.
137. Total bed capacity fell from 154,000 to 32,400 between 1954 and 2004. See L. Warner, Acute care in crisis, in The Sainsbury Centre for Mental Health, *Beyond the Water Towers: The Unfinished Revolution in Mental Health Services 1985–2005*, p. 37.
138. [1985] 3 All ER 775.
139. *Ibid.*, at 1107.
140. *Ibid.*, at 1110.
141. On the relationship with CTOs, see M. Kinton, Towards an understanding of supervised community treatment, *Journal of Mental Health Law*, **17** (7) (2008), pp. 7–20.
142. See note 13 above, p. 4.
143. Community treatment orders, in *Principles of Mental Health Law and Policy*, note 2 above, pp. 514–5.
144. See note 4 above, at para. 25.8.
145. *Ibid.*, at para. 25.9.
146. *Ibid.*, at para. 25.11.
147. *Ibid.*, at para. 25.14.
148. In this respect, the criteria of 4A mirror those of Part IV. See section '9.1.2.2 Treatment under section 58' above.
149. *MHA Code of Practice*, note 4 above, at para. 23.16.
150. *Ibid.*, at para. 23.14.
151. *Ibid.*, at para. 25.34. Any conditions should be recorded in the patient's note: at para. 25.35.
152. *Ibid.*, at para. 25.11.
153. *Ibid.*, at para. 25.36.
154. *Ibid.*, at para. 25.33.
155. More likely routes to discharge are non-renewal of the CTO following expiration of the current term (under section 20B(1B)), or discharge by the RC following recall to hospital (section 17G).
156. The extent of the entitlement varies. A community patient or patient detained for treatment in hospital is entitled to a hearing before a tribunal judge, a medical member and a lay member once during the first and second six months of detention, and once in every 12-month interval thereafter. Restricted patients are entitled to apply for a hearing once within the second six months of the making of the restriction and once within every 12-month period thereafter. See section 69(1)(a). A patient detained in hospital for assessment (under section 2) should apply within the first 14 days, owing to the shorter 28-day period of detention. See section 66(2)(a).
157. The First-tier Tribunal (Health and Social Care Rules Chamber) Rules 2008, rule 15. Precise details of what must be included in the documents and reports are contained in Practice Direction (Health and Social Care Chamber) Mental Health Cases.
158. *Ibid.*, at paras 5, 8.
159. *Ibid.*, at paras 18–19.
160. [1979] 2 EHRR 387, at 37. To ascertain whether this is the case, nurses are increasingly called upon to make representations as to whether or not the continued deprivation of liberty is justified.

161. The barring of discharge in respect of hospital managers is authorised by presentation of a barring certificate by the RC, who will have certified that the patient would, if released, constitute a danger to self or others (section 25). This can, however, be overridden by the Tribunal.

162. *Monitoring the Use of the Mental Health Act in 2009/10*, p. 62.

163. *Ibid*.

164. *12th Biennial Report 2005–2007*, note 46 above, at para. 4.89.

165. *AA* v. *Cheshire and Wirral Partnership NHS Foundation Trust* (2009) UKUT 195.

166. See *R (on the application of Von Brandenberg (aka Hanley)* v. *East London and the City Mental Health NHS Trust, ex parte Brandenberg* [2003] UKHL 85, at 10.

167. First-tier Tribunal (Health and Social Care Rules Chamber) Rules 2008, rule 5.

168. See note 164 above, p. 62.

169. First-tier Tribunal (Health and Social Care Rules Chamber) Rules 2008, rule 34.

170. Elizabeth Perkins, for instance, found that it was not uncommon for the medical member to '. . . have a word with the [patient's doctor] at some point before the meeting if possible'. See *Decision-Making in Mental Health Tribunals* (London, Policy Studies Institute, 2003), p. 30. See also N. Ferencz & J. Maguire, Mental Health Review Tribunals in the UK: applying a therapeutic jurisprudence perspective, *Court Review: The Journal of American Judges Association*, **37** (1) (2000), pp. 48–52.

171. Following the observation of 50 Tribunal hearings, Richardson and Machlin found that '. . . none of the observed tribunals . . . were reached in the face of opposition from the medical member'. See G. Richardson & D. Machlin, Doctors on tribunals: a confusion of roles, *British Journal of Psychiatry*, **176** (2000), pp. 110–5.

172. *R (S)* v. *MHRT* [2002] EWHC 2522 (Admin), at para. 23.

173. Data Protection (Subject Access Modification) (Health) Order 2000, Article 5.

174. [2008] EWHC 1934 QB.

175. *Ibid.*, at para. 10. For discussion of this judgment, see L. McRae, Withholding medical records without explanation: a Foucauldian reading of public interest, *Medical Law Review*, **17** (2009), pp. 438–46.

176. Supported by the Upper Tribunal in *RM* v. *St. Andrew's Healthcare* [2010] UKUT 119 (AAC).

177. *Dorset Healthcare NHS Foundation Trust* v. *MH* [2009] UKUT 4 (AAC).

B   An Ethical Perspective – Compulsion and Autonomy

Harry Lesser

Honorary Research Fellow in Philosophy, Centre for Philosophy, University of Manchester, Manchester

In mental health nursing two ethical issues predominate. One is how the ethical principle of respect for persons is to be maintained when dealing with people who appear, temporarily or more permanently, to lack full rationality. The other is the ethical problem of when the use of compulsion, whether as compulsory hospitalisation, compulsory treatment or compulsory restraint, is justified. These two issues are closely connected, both involving judgements about a person's competence. For compulsion can presumably be justified only if a client's or patient's mental judgement is so impaired or underdeveloped that they lack the competence to decide for themselves whether they should be hospitalised or how they should be treated. This does occur sometimes in physical illness (for example, in delirium), and also as a matter of course with children, people who are unconscious, and people who are drunk or drugged. However, with mental illness the situation seems more problematic: the decisions can be very difficult to make, because of uncertainty whether the client is or is not competent. Moreover, as well as the decisions being made on the facts, in so far as they can be determined, it is also vital that they be made in the proper ethical spirit and on ethically justifiable grounds.

The law regarding mental health is, as has been explained in Part A of this chapter, to be found in the Mental Capacity Act 2005 and the Mental Health Act 1983, as significantly amended by the Act of 2007. To these one may add the very substantial Codes of Practice that have been issued for both of these Acts. They are in a sense also part of the law, in that, though they give only guidance, it is made clear that the Courts will expect health professionals to comply with this guidance, unless there is some good reason to depart from it. This body of law is now in at least three ways very much in line with ethics: it sees respect for persons as something to be always maintained; it supports the view that the initial presumption should, with adults, be that a person is competent and should not be subject to compulsion; and it gives detailed advice and criteria for deciding when compulsion is necessary. That respect for persons should be maintained will probably not be disputed. But to see why, ethically, we ought to presume that a person is competent, and abandon that presumption only on good evidence, requires some further discussion.

9.5   The ethical use of compulsion

There are two reasons for maintaining that in dealing with adults, even if they are mentally disturbed, the presumption should be that compulsion should be avoided if possible, and it is the use of compulsion which requires to be justi-fied. One is that individual autonomy is valuable in itself, and to be preserved unless it thwarts other important values: some people would go so far as to say that it should be preserved except when its restriction is needed to maintain future autonomy, so that people should be left alone unless they propose to do, or appear likely to do, something which will destroy or seriously harm either their own autonomy or that of others. The second reason is that people are nor-mally the best judges of their own interests, even though they are not perfect judges. This is particularly the case when there is no objective answer to what is in their best interests, but only a subjective preference: for example, while some-times it seems obvious that the benefits of medical treatment outweigh the dis-advantages, at other times only the client can decide whether, for them, the pain of the side-effects (for example) is worth enduring for the sake of the improve-ment in their condition. Hence the conclusion, for both ethics and the law, that competent adults must not be subjected to compulsory treatment or compul-sory hospitalisation.

However, it seems clear that not all adults are, in the required sense, compe-tent, and that lack of competence can be caused not only by being unconscious (the paradigm case), or by being temporarily under the influence of drink, or drugs, or delirium, but also by mental illness. Even as staunch a supporter of the freedom of patients as Thomas Szasz, who holds that 'mental illness' is in any case either not an illness at all or a 'brain illness', since the brain, not the mind, is the diseased organ, agrees that some brain illnesses or diseases, such as advanced Alzheimer's disease, leave a patient as incompetent as if they were actually unconscious, so that decisions have to be made on their behalf.[1] Szasz thinks such cases are a tiny percentage of the instances of (as he would say) so-called mental illness. But the evidence is that there are many other cases of this sort, in which a person's delusional beliefs or emotional pressures make it impos-sible for them to make competent decisions: the failure of many anorexics to admit the harm they are doing to themselves is an example of the first; the inabil-ity of people in a deep clinical depression to make any decisions at all is an example of the second.

This also, though, illustrates the problem. To hold beliefs that are false and based on poor, or no, evidence is not peculiar to the 'mentally ill', but statistically absolutely normal, as is having one's judgement distorted by one's emotions. Yet we not only distinguish these normal conditions from such things as delusion or depression, or phobia or addiction, but often the experts, and sometimes even we laypeople, have no difficulty in deciding whether a person is normal or dis-turbed: only a few cases seem to appear as borderline. There are celebrated cases of misdiagnosis, in both directions, involving both the lengthy detention of people who were not mentally ill and the failure to detain people who were ill. But these cases often, perhaps always, involved a failure to consider the evi-dence. Sometimes this was a cynical and deliberate political move, as with the hospitalisation of political dissidents in the Soviet Union.[2] Sometimes it was the result of assuming that 'immoral' or anti-social behaviour of certain types was always a sign of mental illness, and investigating no further, as with the unmarried mothers who were 'put away', sometimes for years, or with the classification of homosexuality as a mental disease. Sometimes very few pieces of evidence were considered, as in the Rosenhan experiment, in which several mentally normal members of a university Psychology Department were admitted as mental patients solely because they complained of hearing voices.[3] Sometimes evidence was discounted for ideological reasons, as when followers of RD Laing (though perhaps not Laing himself) ignored what was said by a person's close family.[4] So the fact that mistakes have been made merely shows that decisions must be properly based on the evidence available.

This in its turn means that, as said above, and as the MCA Code of Practice says (p. 19), we have to start by presuming that a person has the capacity to make their own decisions, that is, to understand, weigh up, retain and use information and to communicate their decision to others (see MCA Code, p. 45). The assessment that they do not have this capacity should be made only after all the relevant evidence has been considered; and the Code particularly notes that the mere fact that a decision is, in the opinion of the health professional, unwise, even seriously unwise, is not enough to establish incapacity. It also should be made only after all practicable steps to help the person in question have been taken, in particular after the relevant information has been given to them in terms they can understand (MCA Code, pp. 29–39). Also, in the case of compulsory admission, the issue is not simply whether the person is competent, but whether their incompetence is likely to result in their injuring themselves or others, that is, whether they have a serious mental disorder which puts themselves or others at risk.

At this point we have to deal, once again, with an objection from Thomas Szasz, who argues that this question is a moral and political one, and not a medical one at all. If people injure others, that is a matter for the law; and if they injure themselves, that is their business. As to whether anyone should intervene merely because people are, supposedly, likely to injure themselves or others, this is a political issue. If one believes that freedom is the supreme political value, one will hold that there should be no intervention merely on the ground of what a person might do, but only when they are actually trying to do it. If one has a different political and moral view, one may support intervention. But the question, according to Szasz, is one of values, not one of medical science.

This, however, is based on the belief that, except when a person is so affected by brain illness that they in effect cannot make decisions at all, their decisions are always competent – their decisions and their behaviour may be wise or foolish, justifiable or wicked, but cannot be classed as 'well' or 'ill'. But there is strong evidence against this, evidence that, even when someone does make a decision, that decision can be the result of, or seriously affected by, such things as a delusive belief or set of beliefs, a deep disturbance in the functioning of memory or perception, an emotional disturbance such as mania or depression, an inability to control acting on one's desires or fantasies, or an abnormal lack of conscience or concern for others. If this is happening regularly, and not simply as a 'one off', and if its effect on that person's behaviour is serious enough, it must be right to regard the person as mentally ill; and sometimes it will also be right to see them as being a danger to themselves or others because their mental functioning is impaired. It is true that all these conditions have analogous states which are normal, in the sense of not preventing a person from being responsible for their actions, so that they may be stupid, or wicked, or both, but not 'ill'. But people in a disturbed condition are nevertheless different from those in these analogous states, sometimes so much so that this is obvious to anyone who deals with them, even if they cannot define the difference in words. Certainty is presumably impossible: but if all the evidence is considered, high probability may be obtained. To repeat, the mistakes are typically made because the evidence is not properly examined, not because diagnosis is impossible.

So what ethics requires is that the decision to detain someone in hospital compulsorily should be made only on the ground that there is good evidence that they have a mental disorder and are dangerous to themselves or others because of it, or in part because of it. Similarly, the decision to administer compulsory treatment should be made only on the ground that the patient is not competent to make decisions about their treatment. Neither decision should be made on punitive grounds, however unpleasant the person's behaviour: and this may require some self-awareness on the part of nurses, since this is the kind of motivation people will reject on the conscious level but can be influenced by without noticing it. Nor should they be made on the grounds of someone's convenience. Here, though, caution is needed, especially when the 'someone' is the family. On the one hand, there are people who have been 'put away', to use the phrase of an earlier time, when they were not mentally ill but merely an embarrassment to their relatives. On the other hand, there are people who were seriously disturbed but nevertheless allowed to make life intolerable for their families, to threaten their lives, and to end by committing murder or suicide, all because what the family kept saying was not taken seriously. So, in saying that people should not be hospitalised merely because it suits their family, or anyone else, one should not deny that in deciding whether they are 'disturbed' and dangerous the evidence of the family, or in general of those in close contact with them, may well be crucial and should never be taken lightly.

It is worth exploring some more examples of failure to consider all the evidence. As mentioned above, there have been psychiatrists who for ideological reasons discounted what was said by the patient's family. On the other hand, what the patient himself or herself actually says may also be wrongly discounted, if it is already assumed that they are mentally ill. There is also the need to interpret words and behaviour correctly, which requires awareness of different ways of speaking and acting: forms of address and ways of behaving which are absolutely normal in one place have sometimes been marked as deviant or inappropriate by interviewers who come from somewhere else.

The other element in handling evidence is not to allow one piece of evidence, or even one sort of evidence, to be too conclusive. Rosenhan (see above) is an example of this: people were diagnosed as mentally ill on only one piece of evidence, that they heard voices, which was in fact a lie! In particular, the fact that a person in general resembles those with a type of mental disorder, or comes from a group in which a particular type of disorder is thought to be common, should not be in any way conclusive. Even someone's behaviour, without evidence of mental disturbance, direct or indirect, is probably not enough. If the behaviour appears bizarre, the person may have unusual tastes: we should be warned by the fact that it is not very long since homosexuality was classed as an illness. If the person's behaviour is cruel and destructive, and not merely unusual, this in itself does not establish that they are mentally ill. It may, after all, indicate that they are morally bad, rather than 'sick'.

For there are at least three kinds of evidence of mental illness. One is the reports of people who know the person, such as family members and workmates. Another is what people say about their experiences, whether perceptual, emotional or both. It is important to note that those such as Szasz who oppose the whole concept of mental illness are wrong to assert that diagnosis is based simply on behaviour: it is very much based on what is learned about a person's experiences from the person themselves. But one has to note that in describing their experience the person may lie, or exaggerate, or misinterpret: malingering (deliberately pretending to be ill) and hypochondria (exaggerating the significance of symptoms) are not confined to physical illness.

The third kind of evidence comes, roughly, from the style of behaviour. This includes many very different things: compulsive and addictive behaviour, of many different kinds; behaviour that is the result of a phobia (some phobias are mild enough not to present a great problem, but others, such as extreme agoraphobia, may prevent normal living); and behaviour which is bizarre and/or harmful to the person themselves or to others. It is especially this last which raises problems; if the behaviour is harmful to others, is it the result of mental illness or simply of an indifference to the needs and rights of other people. As the question is sometimes phrased, is the person mad or bad?[5]

For example, to steal is not in itself a sign of mental illness: it may simply indicate dishonesty and lack of concern for others. But to steal objects of no use or value, or only objects of a very specific type, or to steal when one is bound to be caught, is evidence, though not always conclusive, of a mental problem. Some people would regard the very existence of certain desires, such as a desire to torture, as itself a sickness. But if the person themselves sees that acting on such desires is wrong, and has a normal capacity to control their actions, but fails to do so, there is good ground for saying that they are not ill, but behaving wrongly and wickedly. Mental illness, one may suggest, exists only if there is not only a bizarre desire, or one harmful, if acted on, to the person themselves or to others, but also an inability to control it. So the behaviour alone cannot settle the question 'Mad or bad?': evidence as to what the person can and cannot control is needed. Once again, one may suggest that, while one perhaps can never be 100 per cent certain whether a particular person has acted wrongly through no fault of their own, but because their mental or emotional faculties are in some way seriously impaired ('mad') or on the other hand has deliberately chosen to do things which harm other people ('bad'), the more the evidence is considered, the more likely one is to find a balance of probabilities in one direction.

However, mention of 'harm' raises another problem. What is being assessed is whether someone's judgement is impaired in such a way as to make them a danger to themselves or to others. But it might be objected that what is actually the case is that this person is judging values and priorities differently from the person assessing them and acting on these judgements. To say that their judgement is impaired and that what they are going to do is harmful (which is what 'being a danger' means) is simply to impose the different values of the assessor.

However, this is needlessly pessimistic. First of all, one can have a more objective notion of 'harm'. Anything that in general reduces a person's capacity for action may be said to harm them objectively, because whatever one thinks they ought to be doing and whatever aims one believes to be good and right, it will interfere with the pursuit of them; and therefore, whatever one's values, will be undesirable. Death is the supreme example of something harmful in this sense; examples which can be mild or serious are injury, disease, being deceived, losing or being deprived of one's property, being imprisoned or tied up, and so on. Now any of these, even death, can be, under some circumstances, intelligibly endured for the sake of some good, for oneself or for others, or to avoid something worse: it was rational, though arguably not right, for a man to cut off a finger to avoid military service. But when a person cannot see or admit that something reasonably serious of this sort is happening or going to happen, or simply likely to happen, to themselves or to others, unless they change their behaviour, or is apparently indifferent to its happening, then they may quite appropriately be said to be mentally ill in a way that makes them a danger to themselves or others, and to require compulsory admission to hospital.

One objection to this remains. It might be said that when the danger is to oneself, then being unable to see it, or admit it, or consider it to be a danger, is indeed a kind of illness, as being an involuntary condition that interferes with proper mental functioning. But if the danger is to others, is the term 'illness' appropriate? That is, is it justifiable to bring in personality disorders as a type of mental disorder? The problem posed is not just that they are currently untreatable, but that they may be untreatable in principle. Loss of memory, distortions of perception, mania and depression, addiction, phobia might all fairly be called illnesses; but can lack of self-control and lack of a conscience be put in the same category? (Anthony Flew[6] is an example of a philosopher who raised this problem some years ago.)

There are three reasons why one might wish to make a distinction here. First, the conditions in the first list can all sometimes (admittedly not always) be fairly clearly distinguished from their 'normal' analogues, whereas to distinguish an involuntary mental disorder of having no self-control, or no conscience, or no empathy for others, from plain selfishness or wickedness, is appreciably harder: can one be sure one is not dealing with ordinary wrongdoing? Second, other illnesses are a danger to the person who has them, whereas these are dangers, in the first instance, to other people. Third, are lack of a conscience and lack of self-control involuntary, as these other conditions are? (Addiction may be produced by voluntary self-indulgence, but is itself an involuntary state.)

As regards the first objection, one may say that it is harder but still not impossible. As regards the second and third, one may say that to apply the notion of 'illness' or 'disorder' to these cases is indeed to extend the concept, which has already been extended by being applied to mental illness. But there is nothing wrong with extending a concept, if there are good reasons for doing so: the fact that the concept of mental illness has been wrongly extended does not show that it cannot be rightly extended. So why in this case might it be right?

First, it is being extended to people who are dangerous. Second, they are dangerous because of a mental abnormality. To fail, sometimes, to control oneself, and to let one's own interests override those of others are, very regrettably, 'normal', that is, failings for which a person is fully responsible. But to be radically unable to control certain desires or emotions, or to be unable to see the point of morality at all (as opposed to having different moral ideas from one's own society), or to be unable to see that other people even matter, is abnormal. It is, indeed, radically abnormal, not simply statistically: a person in one of these conditions is cut off, to some extent, from normal human understanding and relationships, except in so far as they learn to conceal it.

It might still be objected that there are 'normal' people who are even more dangerous, and that there is the threat of the law to control both the normal and the abnormal, so that it cannot be right to lock people up who have committed no crime, on the ground that they might commit one. But this is a largely (though not of course totally) identifiable group (identification may be difficult but is certainly possible and is done), and particularly unlikely to be deterred by the law: and it is highly desirable to prevent them committing, for example, assault or murder, rather than simply punishing or incarcerating them after the event. So it is better to stretch the notion of illness to include them, as has now been done in the law, and to hope that treatments, whether physical or involving psychotherapy, can be found, rather than to accept, in the name of freedom, murders and assaults. But this does require resisting the temptation to sweep 'innocent' and 'normal' people into the net, in the interests of being on the safe side.

So we may finally summarise the ethical position regarding compulsory admission to hospital. The aim is that all and only those who are dangerous to themselves or others because of a mental disorder should be compulsorily admitted (if they will not go into hospital voluntarily). I have argued, against Szasz and others, that this aim is both intelligible and ethically sound, even if, as is now legally the case, it includes those with a personality disorder. So the law, as it now stands, is ethically sound. To administer it ethically, with regard to compulsory hospitalisation, requires two things. First, the decision to admit must be made solely on the grounds that the person in question has a mental disorder which renders them dangerous. Second, this must be decided solely on the evidence, and using as much evidence as possible.

9.6 Compulsory treatment

As regards compulsory treatment, as opposed to compulsory admission, there are four main ethical issues. The first of these is once again the issue of competence: only if the patient or client is genuinely unable to decide issues concerning their treatment should this be imposed by compulsion, and the presumption should be that they are competent, unless the evidence shows otherwise. What is involved in deciding whether someone is competent has already been discussed. But what is very important is to note that the fact that someone has been compulsorily admitted does not of itself show that they are incompetent as regards treatment. They might indeed have a mental disorder, and be a danger to themselves or others; but they might still be able to decide competently whether they should have treatment and how they should be treated. So the question of compulsion needs to be reconsidered; it is not settled by the fact that the admission was compulsory. This issue has been very well explained in an article by Simona Giordano[7]: the conclusion may appear surprising, and indeed it is not the view so far taken by the Courts (see the opinion of Baroness Hale, quoted in section 9.1 above), but once one recognises the fact that incompetence in one area is not in itself proof of incompetence in another, even if the two are closely related, it can be seen as appropriate. It will, no doubt, often be the case that a patient or client has both kinds of incompetence, but not always and not automatically – further tests are needed to establish that a person should be compulsorily treated. It is after all already the case that competence has to be reassessed if the medication is to be continued after three months (section 9.1.2 above): this would be a different kind of application of the same principle that one assessment cannot be relied upon to be valid indefinitely and in all areas.

Second, any treatment prescribed must be in the 'best interests' of the patient: here ethics and law are in total agreement. From the point of view of ethics, what is particularly important is that 'best interests' is defined by the law not purely 'objectively' but also with regard to the tastes and values of the patient, in so far as these can be discovered if the patient is not in a condition to be asked and reply. It means, in effect, what they would choose if they were able to make the decision themselves, while being free from the mental characteristics that are merely the result of their illness, but in other respects as they are now, that is, if they were free from any mental disorder but had the same tastes, aims and values that they have currently, especially those that involve long-term commitments. In Chapter 9A Leon McRae points out that anyone over 18 can, as regards refusing treatment, circumvent all this by making an advance directive as to what should be done if in the future they lose competence; and in a sense, determining a person's 'best interests' is trying to determine what they would have put in an advance directive if they had made one.

There is, though, an objective element in the law's definition of 'best interests'. This objective element is set out in section 9.1.2 above with reference to *R(B)* v. *Dr SS and others*. Whatever is necessary to save life, to prevent a serious deterioration in health, to prevent or end serious suffering (if it is not at the cost of making an irreversible change which could be seen as harmful) or to prevent violent behaviour which would injure the person or someone else, is seen as being in the patient's best interests. This seems in most cases to be ethically right, since what is being prevented is something which, irrespective of what their desires and values happen to be, will either prevent them acting on them altogether (as death does!) or seriously interfere with their capacity to act. It is thus, regardless of their tastes, wants and values, in their interest to take this action, even if it requires compulsion.

Nevertheless, this raises further ethical problems. First, does the same apply to treatment which is not strictly medical, such as force-feeding people who will otherwise starve themselves to death, or compelling someone to have a Caesarian section who will otherwise die or be seriously injured if she gives birth naturally? (see section 9.1.2 above). The law, at least as regards force-feeding, has held that it does, and this seems normally to be right. Similarly a Caesarian section, under these circumstances, would be in the best interests of the mother, and it should be legitimate, if the mother is genuinely not competent to make decisions, to compel her to have one, although presumably an enforced Caesarian section is something that should be avoided if this is at all possible.

However, though the mere fact that the treatment is not medical does not seem to alter the ethical position, provided the consequences of withholding it are genuinely very serious, there are other relevant considerations. One is that it can be in a person's best interests to die, if to continue living involves permanent and serious mental or physical suffering which cannot be relieved in any other way. Here the balance shifts, and, if it is clear that the person wants to die and wanting to die is perfectly reasonable in their circumstances, humanity requires not only that there be no forced feeding but also that medical treatment be avoided, if its effect is simply to prolong life without relieving the pain. What is important is that as far as possible the decision to treat or not to treat should be made in accordance with the person's own wishes, or the best possible assessment of what they are. It should not be automatically assumed, merely from looking at their situation as it appears to others, either that it must be worthwhile for them to continue living or that it cannot be worthwhile.

The most difficult moral problem seems to be in the situation in which permission for a Caesarian section is being refused by the mother, when it is not needed in order to preserve her health but is needed for the sake of the child. It may be that this can be regarded as still in the mother's long-term best interests, given how much she will suffer, and how much her opportunities will be limited, if she gives birth to a brain-damaged child. So once again it would seem that it is legitimate, and in her best interests, to require her to have a Caesarian section, if there is no other way of preventing the birth of a seriously damaged child, and if she still refuses consent; but that this should, once again, be a decision of last resort, to be avoided if at all possible.

So there can be situations in which, both in law and in ethics, a person's best interests can be different from what they currently want, though not from what they would want in the long term. Both legally and ethically, the crucial thing is that this be properly assessed, using all the evidence. In the cases discussed so far, this is in one way made easier to assess, because the question is not what their long-term wants and values are, but whether the treatment is needed to reduce or prevent interference with meeting those wants and values, whatever they may be. However, often it will be necessary to go beyond this, and to try to determine a patient's specific long-term desires and values. The MCA Code of Practice particularly mentions, in this connection, taking into account the person's expressed views, what is known about their circumstances, and what other people who know them have to say (p. 65), and not making automatic assumptions about their quality of life (ibid) or automatic inferences from their age, appearance, general condition or behaviour (p. 71).

There is also an emphasis on consulting other people who know the patient or client. The law (see section 9.2.3 above) requires four kinds of person to be consulted: anyone specifically named by the patient; anyone to whom they have delegated power of attorney; their carers; and anyone appointed by a Court as a deputy. The Code of Practice goes beyond this, in effect requiring anyone whose evidence is likely to be helpful to be consulted. We may say, in fact, that the law and ethics are in agreement about how to determine best interests, as they are about the criteria for compulsory treatment: in both cases what is needed is, as far as time commits, proper attention to all the evidence, and not just selected parts of it.

The third issue regarding compulsory treatment is one that applies equally to voluntary patients. It is the issue mentioned at the very beginning of this section, of maintaining respect for the patient or client at all times, whatever form of treatment or restraint may be necessary. Ethically, there is a requirement to maintain this at all times, even if the patients fail to treat the nurses with the respect that they ought to accord them, and even if they are morally responsible for this failure. (Some mental health patients are too ill to be responsible for their actions; but others still have moral obligations.) The right to respect, unlike some other rights, cannot, one may suggest, be forfeited.

As regards putting this into practice, it is important to note that this is not only a matter of individual nurses dealing with individual patients. It is also a matter of designing procedures which maintain respect for patients and are not geared only to staff convenience. Even more importantly, it requires fostering a culture of respect, through such things as the education of new staff and the example set by senior staff. The worst abuses seem to arise when a ward, or even an institution, develops a culture with no respect for patients. Ethics here requires, within reason, a more detailed consideration of what is needed both in the general organisation of a ward, or, for example a surgery or day centre, and in dealing with individual patients, than is provided by the law and the Codes of Practice. The general principle is there; but the nurse still has to think how to apply it to the particular situation. This can be hard work; but one consequence may well be that, because the patients feel that they are respected, there is less 'trouble', and of a less serious sort, so that, as well as this being an ethical duty, it has practical benefits for both nurses and patients.

Fourth, there are the ethical issues regarding physical treatments. By far the commonest physical treatment is the administration of drugs. But there are also electro-convulsive therapy, neurosurgery and the surgical implantation of hormones. The last three all involve special legal safeguards before they can be used (see section 9.1.2 above). They are also becoming rare (see section 9.1.2 again): implantation of hormones seems to have stopped altogether; neurosurgery to have become very rare and perhaps about to cease altogether, at least as compulsory treatment; and ECT to be limited to patients particularly likely to benefit. These treatments, which are particularly invasive, nevertheless do not raise ethical problems other than those raised by physical treatments in general (which will be discussed shortly). For, if it is clear that it really will benefit the patient, a treatment of this kind is as justifiable as any other. The special feature concerning invasive treatments, as regards ethics, is that the checking beforehand that the treatment really is likely to do good and not harm needs to be particularly thorough and careful: we know that in the past appalling mistakes have been made through the careless use of invasive treatments. But since treatments of this sort are becoming rare, and sometimes ceasing to be used, and since the law recognises the need for special care in deciding whether they should be used, ethics here requires essentially a strict and careful application of the law.

However, as regards physical treatment in general, including the administration of drugs, there are three ethical objections to be considered. The first is that physical treatments can tackle only the symptoms of mental illness, and not the underlying condition which is producing the symptoms. They may relieve a depression, or an addiction or compulsion (such as alcoholism), or a phobia, but do not affect the psychological or social conditions which are causing the problem. However, even if this is true, to relieve the symptoms is to do some good, sometimes much good. Still more importantly, the symptoms may have to be relieved before the person can begin to tackle the underlying problem. For example, a clinically depressed person may be depressed for very good reasons – such as having no job, lousy accommodation, a violent partner or all three – but the depression may need to be lifted by medication before they feel able to do anything about its causes.

Second, it has been argued that it is inherently wrong to try to alter a person's mental state by physical means rather than by rational argument. But the proper use of physical treatments is precisely to remove obstacles to rational thinking. For these obstacles are often (not of course always, by any means) either physical in origin or made worse by the physical state of the brain and nervous system. To use drugs to enable a person to stop hearing voices or experiencing other sorts of hallucinations or disturbances of perception or memory, or to be no longer subject to sudden frightening changes in personality, or no longer so clinically depressed that making any decision is impossible, is to restore, not to remove, the capacity to think rationally. The same can be said of behaviourist therapy: if it helps to free a person from, for example, compulsive gambling or alcoholism, it is helping to increase rationality.

The third objection is that physical treatments are misused in order to bring a person into line socially and to try to alter behaviour which is statistically unusual but harmless – for example, in the past, by trying to 'cure' homosexuality by hormone treatments or by aversive therapy. But this is not an objection to the kind of treatment but to the use to which it is being put. All treatments are objectionable if they are forced, whether by actual compulsion, threats or social pressure, on competent patients, or if they are not in the patient's best interest (as defined above).

Indeed, psychotherapy and 'talking' cures raise similar ethical problems to those raised by physical treatments, with regard to the uses to which they may be put. In one sense, it is not possible to impose psychotherapy: a person can be forced to attend one-to-one or group sessions, but cannot be forced to permit them to have any effect. But all kinds of covert manipulation are possible: it may be true that 'brainwashing', in the sense of using psychological techniques for planting ideas in the mind, is a myth, but persuading people to conform to what is expected of them, and at least to say in public what is acceptable to 'authority', whether of the group or the therapist, is very far from a myth.[8] This situation, in which lip-service is given to the idea that the therapist is non-directive and non-judgemental, but there is in fact considerable pressure, whether from the therapist, the group, or both, to adopt certain views and ideas, may be objectionable in two ways: that it is in fact coercive, and that it is not in the best interests of the patient or client to adopt these ideas, especially if false beliefs are involved. The extreme example of this is 'false memory' syndrome: there is evidence that, though many 'memories' of being sexually abused as a child are genuine, others are the result of being persuaded that this happened when it did not.

This brings out, once again, the point that physical treatments are not special from the point of view of ethics, but that the same criteria operate with regard to all treatments, that they are in the best interests of the patient, that they are not forced, whether by actual compulsion or by undue psychological pressure, on competent patients, and that respect for the patient as a person is maintained throughout the treatment. A fourth point emerges from this discussion, that the treatment should be used honestly: if the patient can understand the aim of the treatment and its likely consequences, they must be informed of what they are. And here physical treatments have a slight advantage: it is less easy to be dishonest or to conceal what is really going on than it is with 'talking' methods of treatment.

In conclusion, the point should be made once again that, as regards compulsory treatment, the law, as it stands, is now very much in line with these ethical criteria, and what ethics requires is a really thorough and careful application of the Codes of Practice. In particular, this requires two things. The first is proper examination of whether the patient is competent, and, if they are not, of what is genuinely in their best interest. The second is maintaining an ethos of always treating patients with respect and with honesty. This, incidentally, brings out an important general point, that nursing ethics, and health care ethics in general, is largely not about developing a special set of ethical principles, but about applying the general principles of ethics to the nurse's situation.

9.7   Seclusion and Community Treatment Orders

Two contrasting ethical issues, both discussed from the legal point of view in section 9.3 above, remain. They are the use of seclusion to deal with violent or aggressive patients, and the use of Community Treatment Orders (CTOs). Seclusion, or 'supervised confinement', is not specifically mentioned in the law itself, but is discussed in section 15 of the MHA Code of Practice; and the attitude of the law is, once again, very much in line with the ethical position. There have, as Leon McRae notes (see section 9.3.2 above), been a number of people who have objected to seclusion being used at all; but the evidence seems to be that, though the necessity to use it can be rare, it is not always possible to deal with violent patients in any other way.

Ethically, the most important point is that restraint, whether by medication, physical restraint or actual seclusion, should always be the last resort. This means not only that other methods of calming a tense situation or an agitated patient should be tried first, unless there is already an immediate need to prevent someone from injuring themselves or others. It also means that much attention should be given to ways of preventing such a situation arising in the first place, that there should be procedures for defusing situations of potential violence or conflict, and nurses should learn these procedures and develop an ethical attitude that emphasises 'defusing' and thinks of restraint, and especially seclusion, as to be used when all else fails. If this were done in every ward, seclusion would still be needed sometimes, but not often.

The other crucial element in the ethical use of seclusion is the importance of maintaining respect for the patient, even under very difficult circumstances. This means that seclusion should be used only when necessary, and not as a punishment or for staff convenience; that the room used should be safe and not unnecessarily uncomfortable; that the period of seclusion should be the minimum needed; and there should be no unnecessary humiliation of the patient. And, to repeat a point already made, if respect for patients is the rule, then the sort of behaviour that requires seclusion of the patient will be relatively infrequent. Once again, what ethics requires is a really thorough and careful operation of the law and the Codes of Practice.

The use of Community Treatment Orders (see section 9.3.3 above) contrasts in two ways with the use of seclusion: it is increasing, and it can be seen as giving clients more freedom rather than less. Ethically, CTOs should be used to enable people who would otherwise be detained in hospital to live in the community, provided they continue to attend for treatment, take prescribed medication, and fulfil any other required conditions: it is desirable (see section 9.3.3 again) that these be kept to a minimum. The treatment is in one sense not compulsory, since it is not administered by force. But in another sense it is compulsory, since if the patient or client refuses or neglects it, and this is reported, they can be compulsorily admitted or returned to hospital. Normally, moreover, there is a clear ethical as well as a legal duty on the nurse to report any failure by a patient to comply with the conditions: this is so both because a patient who fails to take the medication may become a danger to themselves or others, and because they are helping to operate a system which is increasing rather than decreasing freedom. It is possible, of course, that CTOs will sometimes be used unnecessarily, for patients who do not need the medication, and whose freedom is therefore being interfered with rather than enhanced. Whether this could justify a nurse in deliberately not reporting the patient is a difficult question: one can say, though, that the nurse would need to be very sure that the CTO was unnecessary and harmful, and that this situation is, mercifully, likely to be uncommon.

9.8   Conclusion

All this is summed up in paragraphs 16 and 17 of the NMC Code of Practice: 'You must be aware of the legislation regarding mental capacity, ensuring that people who lack capacity remain at the centre of decision making and are fully safeguarded' and 'You must be able to demonstrate that you have acted in someone's best interests if you have provided care in an emergency'. Essentially, to repeat this point for the last time, in this area the law and ethics are in agreement, but ethics requires that the law and the Codes of Practice be followed in a very detailed and intelligent way, working out from the evidence available whether a patient is or is not competent (and starting from the presumption that they are), considering carefully (in so far as time permits) what is in their best interest, and working out the implications of treating all patients with respect. Much of this is work for the team rather than the individual, and relates to both practices and attitudes; but it must be remembered that all members of the team are responsible for what it does.

In connection with this, paragraph 32 of the Code needs to be kept in mind: 'You must act without delay if you believe that you, a colleague or anyone else may be putting someone at risk'. Thus if the practices and attitudes in a particular ward are not satisfactory in these respects (as has been all too often the case in the past), it is the duty of a nurse to try to improve them, if they can. It may even be their duty to report the matter to a higher authority, if they are sure of their facts and there is no other way of dealing with the situation: this could apply to the treatment of one particular patient or to general standards. It is to be hoped, though, that the need for this will not occur often. For in the area of mental health nursing we may say that the law and the Codes of Practice, if carried out thoroughly and intelligently and properly applied to particular situations, are now genuinely in line with best practice; and what is required is for this to be maintained if it is already taking place and aimed at if at the moment it is not.

9.9   Notes and references

1. Jonathan Miller, *States of Mind: Conversations with Psychological Investigators* (London, BBC publications, 1983).
2. Peter Reddaway & S. Bloch, *Soviet Psychiatric Abuse: the Shadow over World Psychiatry* (Barnes and Noble, 1985).
3. D.I. Rosenhan, On being sane in insane places, *Science*, **179** (1973), pp. 250–8.
4. Caroline Dunn, *Ethical Issues in Mental Illness* (Aldershot, Ashgate, 1998), pp. 43–59
5. Michael Bavidge, *Mad or Bad?* (Bristol, Bristol Classical Press, 1989).
6. Anthony Flew, *Crime or Disease?* (London, Macmillan, 1973).
7. Simona Giordano, For the protection of others, *Health Care Analysis*, **8** (2000), pp. 309–19.
8. J.A.C. Brown, *Techniques of Persuasion: from Propaganda to Brainwashing* (Harmondsworth, Penguin Books, 1963).

10 The Critically Ill Patient

A The Legal Perspective

Jo Samanta

Principal Lecturer in Law, Leicester De Montfort Law School, De Montfort
University, Leicester

10.1 Introduction

Caring for critically ill patients can engage a range of legal, ethical and practical
challenges. This is significant in that over 110,000 patients are admitted to NHS
critical care units every year.[1] In England there are currently 3,730 adult critical
care beds, 405 paediatric and 1,368 neonatal intensive care cots with occupancy
rates of 82 per cent, 73.6 per cent and 70 per cent respectively.[2] In fact, these
figures are likely to underestimate the true prevalence, since critical care is not
invariably administered in intensive care or high-dependency units and the location of care will depend upon need.

Delivery of high-quality care to these vulnerable patients can be compromised
by ancillary factors such as resource constraints, which may impact negatively
upon bed availability and access to specialist staff. The legal framework that

Nursing Law and Ethics, Fourth Edition. Edited by John Tingle and Alan Cribb.
© 2014 by John Wiley & Sons, Ltd. Published 2014 by John Wiley & Sons, Ltd.

governs the care of critically ill patients is potentially extensive and incorporates the civil law (e.g. negligence actions), criminal law (physician-assisted suicide and euthanasia), public law (judicial review) and European law (clinical research). All these aspects are underpinned by human rights and equality jurisprudence. Additional areas of governance include the formal complaints system and professional regulation.

Part A of this chapter considers the legal framework that pertains to nursing the critically ill patient, and Part B explores its ethical underpinnings. Part A is divided into two main sections: a) competent patients with capacity and b) patients who lack decision-making capacity whether adults, children or infants (incompetent patients). Many adults who are critically ill will fall into the latter category on account of their infirmity, impaired consciousness and pain syndromes, in addition to their possible inability to communicate. Young children and infants will lack decision-making capacity because of their age.

10.2   The competent adult

Many severely ill patients will lack capacity but others will be capable of deciding for themselves. Older children may also fall into the latter category.

10.2.1   Assessing capacity

In English law the rebuttable presumption is that adults have capacity until, and unless, proved otherwise (section 1(2) Mental Capacity Act 2005). However, in critical care situations it may be apparent that a patient lacks capacity due to a low Glasgow Coma Score or because of deep sedation. In other situations the question of capacity will be less certain. The assessment of capacity is a two-stage process. First, does the patient have an impairment of, or a disturbance in functioning of, the mind or brain? Second, does that impairment or disturbance mean that the person is unable to make the decision at the time it needs to be taken? The assessment of capacity is therefore decision and time-specific and needs to be made by the person responsible for providing the treatment, or care. That person must hold a 'reasonable belief' that the patient lacks capacity and the rationale for his or her decision should be documented.

Section 3(1) of the Mental Capacity Act 2005 provides that persons are unable to make relevant decisions if they cannot understand and retain the required information and they are not able to weigh that information as part of the decision-making process. Capacity also requires that an individual is able to communicate the decision made. The ability to retain information for short periods only will not necessarily indicate a lack of decision-making capacity. This may be an important consideration for those receiving medication, or sedation that interferes with mental acuity. Unless an urgent decision is required engaging patients in decision-making should be arranged to coincide with their most lucid moments.

When patients are severely ill factors such as pain, fatigue and the effects of medication can all temporarily interfere with their ability to decide. Fear, shock and anxiety can also induce loss of capacity. The courts recognise that unusual or bizarre decisions might trigger doubt about a patient's competence. A choice that is contrary to that expected from most individuals might be relevant, particularly if there are other grounds for doubting capacity,[3] although a person who fully comprehends a situation should not be treated as lacking in capacity merely because of an unwise choice, as objectively assessed.

The Act requires that patients are not considered to lack capacity 'unless all practical steps' to achieve capacity 'have been taken without success', although in urgent situations opportunities are likely to be limited. Section 3(2) states that: 'A person is not to be regarded as unable to understand the information relevant to a decision if he is able to understand an explanation of it given to him in a way that is appropriate to his circumstances' (using any means to enhance communication). Patients must also be informed of the consequences of their decisions, including their failure to decide (section 3(4)). Where there is uncertainty about capacity, the senior clinician responsible for the overall care of the patient will need to make the decision (usually with input from the multi-disciplinary team).

Patients with capacity have the right to exercise their self-determined choice by consenting to, or refusing, clinically indicated treatment. A competent person's valid consent is decisive and adults may refuse life-saving care, even if this is against their best interests as objectively assessed. To continue treatment in these circumstances could amount to an offence or civil wrong. Persons who lack capacity receive clinically indicated treatment administered in their best interests, or on the doctrine of necessity (see section 10.5 below). The decision that an adult lacks decision-making capacity therefore has considerable implications for that person's subsequent care.

10.2.2   Refusal of treatment

The temptation to make decisions on behalf of critically ill patients, irrespective of their capacity, can be hard to resist. However, even the presence of a life-threatening condition will not validate non-consensual treatment.[4] If a competent patient refuses potentially life-saving interventions, health professionals will need to give 'very careful and detailed consideration to the patient's capacity to decide' and 'the graver the consequences of the decision, the commensurately greater the level of competence required to take the decision'.[5] In this eventuality, and after the patient has been fully informed of possible consequences, a record of the discussions and decision reached should be made.[6]

10.2.3   Requests for treatment

Patients influence the care they receive by agreeing to, or refusing, clinically indicated treatment. Although a patient (or his or her advocate) is free to ask for specific treatment, such requests will be conceded only where these align with clinical judgement.[7] For this reason autonomous choice, as the substantive exercise of free will, is often considered to be a negative right to refuse clinically indicated options, rather than a positive right to choose.

10.3   The competent child

In English law childhood extends to the age of 18 years. Nevertheless, children may give valid consent to treatment prior to this under legislative, or common law, authority.

10.3.1   Children over the age of 16

For the purposes of therapeutic interventions section 8(1) of the Family Law Reform Act 1969 provides that:

> The consent of a minor who has attained the age of sixteen years to any surgical, medical or dental treatment which, in the absence of consent, would constitute a trespass to his person, shall be as effective as it would be if he were of full age; and where a minor has by virtue of this section given an effective consent to any treatment it shall not be necessary to obtain any consent for it from his parent or guardian.

Thus, consent to medical treatment by a competent child of 16 or 17 is as effective as that given by an adult with capacity.

Section 8(2) provides that 'surgical, medical or dental treatment' includes any procedure undertaken for the purposes of diagnosis, as well as other procedures that are ancillary to any treatment being given. This includes, for example, the administration of an anaesthetic which is a necessary precursor to a procedure. The statutory presumption can be set aside if the young person is unable to believe, retain and weigh the information and communicate the decision that is made. In these circumstances the provisions of the Mental Capacity Act 2005 will apply.

Although section 8 of the Family Law Reform Act 1969 applies to consent for diagnosis and treatment, it does not provide for purposes such as transplantation or research participation. Section 8(1) displaces the need for parental consent, but does not render ineffective any consent that would have been effective, but for the Act. This means that parental rights to consent are not precluded, and these can override a child's refusal. The common law applies to children under the age of 16.

10.3.2   Mature children under the age of 16

Children below the age of 16 may possess sufficient maturity to consent based on their knowledge and understanding of the implications of the decision to be made (*Gillick v. West Norfolk and Wisbech Area Health Authority* (1985)). As young people mature and develop they acquire greater autonomy to decide for themselves. Once a young person is considered competent to consent, parental involvement changes from a requirement to a recommendation. A finding of 'Gillick competence', however, will not preclude health authorities, social services, or relatives from referring dilemmas to the court for adjudication.

If a child insists on confidentiality, this ought to be respected. This view was challenged in *R (on the application of Axon) v. Secretary of State for Health* [2006] on the grounds that *Gillick* undermined respect for family life, thereby infringing parental rights under Article 8 of the European Convention. It was argued that if parents were to discharge their responsibilities for the physical, mental and moral welfare of their children, they would need all relevant information in order to do so. The court, while sympathetic to these arguments, felt bound to respect the autonomy of mature young people. The Article 8(1) right to family life owed to a parent (as the right to be notified of medical advice given to a child) will diminish as the child matures and will cease once a child is able to make his or her own decision.

In critical care situations obtaining consent from competent young people is not usually controversial. When medical advice is accepted and followed, no conflict will arise. Difficulties and dilemmas tend to accompany treatment refusals.

10.3.3   Refusal of treatment

Although 'Gillick competence' has wider application than consent to treatment the law has been reluctant to permit young people to refuse recommended clinical care. The case of *Re W (a minor) (medical treatment: court's jurisdiction)* [1993] confirmed that children, whatever their age or personal maturity, lack authority to override the consent of those with parental responsibility (provided that the recommendation is in the child's best interests). If parents refuse consent to clinically indicated treatment, consent may be given by a court order.

W was 16 with severe anorexia. She was close to death at the time of the court hearing. The local authority (which had parental responsibility) sought a declaration that it would not be unlawful to compel W to receive treatment at a clinic that she refused to attend. While emphasising that the views of young people must be given due weight in accordance with their age and maturity the Court of Appeal overruled W's refusal, holding that neither section 8 of the Family Law Reform Act 1969 nor 'Gillick competence' applied in the circumstances. The judges, mindful of family conflicts that might ensue when teenagers and their parents disagreed about treatment, suggested that health professionals ought to refer intractable disagreements to the court.

The guidance in *Re W* was subsequently applied in *Re M (child: refusal of medical treatment)* (1999). M was 15 and required an urgent heart transplant following sudden heart failure. She refused consent on the grounds that she could not face life with a cadaver's heart. Although her parents were in favour of the transplant, the health authority referred the case to court on the basis of *Re W*. The desperate urgency of the situation meant that a duty judge had to be contacted and a decision was made overnight. M's views were conveyed to the judge via her solicitor; although they were overridden the judge prepared a careful record of his reasoning for M's benefit.

Decisions such as *Re W* and *Re M* would have little effect if they could not be implemented. The courts recognise that restraint may be required if treatment is to be given to an unwilling young patient. Although orders authorising a minimum degree of restraint are issued sparingly and cautiously, they are available on application to the court.[8] The Royal College of Nursing has published guidance on the problems related to forcing young people to undergo treatment.[9] If the restraint amounts to deprivation of liberty then additional safeguards may be necessary, such as those under section 25 of the Children Act 1989, or use of the Mental Health Act 1983.

For nurses caring for young persons who refuse clinically indicated treatment, the law may seem to provide inadequate protection for their self-determined choice. However, the limited opportunity for teenagers to refuse consent has acquired new potential under the European Convention on Human Rights. The emphasis of the Convention on the right to life (Article 2), the right not to be deprived of liberty (Article 5), of due process (Article 6) and the right to protection of family and private life (Article 8) may serve to enhance respect for young people's rights to participate in decision-making processes.

Another possible avenue for protecting self-determined choice is the Convention on Human Rights and Biomedicine 1997. Although the United Kingdom is not a signatory to this Convention, it nevertheless exerts persuasive influence over English courts. The Convention resolves 'to take such measures as are necessary to safeguard human dignity and the fundamental rights and freedoms of the individual with regard to the application of biology and medicine'.[10] More specifically, Article 6(2) insists that 'the opinion of a minor shall be taken into consideration as an increasing determining factor in proportion to his or her age and degree of maturity'. Taken together these provisions would seem to provide useful support for the protection of the autonomous rights of mature young people. Furthermore, while breach of a Convention right conveys no direct cause of action, it may be used as an indirect cause of substance under actions brought under the Human Rights Act 1998.

It appears that the law that pertains to treatment refusals by competent minors is more pragmatic than principled. If a child has sufficient competence and maturity to consent to treatment then, arguably, those qualities ought to apply equally to treatment refusal. In sum, there is a period when young persons may consent for themselves but if they refuse treatment that is objectively considered to be in their best interests, then the court, or those with parental responsibility, may consent on their behalf.

10.4   Patients who lack capacity

Critically ill patients often lack capacity to make healthcare decisions and treatment must be given in their best interests. The Mental Capacity Act 2005 provides the legal framework for patients over 16, whereas the common law applies to younger children and infants. Nurses, with their unique insight and knowledge, can provide an invaluable perspective as part of the multi-disciplinary team in determining best interests.

10.4.1   Best interests: guiding principles

The principle of 'best interests' is used to determine which course of action, or decision, is best for the patient who lacks capacity, all things considered. It encompasses more than clinical aspects and includes wider welfare, social and emotional interests.

For adults, section 4(6) of the Mental Capacity Act 2005 provides a checklist of relevant factors to be considered. These include (as far as reasonably ascertainable):

(a)   the person's past and present wishes and feelings
(b)   the beliefs and values that would be likely to influence his decision if he had capacity
(c)   other factors that he would be likely to consider if he were able to do so.

Assumptions must not be made on the basis of irrelevant or discriminatory factors such as appearance, disability or behaviour, and decision-makers must consider the likelihood of the patient regaining capacity at some time in the future. There is a duty to consult others and to consider, as far as practicable, the views of anyone identified by the patient as someone who ought to be consulted on matters of this kind. Adults may have appointed a personal welfare attorney who can consent to, or refuse, treatment on their behalf following their loss of capacity (see section 10.5.6 below). Specific rules will apply where the patient has made an advance decision (see section 10.5.5 below).

For children who lack capacity, those with parental responsibility (see section 10.6.1 below) can consent to clinically indicated treatment that is in the child's best interests. A balancing exercise may be required where there are competing medical, emotional and welfare interests and the choice of treatment, if there is more than one, should be that which is least restrictive on the child's future options.

Where achievable, attempts to prolong life will usually be in a patient's best interests. However, this is not definitive and where the prognosis is hopeless account must be taken of the benefits, burdens and risks of treatment. In certain situations where initiation or continuance of treatment will achieve no medical effect it may be lawful to withdraw or withhold treatment, if such a decision is in the patient's best interests.

10.4.2   Disputes

Tensions can arise in critical care situations when relatives and health professionals disagree fundamentally about what is best for a patient. In these situations it might be worth delaying action until the dispute is resolved. The involvement of independent advocates, such as independent mental capacity advocates for adults (see section 10.5.8 below), or an external second opinion, may be helpful. In urgent situations, however, processes such as these can cause delays which are not in a patient's best interests and for these reasons a judgement call by the senior clinician may be required.

English law recognises that in the event of a dispute the role of the doctor is to determine the range of clinically indicated options while the role of the court is to ascertain the patient's best interests. Doctors are not compelled to provide specific treatments on the basis that they should not have to choose between their professional judgement and a court order (*Re J (aminor) (wardship: medical treatment)* (1990)). There is, however, an obligation to keep the patient's condition under regular review (*Wyatt* v. *Portsmouth NHS Trust* (2005)).

10.4.3   The Court of Protection

In the event of uncertainty, or dispute, the Court of Protection has authority to declare on the lawfulness of any act done, or to be done, in the best interests of an adult who lacks capacity (Mental Capacity Act 2005 section 15(1)(c)). For children, the court will use the statutory welfare checklist of section 1(3) Children Act 1989. A declaratory order permits the court to state the legal position in advance of an intervention, rather than passing judgment after the event.

Some healthcare decisions are of such significance that these can only be made by the Court (unless the patient has a personal welfare attorney (see section 10.5.6 below) or a valid advance decision (see section 10.5.5 below)). This includes the proposed withholding or withdrawal of fluids and hydration from a patient in a permanent vegetative state (PVS).[11]

10.5   Incompetent adults

Adults who lack capacity cannot give valid consent and in the absence of a valid and applicable advance decision, clinically indicated treatment is given under the doctrine of necessity in the patient's best interests.

10.5.1   Restraint and deprivation of liberty

Patients in critical care settings may require physical restraint or, more commonly, restraint by sedation either for their personal safety or to permit treatment to be given. In order to be lawful, health professionals who administer restraint must reasonably believe that this is necessary and that the length of time and amount used is proportionate to the likelihood and seriousness of harm (Mental Capacity Act 2005 section 6). If the level of restraint amounts potentially to a deprivation of liberty with the meaning of Article 5(1) of the European Convention on Human Rights, then additional safeguards are needed.

The deprivation of liberty safeguards are part of the legal framework of the Mental Capacity Act 2005 and are intended to protect people who lack capacity from being arbitrarily deprived of their liberty.[12] In critical care situations restraint will most often be used for therapeutic purposes in the patient's best interests, but where restraint is required to control the movement of patients, an early formal application according to institutional policy should be sought (*Cheshire West and Chester Council* v. *P* [2011]). Use of excessive restraint could leave health professionals open to a range of criminal or civil penalties or referral to the professional regulators.

10.5.2   Vegetative states

Patients who are in a vegetative state (VS) may not be 'critically ill' since appropriate care and the maintenance of nutrition and hydration (often by percutaneous endoscopic gastrostomy) can keep them alive for many years. The ethical and legal issues that can arise during care, however, reflect those associated with nursing critically ill patients more generally. Furthermore, in the event of a life-threatening emergency a decision whether to withdraw or withhold life-saving treatment may be required.

In *Airedale NHS Trust* v. *Bland* (1993) the House of Lords upheld a declaration that it would not be unlawful to withdraw nutrition and hydration from a teenager who had been left in a PVS following a hypoxic cerebral injury during the Hillsborough football stadium disaster in 1989. Although he could breath unaided, Anthony Bland's life was sustained by nasogastric feeding. A declaration was granted that it would not be unlawful for doctors to withdraw life-sustaining treatment, including tube feeding, on the grounds that there was no therapeutic, medical or welfare benefit in continuing treatment. It was held that although the sanctity of life was an important criterion, it was not absolute and would not compel continuation of treatment in all circumstances.

Nurses often regard the administration of nutrition and hydration to be aspects of basic care and which, by definition, should be provided unless a patient refuses, or where death is imminent. Nasogastric feeding, however, could be distinguished from basic care, since the former involved the application of a medical technique (*per* Lord Keith in *Bland*). The decision to withdraw nutrition and hydration was therefore a clinical decision, and doctors have no duty to provide futile medical treatment. The House of Lords recommended that the moral, social and legal issues raised in *Bland* ought to be reviewed by Parliament and that in the interim, life-sustaining treatment should be withdrawn from adults in VS only with the support of an anticipatory court declaration.

Following *Bland* a series of cases were heard. In *Frenchay NHS Trust* v. *S* (1994) the Court of Appeal heard arguments that questioned the diagnosis of a deeply unconscious patient following a severe drug overdose. His nurses were convinced that S suffered pain and there was some clinical evidence of voluntary behaviour. The hospital's application for a declaration was triggered following the disconnection of his nasogastric tube which required urgent replacement for his continued survival. Although the Official Solicitor appealed on the grounds of the uncertain diagnosis, the appeal was lost due to pressure of time. The court distinguished *Frenchay* from *Bland* in that an urgent decision was necessary. In the view of the court an emergency such as this meant that it was not possible to comply fully with the guidance in *Bland*. This decision is controversial on two counts: first, the diagnosis of PVS was equivocal, even though substantive diagnostic guidance has been available since 1996.[13] Second, the nasogastric tube could arguably have been reinserted to permit a more considered analysis of the issues. Since the law views withdrawal and withholding as being equivalent, there would have been little detriment in reinserting the tube to permit full consideration of the case followed by withdrawal, if indeed that decision was correct. Since *Bland*, the state of PVS has received considerable attention. Following the House of Lords' Select Committee on Medical Ethics recommendation, the Royal College of Physicians published *The Permanent Vegetative State*,[13] which was subsequently endorsed by the British Medical Association and the Official Solicitor.[14] The guidance includes several safeguards designed to protect the best interests of patients.

The cases that followed *Bland* revealed a willingness to permit withdrawal of treatment for conditions that fell progressively short of the guidance. In *Re D (medical treatment)* [1998] the court departed from the safeguard that an interval of at least twelve months ought to pass between the initial injury and diagnosis. D sustained a cerebral injury following an accident in September 1995 and in March 1996 was diagnosed as being in a PVS. The hospital's application that it would be lawful not to reinsert the dislodged nasogastric tube was granted even though the Official Solicitor's evidence suggested that D's condition did not satisfy the criteria for definitive diagnosis of PVS. The requirement that diagnosis of PVS should be confirmed by two independent doctors was breached in *An NHS Trust* v. *G* [2001] where the court relied on the evidence of one expert witness alone. The final safeguard expressed in *Bland* that significant weight should be given to the wishes of relatives was ignored in *Re G (Persistent Vegetative State)* [1995] where the court held that the mother's objections would not operate as a veto against a declaration that withdrawing life-sustaining treatment would be lawful.

10.5.3   The minimally conscious state

The minimally conscious state (MCS) describes those patients who show minimal, but definite, evidence of awareness albeit with profound cognitive impairment. In these situations cessation of treatment (which, according to *Bland*, includes nasogastric fluids and hydration) will be harder to justify than in VS. The decision made will depend upon expert opinion and the specific facts of each case. In assessing where a patient's best interests lie, the court will tend to adopt a balance sheet approach similar to that taken when deciding for infants (see section 10.6.2 below).

These principles were tested in *W and M* v. *An NHS Trust* [2011].[15] The Court of Protection was asked to declare on the lawfulness of withdrawing artificial nutrition and hydration from a woman who became minimally conscious after contracting viral encephalitis. According to relatives, M had always maintained that she would never want to be kept alive in such a condition. Although the law requires that account must be taken of previous wishes and feelings in the determination of best interests, M had not made a valid and applicable advance decision. Had she done so, the court would have abided by that decision. According to evidence, M's informal statements had not specifically addressed the question that the court had to consider. In these circumstances the factor which carried most weight was the preservation of life. The court held that while it was apparent that M experienced pain and discomfort, and she was severely restricted in what she could do, there was evidence that she had positive experiences and there was a reasonable prospect that those could be enhanced by a planned programme of stimulation therapy.

Recent evidence suggests that some patients who are in a VS or MCS may be able to communicate by means of functional imaging that detects covert cognitive processing. Experience with such techniques is still in its infancy but could have profound implications for the care of such patients.

10.5.4   Locked-in syndrome

Locked-in syndrome follows injury to the brainstem which interferes with voluntary control of movement, leading to complete paralysis of all (or almost all) voluntary muscles. Although consciousness is not usually interfered with, the Mental Capacity Act provides that if persons cannot communicate their decision, they must be treated as if they lack capacity. Recent developments in computer technology, in combination with eye-tracking devices, mean that some patients in locked-in syndrome are able to communicate, albeit slowly.

In *R (on the application of Nicklinson)* v. *Ministry of Justice* [2012] and *R (on the application of AM)* v. *Director of Public Prosecutions* (2012) two claimants with locked-in syndrome wished to end their lives but required the assistance of others in order to do so. In English law active measures taken with the intention of ending life are prohibited and amount to active euthanasia, or assisted suicide. Tony Nicklinson's argument was that in his circumstances voluntary euthanasia could be legitimately defended on the grounds of necessity. The other claimant, Martin, argued (on human rights grounds) that the Director of Public Prosecutions (DPP), the Solicitors Regulation Authority and the General Medical Council had a duty to clarify, in advance, their policies for prosecution and disciplinary action in cases of assisted suicide. The cases both failed on the basis that an affirmative decision would have had very significant consequences and would represent a major change in the law. It was therefore a matter for Parliament to decide, rather than the court. It was also held that the neither the DPP nor the regulatory bodies were under a legal duty to clarify their policies.

10.5.5   Advance care plans

Patients who are admitted to high-dependency units may have prepared for their own incapacity by producing anticipatory instructions to indicate the treatment they would seek to avoid in that eventuality. This is particularly likely for patients with chronic conditions such as progressive neurological disease or malignancy. These anticipatory instructions are known as 'advance care plans' and include advance decisions, statements of wishes and the instruction of personal welfare attorneys. Statements of wishes are not binding on health professionals, but they can provide useful evidence of the previously competent patient's values and choices.

Advance decisions can be made by competent adults to refuse medical treatment in the event of their future incapacity. Following a person's loss of capacity, a valid advance decision will be binding to the same extent as a contemporaneous refusal of treatment, provided that decisions to refuse life-sustaining treatment are in writing and have been signed and witnessed. Sections 24 and 25 of the Mental Capacity Act 2005 govern advance decisions, subject to a range of statutory requirements. First, in order to be valid, the person making an advance decision must be competent and over the age of 18. Second, the advance decision will be relevant only in those situations where the person lacks capacity to decide. Third, an advance decision will be binding in respect of refusals of care, but not in respect of positive requests for treatment. An advance request might provide a useful indication of which course of action will be in a patient's best interests, but it will not be decisive. An advance decision will not be valid if a lasting power of attorney has been created with authority over the same treatment to which the advance decision relates, or where the person has done anything else that is inconsistent with the advance decision remaining his or her fixed decision. Advance decisions can be revoked at any time provided that the person has capacity to do so.

It is the responsibility of the lead clinician, in collaboration with the multidisciplinary team, to decide whether an advance decision is valid and applicable. Where there is doubt, a declaration can be sought from the Court of Protection (section 26(4) Mental Capacity Act 2005). In the interim life-sustaining treatment can be commenced, or steps taken to prevent deterioration of the patient's condition in his or her best interests.

The case of *A Local Authority* v. *E and others* [2012] concerned an anorexic woman, E, who was dying imminently from her condition. She had twice attempted to make an advance decision to refuse life-sustaining treatment by way of force-feeding. The court found that E's obsessive fear of weight gain meant that she lacked sufficient capacity to make a valid advance decision and force-feeding would be in her overall best interests.

Following implementation of the Mental Capacity Act 2005 the first reported case on the validity of an advance decision was *X Primary Care Trust* v. *XB and YB* [2012]. XB had motor neurone disease and was maintained by an invasive ventilation device. Although he was unable to talk, he was able to use a communication board. In 2011 he made an advance decision (based on a pro forma downloaded from the internet) to refuse life-sustaining treatment in the event that he lost the ability to communicate. The document referred to the date of 2 May 2012 for the purposes of review. In 2012, after XB had lost the ability to communicate, two issues arose. First, concerns were raised by a carer that XB has not expressly consented to the advance decision. On the basis of the carer's concerns and the date for review, the primary care trust sought a declaration as to the validity of the advance decision. On the evidence it was apparent that the advance decision was valid. The carer had not been present at the time that the decision had been made and the date for review had not been consented to, nor discussed, with XB. The case finished on 1 May 2012 and Theis J. made the following observations:

(a) Issues that pertain to the validity of advance decisions should be investigated as a matter of urgency.
(b) There is no prescribed format for an advance decision but guidance from the Mental Capacity Act 2005 Code (paragraphs 9.10 to 9.23) should be followed.
(c) The implications of review dates in pro formas needed full consideration since these could inadvertently frustrate intentions.

10.5.6   Personal welfare attorneys

The Mental Capacity Act 2005 permits the appointment of proxy decision-makers to make health and welfare decisions for individuals following their loss of capacity. The authorising instrument is known as a healthcare and welfare lasting power of attorney (section 9(1)(a) Mental Capacity Act 2005). The formalities of conferring a lasting power of attorney are detailed in Schedule 1 of the Mental Capacity Act 2005 and the power will be ineffective unless these provisions are complied with. As with other proxy decision-makers, attorneys must make decisions in the best interests of the patient, while taking into account the likelihood of the patient regaining capacity at some time in the future. Attorneys can be empowered to take decisions about life-sustaining treatment if this is expressly included in the document. In critical care situations the personal welfare attorney will, for decision-making purposes, 'stand in the shoes' of the patient who lacks capacity.

10.5.7   Deputies

If a person lacks capacity in relation to a matter concerning personal welfare, and where time permits, the court may appoint a deputy (usually a relative or an official of the court) to make decisions that are in the person's best interests. The deputy may not refuse consent to life-sustaining treatment and may only act if the patient lacks capacity in respect of the decision to be made.

10.5.8   Independent mental capacity advocates

The role of the independent mental capacity advocate (IMCA) is primarily to support the 'un-befriended' patient who lacks capacity in circumstances where only a professional caregiver is available to determine his or her best interests.

In these circumstances an IMCA must be consulted when a decision needs to be made about serious medical treatment.

The instruction of an IMCA will also be necessary where carers believe that relatives or representatives are not acting in the best interests of a patient and that safeguards are needed to protect the patient from potential abuse. The IMCA process does not apply if treatment decisions are urgent. In these situations treatment must be given in the patient's best interests.

10.5.9   Do not attempt resuscitation orders

In the event of a cardiopulmonary emergency a decision must be taken as to whether to attempt one or more forms of resuscitation. Guidance is available from the Resuscitation Council *Resuscitation guidelines*.[16] If no explicit anticipatory decision has been made about whether cardiopulmonary resuscitation should be attempted, and the wishes of the patient are unknown, the presumption is that health professionals should make reasonable attempts to revive the patient.

In situations where a cardiac, or respiratory, arrest is anticipated the patient who is capable should be involved in the decision-making process. Summaries of the discussions and the outcome should be recorded in the patient's notes. If a decision is taken not to involve the patient, the rationale for doing so should also be documented carefully.

For the patient who lacks capacity the decision about whether to attempt resuscitation is based upon best interests (Mental Capacity Act 2005 section 4) and whether or not such efforts would be futile. Standard proforma documents are most commonly used in compliance with internal organisational governance policies and arrangements. Do not attempt resuscitation decisions should be the outcome of discussions with the multi-disciplinary care team (and the patient where possible) although responsibility for the decision lies with the lead clinician.[17] Factors that necessarily engage in the determination include human rights, equality legislation and organisational policy.

10.6   Incompetent children and infants

Young children and infants invariably lack decision-making capacity for treatment decisions and consent will be provided by a proxy who acts in the child's best interests.

10.6.1   Parental responsibility

The concept of 'parental responsibility' refers to the rights, duties, and powers that most parents have in respect of their children. Although parental responsibility may encompass the right to consent to treatment this is not invariable. In certain circumstances parental responsibility permits delegation of decision-making responsibility to others and in an emergency the person responsible for a child's care may do what is reasonable in order to safeguard, or promote, the child's welfare.[18] For a critically ill child consent will not be required to authorise urgent interventions although, where time permits, the consent of a person with parental responsibility should be obtained (*Gillick* v. *West Norfolk and Wisbech Area Health Authority* (1985); *Glass* v. *UK* (2004)).

Determining who has parental responsibility is not always straightforward. A woman acquires parental responsibility automatically following the birth of her child. The child's father may attain parental responsibility depending on when and where the child's birth was registered. He will acquire this automatically if he was married to the mother at the time of the child's birth, or subsequently. By comparison, an unmarried father cannot acquire automatic rights. Parental responsibility will be obtained if his name is recorded on the birth certificate (at registration, or re-registration),[19] if he acquires a parental responsibility order through the courts, or by virtue of a court-registered parental responsibility agreement with the child's mother.[20] The form of agreement is prescribed by law and must be recorded at the High Court in order to be valid. Civil partners acquire parental responsibility by the same routes and divorce does not extinguish parental rights. Parental responsibility may be acquired by a second female parent using equivalent procedures.[21] If both parents have parental responsibility the consent of either is usually sufficient in law, although consent from both may be necessary for procedures considered to fall within 'special categories', such as non-therapeutic interventions.

The implications are that an unmarried father's capacity to act as proxy for his child should be confirmed before his instructions are followed. If this seems officious it may help to remember that schools too have to explore this issue before accepting a father's authority over a pupil.

10.6.2   The best interests of infants and young children

The court's approach to determining a critically ill child's best interests has not always been consistent. Parental responsibility (see section 10.6.1 above) must be exercised in child's best interests with the guiding principle being the welfare of the child. Advances in clinical care means that restoring the health or sustaining the lives of young children and infants may be possible in situations previously considered to be hopeless. While respect for the sanctity of life is an overriding criterion when assessing a child's interests in some situations a palliative, rather than curative, approach might be best for a child.

In *Withholding and Withdrawing Life-prolonging Medical Treatment*[22] the British Medical Association asserts that the criteria for determining best interests for paediatric and adult patients are equivalent and include: the potential to develop awareness the patient's capacity and ability to interact with others; and whether the patient will suffer severe and unavoidable pain and distress. The guidance emphasises that the value of proposed treatment is to be assessed and not the value of the child.

The Royal College of Paediatrics and Child Health in *Withholding or Withdrawing Life sustaining Treatment in Children*[23] identifies five situations in which palliative, rather than life-sustaining, care might be considered. Where a child is brain dead or in a vegetative state (see section 10.5.2 above) this would be permissible as well as in circumstances where there was 'no chance,' 'no purpose' or where further treatment would be 'unbearable'.[23] While the first and second categories seem relatively uncontroversial, the latter presents considerable scope for disagreement between health professionals and relatives. Although guidelines are not law, they have had direct influence on judicial thinking in several cases. *Re C (a minor) (medical treatment)* (1998) concerned a severely ill infant with spinal muscular atrophy, a terminal condition characterised by recurrent respiratory arrest. She nevertheless appeared to interact meaningfully with her parents. Medical opinion was that further ventilation was futile and not in her best interests and that further resuscitation would inflict needless suffering. C's parents, who were orthodox Jews, consented to the withdrawal of ventilation provided that this would be recommenced if their daughter suffered respiratory distress, a precondition which was not agreed to by the clinical team. To resolve the dispute the health authority applied for a declaration that treatment withdrawal would be lawful. In granting the declaration the court held that although the sanctity of life was a fundamental consideration, it was not determinative in the context of a child's suffering.

A body of case law has developed on account of 'no purpose' situations. Patients typically include children who may survive indefinitely with medical intervention but whose continued survival is believed to be accompanied by severe pain and suffering. An early decision was *Re J (a minor) (wardship: medical treatment)* [1991]. J was profoundly disabled and his doctors believed that he was blind, deaf and would be unable to develop speech. He had a limited life expectancy and was likely to develop spastic quadriplegia. J would, however, experience pain and discomfort to the same extent as other infants. In assessing whether the withholding of further aggressive treatment would be in J's best interests, the court considered the distress caused by re-ventilation, the likelihood of further deterioration and his general prognosis. The 'critical equation' was the child's quality of life as balanced against the very strong presumption in favour of life preservation. The court granted the declaration on the basis that prolonging life was considered to be intolerable to J.

This judgment, and others like it, can be criticised for the relative importance given to doctors' opinion about an infant's quality of life. Psychologists, physiotherapists, teachers and respite centre staff are among those who could, arguably, have been better placed than neonatal intensivists as to whether a disabled child might learn to interact meaningfully with others, or at least derive some satisfaction from life. But unless such experts are already involved with the care of a young patient, they are unlikely to be called upon to give evidence to the court. Potentially valuable insights and perspectives might therefore be neglected and the basis for the court's assessment of future quality of life could therefore be incomplete.

For situations where further life-sustaining treatment is considered to be 'unbearable' according to Royal College guidance, the courts have moved away from a frank *Bolam* approach. The concept of 'intolerability' has also assumed less importance. In *Wyatt v. Portsmouth NHS Trust* [2005] a profoundly brain damaged infant, Charlotte, was blind, deaf and unable to move. Her condition was described as 'terrible' and further aggressive treatment was considered to be intolerable. Her parents, however, disagreed and argued that every effort ought to be made to protect the intrinsic value of her life. In granting the hospital's declaration that it would be lawful to withdraw invasive treatment, Hedley J described the concept of 'intolerable to that child' as being a valuable guide to the determination of best interests. Instead of dwelling on the disadvantages of further invasive treatment, he emphasised the intrinsic benefits of withholding aggressive interventions such as increased opportunities for parental contact and the enhanced likelihood of a more tranquil death. The Court of Appeal supported this approach in rejecting that intolerability, or any other single test, should determine what is in the best interests of a patient who lacks capacity. This approach has been followed subsequently (*Re L (medical treatment: benefit)* [2005]; *Re B (A Child) (Medical Treatment)* [2008]; *An NHS Trust* v. *H* [2013].

Since *Wyatt*, it appears that the concept of intolerability will be part of a wider consideration of factors that contribute to a child's overall welfare.[24] In undertaking best interests assessments the perceptions of nurses and others with substantial contact with the child will be vitally significant. The case of *An NHS Trust* v. *MB* (2006) concerned a two-year-old with severe spinal muscular atrophy, a degenerative and progressive condition. At the time of the proceedings MB was unable to use his muscles in an age-appropriate way, although he was capable of barely perceptible movements of his face and extremities. In assessing his best interests the court used a 'balance sheet' approach and included the analysis in the judgment. It was held that at present the balance lay in favour of continued life-sustaining treatment on the grounds of a net balance of benefit from continued life which included a relationship of value with his parents. In the future, when the benefits of treatment withdrawal outweighed the benefits of continued life, MB should be allowed to die. Labelling his life as 'intolerable' was considered to be unhelpful, and a careful assessment of where the balance of MB's interests lay was preferred.

In contrast, in *Re K (a minor)* [2006], *MB* was distinguished in that the six-month-old had no accumulated experiences that were comparable with those of MB. The judge considered that in the context of K's pain, distress and discomfort which was unrelieved by the pleasure of eating, there was no realistic evidence of her experiencing the simple pleasures of life. It was therefore held that withdrawal of total parenteral nutrition accompanied by palliative support would be in her best interests. Similarly, in *Re OT (a child)* [2009] no treatment escalation was appropriate for a ten-month-old child who retained little awareness but who nevertheless experienced profound distress caused by invasive life-sustaining procedures. A useful overview of the current law was given in *An NHS Trust* v. *Mr and Mrs H & Ors* [2012].

10.6.3   Family disputes about treatment

Where parental responsibility for a child is shared, to what extent will the consent from one individual suffice for the purposes of the law? Section 2(7) of the Children Act 1989 provides that each of them may act alone and without the other. Nevertheless, the Court of Appeal has ruled that some decisions should not be acted upon unless everyone with parental responsibility agrees.[25] These include non-therapeutic elective procedures such as circumcision, rather than typical treatments that are likely to be necessary for the care of critically ill children. Caution suggests that for non-urgent and irreversible procedures the consent of all those with parental responsibility should be obtained, or else a referral to the court where there is conflict.

10.6.4   Disagreements between relatives and health professionals

Where parents and health professionals disagree fundamentally as to which course of action is in a child's best interests, resolution may be achieved by obtaining a second opinion, involving a neutral third party, an independent advocate, by arranging a multidisciplinary case conference, or review by an independent ethics committee. However, where serious and intractable disagreement concerns life-sustaining treatment, legal advice should be sought by applying to the court for adjudication. The views of the nursing team are likely to be influential.

Although the courts' intrusion into family life could be seen as unjustified state interference, it may be necessary 'for the protection of health or morals, or for the protection of the rights and freedom of others' (Article 8(2) European Convention of Human Rights). The safeguarding of a child's physical, psychological or emotional welfare is considered to be a legitimate basis for court intervention.

The failure of an NHS trust or health authority to refer a case involving disputed treatment might be regarded as an infringement of the Article 8(1) right to respect for private life and the person's physical and psychological integrity. In *Glass* v. *UK* (2004) the European Court of Human Rights reviewed the Portsmouth Hospitals NHS Trust's management of a 12-year-old patient with severe mental and physical disabilities. During an emergency admission for a respiratory tract infection, his doctors concluded that he was in a terminal phase of lung disease and commenced a diamorphine infusion for palliative purposes and made a 'Do Not Resuscitate' order. The judges were not persuaded by the Trust's contention that there had been no time for an emergency application to be made for a declaration of best interests and held that the decision to overrule the mother without court backing was a violation of Article 8.

Disputed treatment decisions that concern critically ill children are frequently litigated. *Re D (wardship: medical treatment)* (2000) concerned a young boy with severe and irreversible lung disease, heart failure, hepatic dysfunction, renal disjunction and learning difficulties. The trust's decision that withholding artificial ventilation in the event of respiratory, or cardiac arrest, would be in D's best interests was strongly disputed. The High Court, in granting the declaration, considered that the benefits of a relatively short extension of life were outweighed by the distress caused by aggressive treatment. By contrast, in *Re T (a minor) (wardship: medical treatment)* (1997) the child's parents objected to medical intervention. T was diagnosed with biliary atresia and doctors recommended a life-saving liver transplant. Previous surgery had been undertaken and the subsequent pain and distress persuaded his parents that further major surgery ought to be withheld. Since no consensus could be reached between independent experts and T's parents (who were also health professionals), the case was referred. The High Court's decision that a transplant would be in T's best interests was overturned on appeal on the basis that a short but happy life, ending in a peaceful death, would not be a worse option than 'a lifetime of drugs and the possibility of further invasive surgery'. The court concluded that the views of the parents should be determinative. Although in *Re T* the persuasive 'broader considerations' were submitted by the parents, it will often fall to the nurse to alert others to relevant factors and concerns.

An example of profound conflict between health professionals and parents was apparent in *Re A (conjoined twins: surgical separation)* [2000]. Jodie and Mary were both considered to be live born individuals despite Mary having a virtually non-functioning heart and lungs and being almost entirely dependent on Jodie for her existence. Surgical separation would allow Jodie to survive but would result in the immediate and unavoidable death of Mary. The health authority sought a declaration from the court following parental refusal of consent based on devout religious convictions. The Court of Appeal ruled that surgery would be lawful even though this would inevitably cause the death of Mary. Although the court stressed that this landmark decision was specific to the unique facts of the case, it remains controversial since surgical separation (a positive act) was the direct cause of Mary's death.

This decision is difficult to reconcile with established legal principle. According to English law active euthanasia is murder and good motives do not provide an excuse. The Court held that Mary's Article 2 right to life under the European Convention of Human Rights was not infringed, since the surgeons did not 'intend' to cause Mary's death. For the purposes of Article 2 the meaning of 'intention' was restricted to those situations where it was the state's purpose to cause death. Instead, the purpose of surgery was to save the life of Jodie.

10.6.5   Neglecting the medical needs of children

Where the medical needs of children are neglected by those with parental responsibility, the latter forfeit their right to make treatment decisions. If time permits, the case should be referred to the court for adjudication and if necessary a referral can be arranged within hours. In more urgent situations treatment may be provided in the best interests of children, since safeguarding and promoting their welfare is an integral aspect of health care. Nurses should be alert to the potential difficulties that can arise in sensitive situations that could result in conflict. Anticipatory reference to policy statements and professional guidance is advised.

Where a decision is made to withhold or withdraw treatment on the grounds of best interests or that continued treatment is futile, the obligation to preserve life will be deemed to be discharged. The well developed communication and interpersonal skills of nurses can be of considerable benefit in defusing the tensions, disagreements and misunderstandings that may accompany these situations. Nurses are often uniquely placed to mediate positively between patients, their families and other health professionals in critical care decision-making.

10.7   Resources

Critical care is a resource-intensive speciality and publicly funded health services cannot provide state-of-the art treatment for all. Priorities have to be set and the courts have been reluctant to become embroiled in decisions that concern allocation of health care resources on the basis that matters of policy ought to be determined by Parliament.

The case law reveals that exceptions are not necessarily made even for critically ill patients whose continued survival depends upon treatment being available.[26] Nevertheless, the courts have often found sufficient procedural irregularities to overturn resource decisions that have been made. At local levels, use of resources should be monitored by nurses as part of their duty to ensure a safe environment of care. Concerns should be reported using appropriate channels and guidance is available from the Nursing and Midwifery Council Code of Professional Conduct.[27] The Code requires nurses to inform those in authority where circumstances are such that nurses are prevented from working to professional standards. Concerns should be raised in writing where environmental issues put patient care or welfare at risk.

Legal issues that are commonly associated with health care can be heightened when caring for critically ill patients. The overarching duty to safeguard and preserve life may at times need to be tempered against a patient's best interests. Being alert to legal and professional developments is a vital component of a competent approach to nursing critically ill patients.

10.8   Notes and references

1. National Institute for Health and Clinical Excellence, 'Critical Illness: Rehabilitation after a Period of Critical Illness' Clinical Guideline 83 (London, NICE, 2009).
2. Department of Health, Statistical Press Notice (London, Department of Health, 2012). (Available at: http://mediacentre.dh.gov. uk/2012/10/26/statistical-press-notice-monthly-critical-care-beds-cancelled-urgent-operations-and-delayed-transfers-of-care-data-england-september-2012-and-revisions-for-january-2012-august-2012/).
3. Re T (Adult) [1992] 4 All ER 649 per Lord Donaldson.
4. This is apparent from a range of authorities: Re C (Adult, refusal of treatment) [1994] 1 All ER 819; Re MB (Adult, medical treatment) [1997] 38 BMLR 175 CA; St George's Healthcare NHS Trust v. S; R v. Collins and others, ex parte S [1998] 3 All ER 673; Re T (Adult) [1992] 4 All ER 649.
5. Re MB (Adult, medical treatment) [1997] 38 BMLR 175 CA.

6. Nursing and Midwifery Council, *The Code: Standards of Conduct, Performance and Ethics for Nurses and Midwives* (London, Nursing and Midwifery Council, 2008). (http://www.nmc-uk.org/Documents/Standards/nmcTheCodeStandardsofConduct PerformanceAndEthicsForNursesAndMidwives_LargePrintVersion.PDF).

7. *R (on the application of Burke)* v. *General Medical Council* [2006] QB 273.

8. See *Re S (a minor) (consent to medical treatment)* [1994] 2 FLR 1065, *Re C (detention: medical treatment)* [1997] 2 FLR 180 and applied recently in *A Primary Care Trust* v. *P, AH and A Local Authority* [2008] 2 FLR 1196.

9. Royal College of Nursing, *Restrictive Physical Intervention and Therapeutic Holding for Children and Young People. Guidance for Nursing Staff* (London, Royal College of Nursing, 2010). (Available at: http://www.rcn.org.uk/__data/assets/pdf_file/0016/312613/003573.pdf).

10. Preamble to the Convention on Human Rights and Biomedicine, 4 April 1997.

11. The Mental Capacity Act Code of Practice provides guidance on the interpretation of the Act. Details of situations that must be referred to the Court of Protection for adjudication are found in para. 8.18. The Code can be accessed at http://www.justice.gov.uk/downloads/protecting-the-vulnerable/mca/mca-code-practice-0509.pdf.

12. The DoLS Code of Practice provides a range of examples and detailed guidance at http://www.dh.gov. uk/prod_consum_dh/groups/dh_digitalassets/@dh/@en/documents/digitalasset/dh_087309.pdf.

13. Royal College of Physicians, The permanent vegetative state. *Journal of the Royal College of Physicians*, **30** (1996), pp. 119–21.

14. Royal College of Physicians, *The Vegetative State: Guidance on Diagnosis and Management* (London, Royal College of Physicians, 2003). (http://bookshop.rcplondon.ac.uk/contents/47a262a7-350a-490a-b88d-6f58bbf076a3.pdf).

15. *W (by her litigation friend, B) and M* v. *An NHS Trust* [2011] EWHC 2443 (Fam).

16. Resuscitation Council (UK), *Resuscitation Guidelines* (2010) http://www.resus.org.uk/pages/GL2010.pdf.

17. Resuscitation Council (UK), *Decisions Relating to Cardiopulmonary Resuscitation: A Joint Statement from the BMA, the Resuscitation Council (UK) and the Royal College of Nursing* (London, Resuscitation Council (UK), 2007). (available at: http://www.resus.org.uk/pages/GL2010.pdf).

18. Children Act 1989, section 3(5).

19. From 1 December 2003 (in England and Wales), from 15 April 2002 in Northern Ireland and 4 May 2006 for Scotland.

20. Children Act 1989, section 4.

21. Children Act 1989, section 4ZA.

22. English V. *Withholding and Withdrawing Life-prolonging Medical Treatment, 3rd end* (Oxford, Wiley-Blackwell, 2007)

23. Royal College of Paediatrics and Child Health, *Withholding or Withdrawing Life-saving Treatment in Children: A Framework for Practice, 2nd edn* (London, Royal College of Paediatrics and Child Health, 2004).

24. Despite what was said about intolerability in *An NHS Trust* v. *MB and Wyatt*, the Nuffield Council on Bioethics report *Critical Care Decisions in fetal and neonatal medicine: ethical issues* (2006) refers to 'intolerable' lives.

25. *Re J (Specific Issue Orders: Child's Religious Upbringing and Circumcision)* [2000] 1FLR 571 at 577 (d).

26. See, for example, *R* v. *Central Birmingham Health Authority, ex parte Walker* [1987] BMLR 32; *R* v. *Cambridge Health Authority, ex parte B* [1995] 2 All ER 12 (CA). *R (Rogers)* vv. *Swindon Primary Care Trust* [2006] 1 WLR 2649, *R (Otley)* vv. *Barking & Dagenham NHS*

Primary Care Trust [2007] EWHC 1927 and *R (Ross)* vv. *West Sussex Primary Care Trust* [2008] EWHC 2252.

27. Nursing and Midwifery Council, *The Code: Standards of conduct, Performance and Ethics for Nurses and Midwives* (London, Nursing and Midwifery Council, 2008). (http://www.nmc-uk.org/Documents/Standards/nmcTheCodeStandardsofConduct PerformanceAndEthicsForNursesAndMidwives_LargePrintVersion.PDF).

B   An Ethical Perspective

Robert Campbell

Pro Vice Chancellor (Academic), University of Bolton, Greater Manchester

10.9   Introduction

Why does the treatment of critically ill people pose particular problems? Patients with a strong chance of recovery and a clearly indicated and effective treatment present us with few ethical issues. What challenges us are cases where it is unclear what treatment will be effective or, indeed, if any treatment would be. Unfortunately, it is often in those very cases where we need to communicate clearly and sensitively with patients that we also find that they are too ill, frightened or bewildered to hear and understand what is being said. Sometimes this can be compounded by the patient's situation; the very young, the very old and those with communication or learning difficulties all pose particular challenges for those whose responsibility is to care for them.

As has rightly been noted, the responsibility of care can also create legal liability, and nurses and other related professionals owe a duty of care to their patients which, legally and, arguably, morally, goes far beyond what we normally owe each other as a matter of course. This can mean that our liability extends far beyond what we may feel comfortable with into areas with which our training has not really equipped us to deal. Ethics can help to shed some light on these areas, make them a little less unreal and give us opportunities to rehearse our responses to them.

10.10   Consent

We begin with consent because it is absolutely basic to medical care. In law to touch someone without their consent is a battery, and hardly any medical or nursing care or treatment, is possible without physical contact. For everyday treatments like having a tooth filled or an eye examination, consent is both presumed and implicit in the patient's simply being there. For more complex, unusual or potentially dangerous interventions, more formal procedures are needed to establish consent. This is because both the law and morality (and common sense) assume that consent involves more than just saying 'yes'. To consent in any real sense you must know what you are consenting to and your consent must be genuine, that is, unforced. In the case of *Re T (adult: refusal of treatment)* (1992) T had signed a form of refusal of consent to blood transfusions (on religious grounds). She'd been told there was an alternative to a blood transfusion, but the form was not read out to her, nor was there any discussion of the possible consequences of her refusal. The court held that this refusal of consent could not be relied on when subsequently T lost consciousness in intensive care and needed a transfusion to survive. It could not be relied upon because the evidence that T really understood what she was refusing was not convincing.

If I were to get you to sign the bottom of a blank sheet of paper on which I then type a deed of gift which transfers all your worldly wealth to me, then no one would suppose that this constituted a genuine agreement. You did not realise that you were agreeing to anything, let alone that you were agreeing to that. In the same way, a patient must understand the nature of the treatment proposed if any verbal or written declarations are to count as genuine consent. What counts as 'understanding the nature of the treatment' is more complicated, but courts have held, quite reasonably, that it involves more than simply being told what will be done. In particular, it also involves having some understanding of the likely consequences of the treatment – and as *Re T* showed, of refusing it – and of how likely they are.

Consent to treatment is problematic for many critically ill patients for two reasons. First because their condition may make it hard for them to express consent, or it may mean that they are not able to give consent at all (because they are unconscious, or no longer capable of full consent – see sections 10.10.2 and 10.11 below). Or second, because deciding on an appropriate course of treatment may not be a wholly clinical issue. Sometimes a particular procedure becomes less and less effective each time it is performed, and the benefit to the patient declines correspondingly. This can be especially true of palliative or symptomatic care, which does nothing to arrest an underlying condition. At some stage a judgement must be made that the benefits are now too negligible or too heavily outweighed by the discomfort of the treatment or its possible side-effects. Equally, a treatment may be uncertain or risky and, although the degree of uncertainty may be a medical matter, the question of whether the risk is worth taking is not. Aggressive chemotherapy may give a patient with advanced cancer an outside chance of a remission, but will it be worth the severe discomfort the treatment will certainly cause? In matters of life or death some might think that any chance, however remote, is worth taking. Others could, quite reasonably, disagree.

10.10.1   Why does consent matter?

The job of the therapeutic team is to do their best for the patient, given the resources at their disposal. It is also, of course, their legal and moral duty once the patient has been accepted as a patient. And it is hard to see how the patient, unless in some way deranged, can object to this. Doesn't everyone want the best for themselves? Why do we need their consent? There are four major reasons.

The first is related to the issue raised at the end of the previous section and has to do with expertise and the authority that goes with it. Most would agree that, normally, medically trained staff are more likely to know what the likely outcome of a given intervention or treatment will be. That knowledge gives them an authority which is the basis of the trust we place in them. However, judgements to do with how much risk is worth taking or how much pain or discomfort may be bearable in order to gain a benefit in the future lie outside that area of expertise. The expertise in these matters, and hence the authority, lies with the person who has to take the decision. (See also the fourth reason below.)

The second is located in the idea of a *person*. Most human beings are persons and most persons are human beings, but the terms do not have the same meaning.[1] A human being is a member of a particular biological species; a person is a moral agent who has plans and purposes and the capacity for free choice. From the point of view of personhood, all persons are morally equal in as much as there is no inherent reason for preferring one person's plans and purposes to another's. It is not possible for everyone to realise each one of their plans. What I want may conflict with what you want, may even make it impossible for you to get what you want. This is why we need mediation, compromise, negotiation and, eventually, law. But such procedures do not ignore a person's moral agency. On the contrary, they only make sense when they are addressed to a person as someone capable of making choices and acting on them.

Disregarding a patient's right to consent to or to refuse treatment ignores the fact that the patient is an agent and assumes that your plan to treat a patient in a particular way is the only plan that matters. It is, in Kantian terminology, to treat the patient as a means to an end and not as an end in herself. It, therefore, fails to accord that patient the respect and dignity due to a person whose moral importance is as great as your own. And if you believe that your plans and choices are important, then you must allow that other people's are equally important. To fail to do so is illogical as well as insensitive.

The third reason why consent matters has to do with human psychology rather than logic or morality. A patient whose agreement to treatment has been sought and obtained will feel empowered in a number of ways. First, they will *own* the treatment as an equal member of the team which has decided on it. They will be acting, rather than acted on. Second, they will be less apprehensive about what will happen since, if the agreement is real and not just stage-managed, they will understand what is involved and its implications. And third, they will have retained control over their situation and, in situations where people are profoundly vulnerable and probably distressed, this is clearly, and in some cases literally, vital. They will feel, and be, *autonomous*; and since that term means no more than being a free moral agent, a person, this second point connects us back to the first again. It is also important to see that this process of empowerment will go on whether the patient agrees with the proposed course of treatment or whether they refuse it.

The fourth reason why consent matters has to do with human fallibility. People can be wrong and, in particular, they can be wrong about what is good for another person. The medical team is composed of experts in various fields, but the only person who is an expert on what is good for me is me. Fallibility can come in here too, admittedly. I can be wrong about what is in my own best interests. We all know that can happen. But I am less likely to be wrong about it than someone else is because I'm an expert on me and I have, as well, an incentive to get it right which no one else has. I will bear the consequences – good or bad.[2] It is, therefore, vitally important that when decisions need to be taken about what will be good for me, I take them, even though I may need expert advice from others. What this means, in practice, is that I must have the opportunity to decide whether to accept the treatment offered, even though others may feel that I am wrong in the decision I come to.

10.10.2   Refusing treatment

It is clear that, in English and US law,[3] I have the right to refuse treatment, however unreasonable this may seem to someone else. Treatment carried out against my wishes would, in theory, ground an action for battery. What is less clear is how far I have the right to decline treatment when such treatment is, or is likely to be, life-saving. For, in practice, the refusal of life-saving treatment is often regarded as *prima facie* evidence of an inability to give or withhold consent on a rational basis.[4]

This is not entirely unreasonable. Declining to have dental treatment or a hip replacement is not only, as I have argued, your business, but it also leaves you around afterwards to change your mind. Declining life-saving treatment does not. This is not just a practical issue. For if the moral importance of consent has to do with autonomy, that is, self-determination, then choosing a course of action which you know is highly likely to result in your death seems inconsistent with this. Self-determination disappears when there is no self left to determine. Perhaps we can merely pass over this as a puzzling oddity, since there are many other examples of it which we accept quite readily: people who risk their lives, and lose them, in the attempt to help others; people who choose death rather than the violation of a principle or value which seems to them more important that their own lives; and people who rationally choose to commit suicide. Counselling this latter category does, however, raise some practical difficulties also thrown up in dealing with those who refuse life-saving treatment. For the general principle that people should make their own decisions and learn from their own mistakes cuts a little too deeply here. If choosing suicide or refusing treatment turns out to have been a mistake, then it is, in the nature of things, too late to learn anything from that. Just as consent can only be genuine if the patient fully understands what she is consenting to so, equally, the decision to refuse life-saving treatment should only be respected if there is no doubt at all that the patient fully understands that and what she is refusing. (See the discussion of *Re T (adult: refusal of treatment)* (1992), above.)

10.11   Capacity

This last point is related to both knowledge and understanding. Clearly, I cannot be said to have consented to something if I am kept in ignorance of, misled about or simply fail to understand its nature. Doctors, like any other group with specialist knowledge, are perfectly capable of explaining something in such a way that no non-specialist could hope to understand it. This is rarer than it used to be and most doctors at least understand that it is something they should strive to avoid. Nonetheless, it is not always easy to explain a complicated matter in terms which are both perfectly clear to the lay-person and, at the same time, both accurate and complete. Nor are patients always very good at admitting that they have not completely understood and would like it explained again. It is *always* possible, in other words, for anyone to give apparent consent which is undermined by lack of knowledge or genuine understanding. There are, however, classes of people for whom consent is problematic not in specific cases but in general. These are people who, in legal terminology, lack the *capacity* to give consent, not because they *don't* understand, but because they *can't* and can't be brought to understand. Small children are an obvious example. It isn't that they cannot make choices, but that they do not understand the world well enough to realise what their choices might imply. Their developing knowledge means that they are gradually better able to understand and, therefore, more and more able to give consent which is real and informed. Capacity is, in other words, not something which either exists or does not. It is a gradual thing. Children can be in a position to be told or consulted about what may happen without being ready to take the final decision for themselves. Or else they may be ready to take decisions in some areas but not in others. In practice, the law's willingness to allow young people under 18 to make treatment decisions will rest on the seriousness of those decisions. Equally with adults, it can be true that capacity can be diminished or partial.

For example, there is the case of *T*, where the court decided that a refusal of treatment was made under the undue influence of the patient's mother and that there was reason to believe that the patient did not fully understand its implications. There might be enormous difficulty in determining this kind of issue. In the US case of Mary C. Northern,[5] she was described by the guardian appointed for her by the court as '. . . 72 years of age . . . [and] . . . in possession of a good memory and recall, responds accurately to questions asked her, is coherent and intelligent in her conversation and is of sound mind.' She was suffering from gangrene in both feet consequent upon frostbite and burns, but refused to have the feet amputated, as her surgeons were urging her to. Though otherwise apparently entirely rational, it emerged in conversation that she very much wanted to live AND very much wanted to save her feet. She did not seem able to grasp that there was only a one in ten chance that both things could happen and resolutely refused to consider, except as abstract hypotheses, that she would have to choose between them. The court decided to authorise surgery, apparently accepting the view that an otherwise apparently competent adult might, nonetheless, be incompetent in the matter of one specific decision. In the light of the transcripts, which are too lengthy to quote here, this would seem to have been the right decision. Mary Northern seems to have combined a general rational competence with a pathological block with regard to the condition of her feet, which she believed had got better and about which her physicians were lying or mistaken.

Consider this, imaginary, case:

Carla, aged 30 and pregnant, has been admitted to hospital with ruptured
membranes and in spontaneous labour. If natural labour is allowed to continue, there is a grave risk of rupture of the uterus due to the position of the
foetus. The life of the foetus is also in danger and the medical team wish to
perform a section immediately. Carla, who is in great pain and very worried
about losing her baby, nevertheless refuses the caesarean on religious grounds.
Carla is an evangelical Christian, but not a Christian Scientist or a Jehovah's
Witness, and none of the chaplaincy team is aware of any other Christian sect
which might object to this procedure.

Is this a rational refusal of consent to treatment? May we characterise Carla as
an otherwise rational patient with a pathological block about Caesarean sections?
We might wish to argue that she is not irrational; she simply has beliefs which
the rest of us do not share but cannot disprove. But Mary Northern's irrationality,
in the end, came down to her refusal to give up a belief about the condition of
her feet which no one was able to prove to her was false. There is no easy answer
to the question of what makes belief irrational. It may help resolve the problem
of distinguishing non-standard religious beliefs from those of people like Mary
Northern that Mary Northern's came from nowhere, that they were ungrounded
by anything apart from what seems to be a desperate attempt to wish the circumstances other than they actually were. Most religious beliefs do form a
system, they are shared by large numbers of people and are culturally transmitted – they have rational validation even if not by those who do not share them.
This is hardly conclusive, but it is persuasive.

10.11.1   Balancing rights and duties

There is another factor here, however, which is disquieting. The mother's refusal
of treatment did not just involve herself, but her unborn baby. The case of *Re S*[6]
raises the issue of how far a person's refusal of treatment can be allowed to
impact on a third party. For it is clear that the judgement arrived at in that case
(where a full-term foetus in a transverse lie threatened the life of both foetus and
mother) turned on consideration of the welfare of the foetus, as well as the
rationality of the mother's decision. Whatever the legal position, this cannot be
ducked. The foetus was at term. The law may not recognise the rights of an
unborn child, but morally it would be curious to assert that a foetus at term is
in any significant way different from a newborn baby. What might be arguable
is whether its life may be saved at the cost of what has been called 'a massive
intrusion into a person's body',[7] that is, a Caesarean section. In a parallel US case,
that of Angela Carder, the original decision to permit the Caesarean section was
overturned on appeal, and Angela Carder's parents won undisclosed damages
from the hospital in a separate action for medical malpractice, wrongful death
and violation of civil rights. In that case neither the mother nor the child survived
the operation. Though the mother was suffering widespread and irreversible
cancer of the bone and lungs, the death certificate listed the Caesarean as a contributing factor.[8]

A Caesarean section is a major surgical intervention, with all the risks and dangers that that involves. It would seem unreasonable to *require* someone to take those risks in order to benefit someone else. In a US case, the courts ruled that someone cannot be forced to donate bone marrow (a procedure considerably less risky than a Caesarean section) even where failure to do so would result in the death of a third party (because only one person could be found who was tissue-type compatible).[9] But it does not follow that that person had no *moral* obligation to be a bone-marrow donor, nor that we may not think badly of them for ducking it. Nor is there an exact carry-over from that case to *Re S*. Those who willingly become pregnant have, in doing so, already accepted a degree of responsibility for the welfare of the child they carry. And a Caesarean section is not so dangerous or unusual an intervention that it is obvious that no one could be expected to risk it. Nor are the declared grounds for refusal as coherent as they may seem. The couple in *Re S* were reported as believing that a Caesarean was against their principles as born-again Christians. According to the *Guardian*, most evangelical Christians would not share the view that a Caesarean section was impermissible and would, indeed, advocate one if the child's life was at risk, and Jehovah's Witnesses do not object to Caesareans as long as they do not involve blood transfusions.[10]

Here there is clearly a balance to be struck between anyone's right to refuse life-saving treatment and the rights of the unborn child (which must have some moral force even if not normally recognised in English law). There must also be a question mark, though perhaps not more than that, over the coherence of the reasons given. These considerations ought to affect what happens when treatment is refused, or indications given that it will be. For a refusal in the circumstances of *Re S* will not be accepted at face value. Efforts will and should be made to explain the consequences of the refusal and to persuade the patient to reconsider. It would be desirable, in such a case, to ask for the patient's spiritual adviser to offer counselling. If the patient is simply mistaken about what his/her religious beliefs require, then the situation could be resolved at this stage without resort to law.

Such a reaction to a refusal of treatment can only be properly understood in terms of our moral disquiet about the decision taken and/or the reasons for it. But though there are good moral reasons for wishing to oppose such a decision, it may well be that there are equally good policy reasons for not giving that opposition legal force. We may, in other words, disagree, perhaps profoundly, with the decision without thinking that it would be right to enforce another course of action on the patient. And, clearly, there are excellent reasons for thinking that a general policy of enforcing Caesarean sections on unwilling women would be an extremely bad thing.

10.12   Advance directives

As mentioned above, it can happen that patients are no longer capable of consenting to treatment. This may be because of mental or physical deterioration or both. In such cases treatment becomes a matter of what the health care team consider to be in the patient's best interests. Ordinarily it might be thought that such a situation would be eased if there exists what has come to be called an 'advance directive'. This could take the form of anything from a simple statement ('If it comes to it, I don't want to be kept alive as a vegetable') to the much more formal 'living will' comparatively common in the USA. A living will can be of two kinds. There is the simpler formal declaration of the circumstances in which you would no longer wish further treatment, for example. There is also a durable power of health care attorney which, effectively, nominates a proxy to take decisions on your behalf should you no longer be able to yourself.[11] A simple living will can be problematic. First of all, it is invariably hypothetical ('this is what I want *if* the following circumstances apply . . .') and also general rather than specific. This is inevitable since, in writing a living will we are trying to anticipate what might happen rather than dealing with an actual situation. What it means, however, is that it may still be difficult to determine how the will was meant to apply since the circumstances will necessarily not be precisely those envisaged. This is especially true if the will maker is not – and most of us are not – medically qualified or knowledgeable. There is also a problem of timescale, and for two quite different reasons. The first is perhaps the most obvious one and it is that treatments may change in the interval between drawing up the will and it coming into operation. Someone who anticipates that they would rather be allowed to die than undergo a particular kind of treatment might well have opted differently had they known the extent to which that treatment had improved. The second has to do with change in personal identity over time. To what extent it is reasonable for a younger version of me to legislate on what will be in the best interests of an older me? I might, by the time it is necessary, come to have taken an entirely different attitude to risk-taking, for example. Or I might have become an entirely different person.

Dworkin[12] cites the case of Margo, someone with Alzheimer's disease who 'despite her illness, or maybe somehow because of it, [. . .] is undeniably one of the happiest people I have known. There is something graceful about the degeneration her mind is undergoing, leaving her carefree, always cheerful.'[13] This is an unusual consequence of Alzheimer's disease which, more often, leaves people anxious, confused and profoundly disoriented. But that is the point. Had Margo considered the prospect of dementia and executed an advance directive, she might well have decided that she would not wish to receive treatment for any other life-threatening illness once she was suffering from Alzheimer's. Had she done so, and the relevant situation had arisen, would it be better to respect the autonomy of the person Margo had once been and comply with the wishes set out in the advance directive? Or would it be better to address the best interests of the person Margo now is, and treat her for any adventitious, life-threatening illnesses unless and until her Alzheimer's deteriorated much further?[14]

10.12.1   A right to die

Is there a right to die? We have seen that a competent patient (i.e. someone who understands his or her situation and can make appropriate decisions) has the right to refuse treatment even where that may shorten their life. Equally, suicide was decriminalized in 1961.[15] However, assisting a suicide is still illegal, the rationale being, presumably, that if it weren't, it would be too easy for someone who intended murder to put this as a spurious defence. This doesn't mean that genuinely assisting a suicide is morally wrong, and one can easily imagine cases where it wouldn't be obvious that it was.[16] But there is the difficult question of what counts as assistance – providing the means, encouraging, giving advice, practical support? This was Diane Pretty's question when she asked the Director of Public Prosecution (DPP) to rule on whether her husband might be prosecuted for helping her to travel to Switzerland where physician-assisted suicide would have been available to her. She suffered from motor neurone disease and feared that, by the time she was ready to travel to Switzerland, she would be unable to do so without the assistance of her husband. Both the House of Lords and the European Court of Human Rights supported the DPP's refusal to give any such assurance,[17] though the DPP's most recent Policy[18] issued in February 2010, makes it clear that, in cases where: 'the actions of the suspect may be character-ised as reluctant encouragement or assistance in the face of a determined wish on the part of the victim to commit suicide', it is unlikely that there would be a prosecution in the circumstances Diane Pretty envisaged. It is ironic, therefore, that she died before this policy was formulated.

It is also perhaps ironic that the growing public acceptance that, in some cases at least, giving assistance of some kind to someone who is determined to die (if that is what the Policy cited above does) is probably attributable to medical sci-ence's ability to keep people alive for much longer than was the case more than 50 or 60 years ago. For it is arguable that in some cases, such as chronic and degenerative illness of the kind from which Diane Pretty suffered, the fact that we are able to defer death is not an obvious benefit, since we cannot restore health, even partially. It is clearly a highly subjective matter whether one prefers an earlier death or more years of life in increasing discomfort, and perhaps the strongest argument for assisted suicide is that it would allow people to make choices which accorded with their preferences.

10.12.2   Withdrawing treatment

Consent to or refusal of treatment is not the only problem in this area. There can be patients from whom treatment can be withdrawn, on the grounds that they are, in fact, dying and it would be considered neither proper nor humane simply to prolong the dying process. Both the American and British Medical Associa-tions endorse this view, as do the Catholic and Anglican Churches, and it is, for the General Medical Council, clearly a part of good medical practice:

> Life has a natural end, and doctors and others caring for a patient need to recognise that the point may come in the progression of a patient's condition where death is drawing near. In these circumstances doctors should not strive to prolong the dying process with no regard to the patient's wishes, where known, or an up to date assessment of the benefits and burdens of treatment or non-treatment.[19]

The cessation of the employment of extraordinary means to prolong the life of the body when there is irrefutable evidence that biological death is imminent is the decision of the patient and/or his immediate family.[20]

In its narrow current sense, euthanasia implies killing, and it is misleading to extend it to cover decisions not to preserve life by artificial means when it would be better for the patient to be allowed to die. Such decisions coupled with a determination to give the patient as good a death as possible, may be quite legitimate.[21]

. . . normally one is held to use only ordinary means . . . that is to say, means that do not involve any grave burden for oneself or another . . . Consequently, if it appears that the attempt at resuscitation constitutes such a burden for the family that one cannot in all conscience impose it upon them, they can lawfully insist that the doctor should discontinue those attempts and the doctor can lawfully comply.[22]

The distinction between deliberate killing and the administration of painkilling drugs or the withdrawal of treatment such as to have the effect of shortening life, though sometimes a very fine one in practice, must remain a guiding principle.[23]

It is widely believed that this position involves drawing a moral distinction between active and passive euthanasia. Many people seem to think, if they think that euthanasia can be justified at all, that it can be more readily justified if it is passive rather than active. Many people also seem to think that, whereas English law strictly forbids active euthanasia, it does, sometimes, allow that passive euthanasia may be permissible. Both doctors and lawyers talk as if they believe that this is so. For example:

A Down's syndrome child is born with an intestinal obstruction. If the obstruction is not removed, the child will die. Here . . . the surgeon might say 'As this child is a mongol . . . I do not propose to operate; I shall allow nature to take its course'. No one could say that the surgeon was committing an act of murder by declining to take a course which would save the child.

A severely handicapped child, who is not otherwise going to die, is given a drug in such amounts that the drug itself will cause death. If the doctor acts intentionally, then it would be open to the jury to say: yes, he was killing, he was murdering that child.

There is an important difference between allowing a child to die and taking action to kill it.[24]

No paediatrician takes life; but we accept that allowing babies to die – and I know the distinction is narrow, but we all feel it tremendously profoundly – it is in the baby's interests at times.[25]

This is potentially most misleading, and should not be taken at face value. I am not a lawyer, and the law in this area is complicated, but it is perfectly clear that being passively responsible for someone's death is, *in itself*, no defence in law to a charge of either murder or manslaughter. Bonnyman was a doctor who realised that his wife was exhibiting all the symptoms of diabetes, and he refrained from telling her. Thinking that she merely had a particularly bad bout of influenza, she did not seek treatment and died. Dr Bonnyman was found guilty of manslaughter by criminal negligence.[26] There are many other such cases. Pitwood was a level crossing keeper who failed to close the gate when a train was approaching and was held to be responsible for the deaths that ensued;[27] Gibbins and Proctor were found criminally responsible for the death of their child whom they had failed to feed;[28] Stone and Dobinson were convicted of manslaughter for the neglect of a dependent relative who died in their care.[29]

English law holds that murder and manslaughter, specifically, are crimes which can be committed either by act or omission. Of course, where a death is caused by someone's action, it is usually relatively easy to identify the responsible agent. He or she is the one who performed the action in question. But who is responsible when someone dies as a result of a failure to act? The responsible agent here is anyone who failed to act *when they had a legal duty to act*. According to one authority,[30] this duty can arise either through a contract, a special relationship (such as parent and child or doctor and patient) or where a person has voluntarily undertaken the care of another. But in a famous case – *Donoghue* v. *Stevenson* – Lord Atkin held that I owe a duty of care to '. . . persons who are so closely and directly affected by my act that I ought reasonably to have them in contemplation as being so affected when I am directing my mind to the acts or omissions which are called in question'.[31] This definition of the duty of care is so much more comprehensive that it is perhaps fortunate that it is only applicable in civil – tort – cases. Either way, it is clear that health care teams owe a duty of care to their patients and that wanton or reckless neglect of that duty which results in death can lead to a criminal prosecution for murder or manslaughter. Why, then, did the House of Lords, in the case of *Bland*[32] authorise the non-treatment of the patient when it was known that it would lead to his death?

Tony Bland was a victim of the Hillsborough football disaster. As a result of his injuries, he was comatose and remained in what is known as a persistent vegetative state until 1993, when his parents applied through the courts for permission for artificial nutrition and hydration to be withdrawn. The courts held that artificial nutrition and hydration was a form of treatment. They also held that, in view of the extreme unlikelihood of Mr Bland's ever regaining consciousness, the treatment was of no benefit to him and withdrawing it would take the form of a legal omission rather than commission, that is, the medical team had no duty to continue to treat Mr Bland.

The arguments were as follows:

(1)   A doctor is under no duty to continue to treat a patient where such treatment confers no benefit on the patient.
(2)   Being in a persistent vegetative state with no prospect of recovery was regarded by informed medical opinion as not being a benefit to a patient.
(3)   The principle of the sanctity of life was not absolute, for example:
  –   where a patient expressly refuses treatment, even though death may well be a consequence of that refusal
  –   where a prisoner on hunger strike refuses food and may not be forcibly fed
  –   where a patient is terminally ill, death is imminent and treatment will only prolong suffering.

(4)   Artificial hydration and nutrition required medical intervention for its application and was widely regarded by the medical profession as medical treatment.

The governing principle here was not that it was permissible to let a patient die so long as he/she was not actually *killed*. It was rather that *caring* for a patient (in cases where cure was not possible and recovery was extremely unlikely) did not require medical interventions which were of no benefit to the patient. But it is also clear that the treatment in question was not a *disbenefit* to Bland. If it did him no good, it also did him no harm. If doctors were under no duty to continue to treat Bland, they were also under no duty not to. But there was a benefit – to Bland's relatives and friends, especially his parents, who were to be spared the grief of continuing to see their son in this exceptionally distressing condition and would, finally, be able to mourn the loss they had suffered two years before. That is not a negligible benefit, by any means, and if, whatever happened, nothing more could be done to harm or benefit Bland himself, it seems right to let the choice of outcome be decided by what would most benefit those closest to him.

But it is interesting to compare the case of Tony Bland with that of Cox. Dr Nigel Cox was found guilty of attempted murder in 1992 for administering a lethal dose of potassium chloride to a patient, Lilian Boyes, who, dying and in acute pain, had pleaded with him to help her die. It is indeed, hard to see how, on the face of it, this case is to be distinguished from that of *Bland*, without invoking the distinction between active and passive euthanasia. The remarks of Butler-Sloss L.J. in the Court of Appeal hearing of *Bland* would seem to do just that.

> The position of Dr Nigel Cox, who injected a lethal dose designed to cause death, was different since it was an external and intrusive act and was not in accordance with his duty of care as a doctor. The distinction between Mr Bland's doctors and Dr Cox was between an act or omission which allowed causes already present in the body to operate and the introduction of an external agency of death.[33]

The *Guardian*'s leader writer called that position a 'philosophical nonsense' (20/11/92) and maybe it is, if taken at face value. What is not true is that there is no other morally relevant distinction to be drawn between the two cases. What follows should not be seen as implying any criticism of Dr Cox who, it would seem, was placed in an extremely difficult situation and, in all good faith, was probably doing what he believed was the only thing he could do to help Ms Boyes. But whether Cox's decision was the right one in the circumstances (and I, inevitably not knowing all the relevant information, am inclined to think it was), the explanation for its rightness must be different from the explanation of the rightness of withdrawing treatment from Tony Bland.

The source of this distinction is an old notion thought by many to be now discredited called 'the principle of double effect'. It should, I think, be seen not as a rule for resolving moral problems but as a guide which can clarify what is at issue in particular cases. It relies on a distinction between what one intends and what one merely foresees as a result of one's actions. The principle suggests that, whereas one is fully responsible for what one intends to do, one is not responsible for foreseen but intended effects of one's actions, provided that:

(1) What is done must be, at the least, morally permissible.
(2) What is intended must include only the good and not the bad effects of what is done.
(3) The bad effects must not be the *means* whereby the good is brought about.
(4) There must be *proportionality* between the good and bad effects of what is done.

Whereas Dr Cox must have intended Lilian Boyes' death as the only way as he saw it of sparing her further pain and suffering, the medical team treating Tony Bland intended to spare him further suffering (or at least to spare his relatives, given that Tony Bland himself may have been aware of nothing at all), while foreseeing that this would probably lead to his death. This distinction may have no practical consequences in those two actual cases, given that both led to the death of the patients concerned. It matters, nonetheless, insofar as they are treated as precedents for action in future cases which may be similar, but will be never be precisely the same.

I do not believe that passive euthanasia is permissible because it is merely a matter of allowing a patient to die rather than acting in order to bring about their death. But I do believe that in cases where the patient's death is imminent or where treatment is painful and offers only a very remote chance of success, then it is justifiable, if the patient and/or her relatives consent, to cease to continue treatment.

Moral responsibility for an event is not determined by whether it came about because one acted or failed to act; it is determined by one's intentions and duties. If there is no duty to treat, and also persuasive reasons for not doing so, it must normally be entirely permissible to withdraw treatment, even if to do so results in the death of the patient.

So what about Dr Cox? Clearly, he cannot be excused on these grounds, for they do not apply to his case. What can be said is that it is possible to imagine circumstances where the suffering of the patient is so great and the possibility of immediate remedy so small that killing the patient is the only available means of preventing the pain. In national disasters or wars such circumstances may arise, or in parts of the world where medical resources are extremely limited. In those circumstances it is possible that acting so as to bring about the death of the patient as easily and quickly as might be would not be wrong. It may be that those were the circumstances in which Nigel Cox found himself. Without being a part of the situation, it is impossible to say. It must be a matter of judgement and one which I hope never to have to exercise. For that reason it cannot be said conclusively that what Cox did was wrong, but, also for that reason, it is also a matter which the law, on policy grounds, can never permit.

10.13   Notes and references

1. For example, it has been doubted whether babies, foetuses, or those who, while still biologically alive, lack any response to the world around them are persons in the strict

sense of the term. (See Robert F. Weir, *Abating Treatment with Critically Ill Patients* (New York, Oxford University Press, 1989), pp. 70–1 and 405–12.) It can also be argued that higher apes and cetaceans (dolphins, porpoises and whales) might conceivably be persons in the required sense. (See Peter Singer, *Practical Ethics* (New York, Cambridge University Press, 1979), passim.) A useful survey of this debate can be found in Hugh LaFollette, *Ethics in Practice*, 3rd edn, (Oxford, Blackwell, 2007), Part II, sec. 14–17.

2. For a more complete, and classic, exposition of this view, see John Stuart Mill, *On Liberty*. (There are many editions of this, but a good recent one which includes critical essays is edited by John Gray and G.W. Smith, *J.S. Mill on Liberty In Focus* (London, Routledge, 1991).

3. This is also heavily stressed in many professional codes of conduct. See, for example, the Nursing and Midwifery Council, *The NMC Code of Professional Conduct: Standards for Conduct Performance and Ethics* (London, NMC, 2008).

4. See Margaret Brazier, *Medicine, Patients and the Law*, 5th edn (London, Penguin, 2011), Chapter 6.

5. John Arras & Nancy Rhoden (eds), *Ethical Issues in Modern Medicine*, 3rd edn (New York, McGraw-Hill, 1989), pp. 72–9.

6. See *Re S (a minor) (consent to medical treatment)* [1994] 2 FLR 1065.

7. Judge John Terry, in the case of Angela Carder (district of Columbia Court of Appeals, 1990), the US case cited in evidence in *Re S*. Compare his remarks with the argument put by Judith Jarvis Thompson, A defense of abortion, *Philosophy and Public Affairs*, **1** (1) (1971), pp. 57–66; that a pregnant woman is no more *necessarily* responsible for the welfare of the foetus she is carrying than she is for anyone else's welfare. She may owe it a duty of care if she is responsible for its being there, but that duty has limits, and she is not obliged morally to risk her life for it. See also Anton Tupa (2009), Killing, letting die, and the morality of suicide, *Journal of Applied Philosophy*, **26** (1) (Feb 2009).

8. See the *Guardian*, 20 October 1992, p. 23.

9. See R. Campbell & D. Collinson, *Ending Lives* (Oxford, Blackwell, 1988), p. 174.

10. See the *Guardian*, 14 October 1993, p. 3.

11. See also the Mental Capacity Act 2005, sec. 9, Shaun D. Pattinson, *Medical Law and Ethics* (London, Sweet and Maxwell, 2006), Chapter 14 and Jean McHale and Marie Fox, *Health Care Law*, 2nd edn (London, Sweet and Maxwell, 2007), pp. 1078–82.

12. R. Dworkin, *Life's Dominion: An Argument about Abortion, Euthanasia, and Individual Freedom* (New York, Vintage Books, 1994), p. 218.

13. A.D. Firlik, Margo's logo. *Journal of the American Medical Association*, **265** (1991), p. 201. Quoted by R. Dworkin (1994), *op. cit.*

14. R. Dresser, Dworkin on dementia: elegant theory, questionable policy. *Hastings Center Report*, **25** (1995). See also D. Degrazia, Advance directives, dementia, and 'the someone else problem', *Bioethics*, **13** (5) (1999), pp. 373–391.

15. Jean McHale & Marie Fox, *Health Care Law*, 2nd edn (London, Thomson, 2007), p. 1001.

16. R. Campbell & D. Collinson, *Ending Lives* (Oxford, Blackwell, 1988), ch.5.

17. Shaun Pattinson, *Medical Law and Ethics* (London, Thomson, 2006), p. 490.

18. *Policy for Prosecutors in Respect of Cases of Encouraging or Assisting Suicide*, CPS 2010.

19. General Medical Council (2002) *Withholding and Withdrawing Life-Prolonging Treatment: Good Practice in Decision-making*, para. 12.

20. *Journal of the American Medical Association* (1974), 227.

21. Church of England National Assembly (Board for Social Responsibility) (1975) *On Dying Well*, Church Information Office, p. 10 and the *Guardian* 20 November 1992, (leading article).

22. Pope Pius XII, *The Pope Speaks*, 4, no. 4, p. 396.

23. Principles endorsed by the House of Bishops of the Church of England in October 1992, as cited by David Sheppard in a letter to the *Guardian*, 27 October 1992.
24. *Obiter dicta* in the case of *Arthur* (1981), taken from trial transcripts cited by H. Kuhse, A modern myth . . ., *Journal of Applied Philosophy*, **1** (1), pp. 21–38
25. Expert testimony from consultant paediatricians in the case of *Arthur* (1981), cited in D. Brahams & M. Brahams, The Arthur case, *Journal of Medical Ethics*, **9**, pp. 12–15.
26. (1942) 28 Cr App 131.
27. (1902) 19 TLR 37.
28. (1919) 13 Cr App Rep.
29. [1977] QB 354, [1977] 2 All ER 341.
30. R Card, R Cross & PA Jones, *Introduction to Criminal Law*, 17th edn (Oxford, Oxford University Press, 2006), p. 32. See also Dennis Barker, *Glanville Williams: Textbook of Criminal Law*, 3rd edn (London, Sweet & Maxwell, 2012), sec. 12.3.
31. [1932] AC 562.
32. (1993) 2 WLR 316.
33. Court of Appeal: *Airedale NHS Trust* v. *Bland*, December 9, 1992.

11 Clinical Governance

A   The Legal Perspective

Vanessa L. Mayatt

Director, Mayatt Risk Consulting Ltd, Cheshire

11.1   The advent of clinical governance

Several decades ago the corporate world on both sides of the Atlantic had to contend with a series of organisational developments that ranged from embarrassing to disastrous. These developments called into question how well companies manage their financial affairs and their businesses in general. Thus the organisational problems encountered at Polly Peck, Maxwell, Enron and others not unexpectedly fuelled the drive for a more rigorous approach to organisational management. This led to the current requirements for governance that are now an integral part of the day-to-day running of large private organisations on both sides of the Atlantic.

In response to this corporate turbulence, a series of reviews were undertaken with the intention of identifying what steps organisations should take to implement good practice in corporate governance. Each successive review built upon the principles of the previous one, so that collectively they helped shape the

Nursing Law and Ethics, Fourth Edition. Edited by John Tingle and Alan Cribb.
© 2014 by John Wiley & Sons, Ltd. Published 2014 by John Wiley & Sons, Ltd.

current approach to corporate governance and the requirements for internal control. These requirements are set out in the Combined Code[1] that companies listed on the London Stock Exchange seek to comply with.

The Combined Code is concerned with the establishment of corporate objectives, identification of the risks to the achievement of those objectives and a system of internal control to ensure that business failure does not happen. It is therefore concerned with the management of risk and the integration of risk management into the day-to-day running of businesses. In simple terms corporate governance is about moving away from firefighting to a more proactive approach to managing risk. While compliance with the Combined Code is voluntary, the pressure on companies to make positive statements in their published annual reports on their arrangements for governance and internal control is sharply felt. The arrangements are subject to close scrutiny by internal and external auditors, as well as by company risk management groups that are usually led by a board member.

To a large extent the developments in corporate governance in the private sector have been mirrored in the public sector. The health care sector has, like the corporate world, experienced a series of high-profile incidents that have called into question how well hospitals, trusts and other health care providers are managed, and how well clinicians are treating and providing care to patients. The circumstances surrounding the death of hundreds of Harold Shipman's patients, the multiple deaths of babies at Bristol Royal Infirmary and the failures in the cervical cancer screening services at Kent and Canterbury hospitals are all evidence of the failure both of individuals and of the health care system in which they work. The lessons from these major incidents, set out in official Inquiry Reports, have, in conjunction with other incidents, shaped the current expectations for clinical governance and the management of risk. These expectations are not unlike those relating to private companies.

The public sector has its own 'Combined Code', in the shape of HM Treasury's Orange Book, *Management of Risk: Principles and Concepts*.[2] The Treasury document recognises the link between the management of risk, the successful delivery of business objectives and meeting the needs of stakeholders. Audit committees in public sector organisations, including the health care sector, use the Orange Book to determine their strategy for managing risk and develop their arrangements for internal control. External auditors, such as the National Audit Office (NAO), also use the Treasury guidance to judge how well public sector organisations are governed.

In the health care sector, governance includes the arrangements for clinical governance. The guidance *Clinical Governance in the New NHS*,[3] published in 1999, defined clinical governance as 'a framework through which NHS organisations are accountable for continuously improving the quality of their services and safeguarding high standards of care by creating an environment in which excellence in clinical care will flourish'. Clinical governance had been described as akin to organisational conscience and the 'beating heart' of care, encapsulating an organisation's responsibility for the delivery of safe, high-quality patient care.[4]

11.2   The development of clinical governance

In the early 1990s, following the formation of NHS trusts, the concept of clinical risk management was taken forward in the UK health care sector. The evidence for the nature and extent of clinical risk came from clinical negligence claims, complaints about clinical experience and patient outcomes, and improving arrangements for clinical incident reporting in NHS trusts. In a typical trust at that time, reported clinical incidents demonstrated the magnitude of drug errors, the multitude of ways that drug errors arose, and poor clinical decision-making and clinical practice, all leading to unacceptable patient outcomes. It was clearly the case that while the vast majority of patients were well served by the health care sector and the dedicated staff it employs, there was clear evidence of some fundamental organisational problems concerning the quality of patient care provision. This evidence fuelled the drive for better quality and clinical governance.

In the late 1990s, the consultation document *A First Class Service: Quality in the New NHS*[5] set out the arrangements for improving the quality of health care provision. The main elements of the document concerned:

- national standards for services and treatments
- local delivery of high-quality health care
- effective monitoring of progress by the newly established Commission for Health Improvement (CHI) – now the Care Quality Commission (CQC)
- a national survey of patient and user experience.

This development was a part of the agenda to modernise the NHS, and clinical governance was viewed as a central part of this strategy. Clinical governance was synonymous with the drive for improved quality in health care. The document stated that the principles of clinical governance were applicable to all involved in the provision or management of NHS patient care. It also set out the accountability of trust chief executives for assuring the quality of service provision on behalf of trust boards.

In 1999 this consultative document[5] was followed by the introduction of a statutory duty for the quality of health care provision under the Health Act. Under the legislation, trust chief executives became ultimately responsible for assuring the quality of health care provision. In the following year, an independent inquiry was established in the light of the Harold Shipman case. Part of the inquiry's remit was to consider what changes were necessary to existing systems to safeguard patients in the future. This led, in 2003, to the General Medical Council requirement for the periodic revalidation of doctors.

11.3   Clinical governance now

In the 1990s, NHS trusts and other health care organisations almost universally developed separate arrangements to manage clinical and other areas of risk.

While this enabled individuals within organisations with relevant expertise to come together to analyse specific areas of risk and make informed decisions about what improvements were necessary, it led to a fragmentation of approach to managing risk and to some duplication of effort. The expectation, in time, for integrated governance was therefore right, as this meant that areas of risk were no longer dealt with in silos and governance arrangements were streamlined as a result.

In 1999 a five-year vision for clinical governance was set out in *Clinical Governance in the New NHS*.[3] This included an expectation that there would be cultural change, a shared commitment to quality, participative working with stakeholders, multidisciplinary team-working and leadership at board level. The guidance set a number of targets for trusts, health authorities and primary care groups. During 1999/2000 these bodies were expected to:

- identify lead clinicians for clinical governance and establish appropriate structures for overseeing clinical governance
- agree a process and timescale for conducting a baseline assessment of capability and capacity for implementing clinical governance and thereafter produce an action plan
- report clinical governance arrangements within their Annual Reports.

These expectations were underpinned by the requirement for a comprehensive programme of quality improvement, which for trusts included the participation of hospital doctors in audit programmes, routine application of evidence-based practice and continuing professional development (CPD) programmes. These are therefore some of the main components of clinical governance.

The National Audit Office summarises the key principles of clinical governance as follows:

- a coherent approach to quality improvement
- clear lines of accountability for clinical quality systems, and
- effective processes for identifying and managing risk and addressing poor performance.

The NAO envisages that this involves putting into place arrangements and systems so that there is early identification and analysis of problems, and action is promptly taken to prevent repetition.[6]

In 2004 the Department of Health (DH) introduced integrated governance as a means of developing a more integrated approach to the management of all risks, while combining the principles of clinical, management, financial and corporate accountability. This was followed in 2006 by the publication of the DH's *Integrated Governance Handbook*.[7] The guidance defines integrated governance as 'systems, processes and behaviours by which Trusts lead, direct and control their functions in order to achieve organisational objectives, safety and quality of service and in which they relate to patients and carers, the wider community and partner organisations'. Integrated governance is therefore concerned with managing risk so that organisational objectives can be delivered and the needs of stakeholders can be met. While the words are not the same, the meaning is no different from HM Treasury's requirements for managing risk or indeed the requirements of the Combined Code.[1,2] The DH guidance contains an expectation that all health care organisations will have best practice arrangements in place for integrated governance and that these arrangements will function across all health care communities and clinical networks.

Following the change of administration, the 2010 White Paper *Equity and Excellence: Liberating the NHS*[8] has taken the quality agenda further forward. The paper sets out the Government's long-term plan for the NHS in England and its overall goal for an NHS which achieves results that are among the best in the world. In relation to quality and governance, the paper:

- enables patients to rate hospitals and clinical departments for quality of care provided
- requires hospitals to be open about mistakes
- requires increased focus on health outcomes and the quality standards that deliver them
- requires the NHS to be held to account against clinically credible and evidence-based outcome measures.

Changes to accountability arrangements are also set out in the White Paper, doubtless driven by the major failings at Mid-Staffordshire of both the trust and the regulatory bodies involved. An independent NHS Commissioning Board will be established and will be accountable for health outcomes and allocation of resources in addition to taking a lead on quality improvement. This Board will therefore play a key role in the governance and quality arrangements within the NHS in England. The paper expands the role of NICE and the Care Quality Commission as can be seen in the next section of this chapter; it also extends the role of Monitor from regulating Foundation Trusts to that of an economic regulator with additional responsibility for safeguarding continuity of service provision.

The Department of Health has created the National Quality Board (NQB) which met for the first time in March 2009. This Board will also play a key role in taking forward aspects of the White Paper requirements, particularly concerning quality. The Board is described as having a role in relation to championing quality and ensuring alignment on quality matters throughout the NHS. The White Paper sets in train major changes to the delivery and commissioning of health care. The NQB has a key role during the transition period. Clearly a particular challenge for the Board will be ensuring that quality and patient safety is not jeopardised during a period of major change for the NHS in England.

In February 2010, the NQB produced a report, *Review of Early Warning Systems in the NHS*,[9] which looked at the way in which the NHS should prevent and take action in relation to serious failures in quality. The reviews into the serious failings at Mid Staffordshire NHS Foundation Trust had unearthed breakdowns in the structure and governance arrangements within the trust which had led to a lack of focus on quality in the organisation. The 2010 NQB report not surprisingly identified the need for further guidance for boards on governance. This further guidance was published by the NQB in March 2011: *Quality Governance in the NHS – A guide for provider boards*.[10] The aim of the publication is to clarify for provider boards what are good governance arrangements so that they can more effectively drive continuous improvement and ensure that levels of quality and safety are met.

There is now a statutory requirement for NHS health care providers in England to produce Quality Accounts. The regulations for Quality Accounts (NHS (Quality Accounts) Regulations 2010) came into force in April 2010. Under the legislation, health care providers are required to publish their Quality Account annually. The first were published in June 2010 and covered activity for 2009/10. For 2010 the requirement related to acute, mental health, ambulance and learning disability NHS trusts. Pilot exercises highlighted the extent of reliance on Primary Care Trusts (PCTs) and Strategic Health Authorities (SHAs) necessary for primary care organisations to produce Quality Accounts to a good standard. The statutory duty for Quality Accounts to be produced by primary care providers was, in consequence, deferred until June 2012 and covered the period 2011/12. Primary care organisations were encouraged to produce Quality Accounts for 2010/2011 but there was no statutory requirement for them to do so.

The Health and Social Care Act 2012 resulted in the abolition of primary care trusts and also strategic health authorities. The legislation in relation to quality accounts has been amended to reflect these organisational changes within the NHS. Parts of the National Health Service (Quality Accounts) Amendment Regulations 2012 came into force on 4 February 2013 and the remaining parts on 1 April 2013. The amended legislation requires that providers send their draft quality accounts to the NHS Commissioning Board or a clinical commissioning group in addition to any local healthwatch organisation.

Quality Accounts are essentially reports about the quality of services provided by a NHS health care provider; they are published electronically both on NHS Choices and on the providers' website and are also sent to the Secretary of State for Health. Quality Accounts are regarded as the means by which trusts:

- demonstrate their commitment to continuous, evidence-based quality improvement
- set out, for the benefit of patients, where they need to improve
- receive challenge and support from local scrutineers on what they are trying to achieve
- are held to account by the public and local stakeholders for the delivery of quality improvements.

A further recent change has been the creation of the National Director for Improvement and Efficiency post. The post-holder has a responsibility for providing advice to help the NHS to deliver its quality (and other) commitments. Another layer to the current quality agenda is the Quality, Innovation, Productivity and Prevention (QIPP) programme. This is essentially an engagement programme for clinicians, NHS staff and patients to address, at local and national levels, the quality and productivity of care provided.

So what are the implications of the current focus on quality for clinical governance? The NQB regards clinical governance as mainly being the focus of clinicians and clinical managers in NHS trusts. It recognises that clinical governance is widely accepted within the NHS and that it concerns the culture, structure and processes necessary to assure and improve the quality of care provision. As the focus of both managers and clinicians is the same – the delivery of the highest-quality health care – the distinction between quality governance and clinical governance is claimed by the NQB to be less relevant.[10] It can, however, be argued that all the elements of quality and clinical governance do not precisely coincide. This point is illustrated by the elements that comprise quality, as set out by Lord Darzi:

- effectiveness of the treatment and care provided to patients
- the safety of treatment and care provided to patients, and
- the experience patients have of the treatment and care they receive.[11]

The NQB correctly regards the boards of provider organisations as ultimately responsible for the quality of the care delivered. It is the responsibility of boards to create the right organisational culture and to have arrangements in place for measuring and monitoring quality. While the words may be different, this is no different from requirements on boards as set out in the Combined Code for the private sector and HM Treasury's Orange Book as discussed at the beginning of this chapter.[1,2]

In government, health policy is, with some exceptions, a devolved responsibility. The structure of the NHS together with the governance and regulatory arrangements does therefore vary; thus the commissioning and provision of health care by the NHS in Scotland, Wales and Northern Ireland is different from England. Similarly accountability arrangements are also different, as are the existence and role of regulators. Legislation that impinges on the health care sector in England has no bearing outside of England. Clearly, there are areas of mutual interest across all countries, such as GP contracts and vaccinations, and such interests are normally addressed by collaboration between the UK health departments.

The country differences can be illustrated by looking at the delivery of health care in Scotland where 14 area NHS boards are responsible for running the NHS in Scotland. There are now no NHS trusts in Scotland. The Boards each have two main structures within them – operating divisions and community health partnerships. The former have taken on the responsibilities of previous NHS trusts in Scotland, and the latter are responsible for planning and delivering primary care and community-based services. NHS boards are held to account by Scottish Government Ministers for:

- 'HEAT' targets
- national guidelines and standards
- annual accountability reviews.

'HEAT' is an acronym relating to **h**ealth improvement, **e**fficiency and governance improvements, **a**ccess to services and **t**reatment appropriate to individuals. HEAT targets therefore include clinical governance.

The arrangements for regulation and inspection are also different in the other UK countries from England. This again is illustrated by the arrangements in Scotland where there are two key bodies – NHS Healthcare Improvement Scotland (HIS) and the Healthcare Environment Inspectorate (HEI). HIS sets standards for care and treatment and then inspects the performance of Boards against the standards. HIS has no enforcement powers other than in relation to independent healthcare providers. The findings of HIS inspections are fed into the annual accountability reviews of Boards. HEI is a part of HIS and is responsible for inspecting hospital compliance with health care-associated infection standards. HEI undertakes two inspections of each Scottish hospital during a three-year period; one inspection is announced and the other is not.

A recent development in Scotland is important to consider in the context of clinical governance. In February 2011, the Scottish Parliament passed a Bill concerning the rights of patients. The Patient Rights (Scotland) Act 2011 received Royal Assent in March 2011 and makes provision for the rights of patients when receiving health care. The Act has yet to be fully enacted but when it is, there will be legal requirements for:

- Scottish Ministers to produce a Charter of Patients' Rights and Responsibilities
- NHS bodies to uphold health care principles
- treatment to be started within the maximum waiting time.

Patient rights under the legislation are for health care to:

- be patient focused
- provide optimum benefit to health and well-being
- allow and encourage patient participation in decision-making.

Patients will also have the right to give feedback, comments, raise concerns or complaints about health care received.

11.4   The role of health care bodies in clinical governance

There are a number of organisations who work in conjunction with the health care sector in England and have a remit for clinical and quality governance. They each have related and in some instances overlapping roles. The following provides a summary of the remit and functioning of four health care bodies:

- Care Quality Commission
- National Patients Safety Agency
- National Institute for Health and Clinical Excellence
- NHSLA.

11.4.1   Care Quality Commission

The Care Quality Commission (CQC) came into being on 1 April 2009 as a Government-funded body. It acts as the independent regulator of health and adult social care in England. CQC replaced three earlier organisations – the Healthcare Commission, the Commission for Social Care Inspection and the Mental Health Act Commission. The Healthcare Commission had a specific role in relation to clinical governance which it delivered by conducting clinical governance reviews and investigations into serious incidents within the health care sector. The main focus of CQC is, however, on ensuring that government standards of quality and safety are met. CQC checks compliance against these standards in relation to services provided by hospitals, dentists, ambulances, care homes and in people's own homes; CQC's remit includes the independent health care sector.

Clinical governance and quality is thread through the standards that CQC enforce. While quality is mentioned, there is, however, no specific mention of clinical governance. There are five essential standards concerning the following:

- patient respect, involvement in care and support, informed about care provision
- care, treatment and support that meets patient needs
- patient safety
- care provided by staff with the right skills to perform their role properly
- routine checking by the care provider of their services.

When CQC inspections reveal that standards are not met, a number of steps may be taken, including imposing a fine or warning, stopping admissions into the care service or suspending or cancelling a care service registration. Annual reports of CQC's activities are published at the end of each March and can be accessed via their website.

There is a memorandum of understanding (MOU) between CQC and Monitor which sets out the respective remit of the two regulatory bodies and how they cooperate. CQC was established under the Health and Social Care Act 2008 and is responsible for the quality of health and social care services. This includes services provided by foundation trusts. Monitor's original role was confined to the authorising, monitoring and regulation of foundation trusts, as set out in the National Health Service Act 2006. The MOU sets out the arrangements for communication between the two bodies on the provision of health care and of the findings of their reviews. It remains to be seen whether there is merit in these two regulatory bodies continuing to operate and whether the NHS in England and governance arrangements would be better served by their responsibilities being merged.

11.4.2   The National Patient Safety Agency

In 2002, the chairman of the NPSA, in the wake of the Kennedy Report on the public inquiry into children's heart surgery at Bristol Royal Infirmary, stated that the Agency had been created to revolutionise patient safety in the NHS.[12] He described the arrangements for collecting information about problems, learning from them and putting in place measures that save lives and prevent adverse events happening again. As such the NPSA has a key role to play in clinical governance.

The NPSA was established in 2001 following the publication of a report, in 2000, led by the Chief Medical Officer for England.[13] *An Organisation with a*

Memory (OWAM) addressed the problems associated with reporting incidents and potential incidents involving patients, and the inadequacy of arrangements to learn lessons and prevent incidents happening again. At that time it was estimated that each year there were 900,000 incidents that either harmed or could have harmed patients in NHS hospitals. The scale of clinical errors and the scope for improving patient safety were becoming increasingly apparent.

One of the first tasks for the NPSA was to set up a national patient incident recording system. The NPSA aims to change the culture within the NHS that acts as a barrier to full incident-reporting and to making improvements to patient care provision. It has therefore focused on the need to remove the blame culture within the NHS and create a culture of openness and learning. As a central body (an arm's length body of the DH), it claims to be able to facilitate learning across health care organisations and the sharing of experience.

The NPSA, like the other bodies, has evolved during its existence and currently has three divisions which cover the UK health service. These are patient safety division, national clinical assessment service and national research ethics service. The first two have a bearing on clinical governance. The focus of the patient safety division is to reduce risks to patients receiving NHS care and improve safety. The national clinical assessment service deals with concerns about the performance of individual clinical practitioners to help ensure that their practice is both safe and valued. For the time being, a continuing role of the NPSA is the analysis of patient safety incidents on a national basis, and the identification of risks and actions to prevent recurrence/reduce severity of outcome. The Government has, however, decided to abolish the NPSA and plans to eventually transfer responsibility for the National Reporting and Learning System (NRLS) to the NHS Commissioning Board. It is to be hoped that this change will not detract from the value of this system in improving clinical governance arrangements.

11.4.3   NICE

The National Institute for Health and Clinical Excellence is also a part of the clinical governance arena. NICE was set up in 2004, as an independent organisation, and preceded an earlier organisation, with the same acronym but a slightly different remit, that came into being in 1999. NICE is currently responsible for producing national guidance aimed at promoting good health and both preventing and treating ill health. In addition to guidance, NICE sets quality standards and manages a national database to improve health and both prevent and treat ill health.

NICE clinical practice guidelines confirm the treatment that is appropriate for particular conditions and are based upon best available evidence. While the purpose of the guidelines is not to override clinical decision-making, they are intended to be used as a guide to best practice. Following clinical guidelines is therefore likely to lead to the avoidance of clinical risk and to good clinical governance.

After clinical guidelines are published, health organisations are expected to review their practice of managing clinical conditions against the requirements of the NICE guidelines. This review is expected to include consideration of the resources needed to implement the guidelines and the system that will be necessary for successful implementation. In situations where clinical practice is markedly different from NICE guidelines, there is likely to be a more significant need for investment, both in time and money, to effect the necessary changes.

NHS Evidence has been developed by NICE to provide easy access by health care professionals to quality and best practice information so that care decisions can be made on best available evidence. Patients too can access this information which they can use in discussion with clinicians on the nature of their care and treatment. Under development are quality standards which address the standards of health care that can be expected. These standards will indicate when a clinical treatment or procedure is highly effective, cost-effective and safe, and a positive experience for patients. As such they are useful tools for both clinicians and patients alike. The Government envisages that NICE quality standards will also be used to inform the commissioning of health care and that regulatory inspections will be against these standards.

11.4.4   NHSLA

The NHS Litigation Authority (NHSLA) is a Special Health Authority established under section 11 of the NHS Act 1977. Its framework document produced in 2002 sets out its role and functioning in some detail.[14] It functions to administer a number of schemes which pool the costs associated with meeting various liabilities, including those associated with clinical negligence. The NHSLA deals with claims for clinical negligence in connection with NHS trusts and other health care organisations; it manages the Clinical Negligence Scheme for Trusts (CNST). This scheme, introduced in 1994, was the first major initiative to be introduced in England to tackle clinical risk. The CNST is essentially a risk-pooling scheme where member organisations pay an annual contribution. Contribution levels are determined by past claims experience, the extent of high-risk health care activity, such as obstetrics, and performance against a number of standards. To progress up through the three compliance levels, CNST members need to be able to demonstrate more complex and robust arrangements for managing clinical risk. Compliance with the standards by CNST members needs to be taken forward within their clinical governance arrangements. As most trust members have not yet attained compliance level 3 and the vast majority remain at level 1, there is still much that needs to be done to improve the management of clinical risk and hence clinical governance.

As part of the drive for integrated governance, the CNST general clinical risk management standards were replaced at the end of March 2006 by the NHSLA Risk Management Standards for Acute Trusts. More recently the NHSLA has marshalled its risk management standards according to type of health care organisation. There are in effect three groups of standards, as follows:

- acute, community, mental health, learning disability and independent sector standards
- ambulance standards
- CNST maternity standards.

It is still therefore necessary for trusts to have an eye to both the residual CNST and newer NHSLA standards in order to identify what they need to do in order to perform well against these standards.

Assessments against the standards are undertaken by an independent specialist auditing and risk management organisation on behalf of the NHSLA. This organisation is also responsible for the routine running of the NHSLA's risk management programme. Evidence templates have been developed to facilitate the assessment process.

The overall aim of the NHSLA is to improve risk management by health care providers. Aside from risk pooling schemes, production of standards and assessment against the standards, the NHSLA also produces publications and holds learning events on good practice. In 2010/11, the NHSLA received 8655 claims of clinical negligence against NHS bodies; this is an increase of over 2000 from the previous year. The reasons for this increase may either be greater awareness among patients and their families of the duty that health care providers owe to patients, or an indication that clinical risk is still not being effectively managed.

In December 2010, the Department of Health commissioned an independent review by Marsh (insurance brokers and risk advisers) of the NHSLA. The review examined the performance of the NHSLA with respect to its risk-pooling functions, whether its performance is linked to rising trends in claims and whether it could be more efficient. The backdrop to the review was that during 2009–10, 62% of the claims referred to the NHSLA were for clinical negligence, and clinical negligence payments during that year totaled £787 million, both indicative of a rising trend. Marsh's review report was published in April 2011.[15]

The review examined claims management and the risk management framework together with strategic and cultural aspects of the NHSLA. The key findings from the review included the following:

- The NHS risk-pooling scheme remains valid, is widely accepted and endorsed.
- The NHSLA maintains effective stewardship and administration of the scheme.
- Use of more commercial practices in relation to claims management and incentivisation with respect to risk management could lead to better performance by the NHSLA.

On strategic matters, Marsh concluded that the NHSLA could play an increased role on patient safety matters. It was felt that this could be achieved by bringing together information on reported claims and incidents which did not give rise to claims (currently dealt with by the NPSA) and greater analysis and communication of root causes of claims so that lessons could be more effectively learnt. It remains to be seen how the Department of Health will take forward the recommendations from the NHSLA review.

11.5   Revalidation and fitness to practice

At the centre of many health care disasters is the question of the competence of the clinicians involved. Comparisons have been drawn with other industries and their arrangements for ensuring the continued competence of professional staff. Outside of health care, auditing performance, being supervised, checking working procedures, re-training and implementation of documented guidelines are an integral part of daily working activity in many organisations. These arrangements elsewhere and the poor quality of health care provision have sharpened the focus on the adequacy of the arrangements to train clinicians.

The most significant change to the regulation of doctors since 1858, when the General Medical Council (GMC) was created, is the revalidation of doctors. Since the late 1990s, it has been argued, and indeed all too clearly demonstrated by the activity of doctors such as Harold Shipman, that the continued registration of doctors based upon past qualifications was no longer sufficient. From 2005 doctors need to demonstrate to the GMC, their governing body, that their clinical practice remains up to date and that they are fit to practice.[16] There are around 200,000 doctors registered with the GMC, each of whom is now required to supply evidence on their fitness to practice in order to secure continued registration with the GMC.

The GMC's *Maintaining Good Medical Practice*,[17] was published in 1998, at a time when major change was under way in the whole area of quality of patient care provision. In this document, the GMC stated:

> In the NHS . . . employers are setting up local 'clinical governance' – formal arrangements to maintain the quality of patient care . . . Along with this, the medical profession and management need to work to set up effective local arrangements for medical regulation . . . Good medical practice and sound local clinical governance are keys to the way forward.[17]

Revalidation is therefore a key part of clinical governance.

Doctors need to continually accumulate a portfolio of evidence to demonstrate that their clinical skills are up to date and that they remain fit to practice. The evidence, together with the views of colleagues, is scrutinised regularly as a part of the local appraisal process. The evidence also has to be submitted to the GMC. In July 2004 the GMC set out its plans for the issuing of licences to practise, which doctors will need to hold in order to practice medicine in the UK. Doctors who fail or refuse to participate in revalidation will lose their licence. Decisions by the GMC, for example from investigations into clinical practice, to limit an individual's practice are now accessible by the public and confirmed on their licence.

It is not just doctors whose professional activities are regulated. In the UK there are eight other bodies that regulate health professionals in addition to the GMC.[18] These bodies cover, for example, nurses and midwives (Nursing and Midwifery Council – NMC), pharmacists (General Pharmaceutical Council – GPC) and dentists (General Dental Council – GDC). The purpose of these bodies is to protect and promote the safety of the public, by setting standards of behaviour, education and ethics that health professionals must meet. Regulators can remove health professionals from their registers and in effect prevent their legal operation.

11.6   The context for clinical governance

The arrangements for clinical governance in the health care sector need to be taken forward against the backdrop of both managing risk (in the broadest sense) and complying with health and safety legal requirements. It is therefore important to understand the relationship between risk management, health and safety legal compliance and clinical governance.

11.6.1   Risk management

All organisations exist for a purpose, whether that purpose is to make a profit and deliver value to shareholders or to provide a service to the public. Additionally, all organisations need to meet the expectations of their stakeholders, whether they are shareholders, partners, purchasers of services, employees or members of the public. In delivering organisational objectives, organisations encounter risks to the delivery of those objectives. Risk management is concerned with the identification of those risks, assessing both their likelihood of arising and impact upon the organisation, and making decisions about how to control them so that the delivery of organisational objectives is not jeopardised.

Organisations control the risks that they face in a number of ways, including the following:

- risk avoidance (ceasing or not engaging in the activity giving rise to the risk)
- risk tolerance (doing nothing more)
- risk treatment (implementing measures to reduce the chance of risk arising and its outcome)
- risk transfer (to another organisation such as an insurer or joint venture partner).

Health care organisations control risk in all four of these ways, as illustrated by the following examples:

- referring patients to health care providers with appropriate clinical expertise – this equates to risk avoidance by the referring organisation
- judging existing arrangements to control (but not remove) risk to be adequate – risk tolerance
- introducing arrangements to increase the competence of staff to undertake a particular clinical procedure and ensuring the presence of experienced staff to supervise the activities – risk treatment
- paying contributions to the NHSLA in connection with the CNST – risk transfer.

The links between clinical governance and risk management will be clear from these examples.

It is not possible for organisations to completely manage out all risk, nor is it desirable for them to do so. Risk management is based upon practical considerations of available resources and the residual level of risk that the organisation is prepared to accept following risk treatment. Running an organisation is an inherently risky process; the nature and extent of that risk depends upon the business of the organisation and its operating parameters. Private sector organisations tend, by definition, to be less risk-averse than those operating in the public sector, as entrepreneurial spirit inherently involves the willingness to take risks. This has been exploited by the previous Government in the Private Finance Initiative (PFI) arrangements that have been established to build new schools, roads and hospitals. PFI deals intrinsically recognise the private sector's greater ability and willingness to accept risk.

Health care organisations have to contend with a diverse range of risks to the delivery of their organisational objectives. These can be categorised into external, operational and those associated with change.[2] The health care sector is beset by significant external risk associated with changes in government and their expectations, performance targets and the need to function within set budgets. In the main, the sector has no control over these risks, but it can take a number of steps to mitigate the associated risks. Operational risks will arise, for example, from the delay in the completion of a new hospital building, inability to attract and retain key staff and the reputation the organisation has with stakeholders. Operational risks will include those that arise from clinical service provision. Change can create risk: for example, when a trust merges with one or more other trusts and when clinical service provision is reallocated between neighbouring health care providers. All of these examples have the potential to block the achievement of organisational objectives to a greater or lesser extent.

11.6.2   Health and safety legal requirements

Despite the drive for integrated governance, it normally comes as a surprise to health care organisations that poor clinical practice can result in criminal prosecution for breaches of health and safety legislation. The requirements of this legislation, and in particular the duty to protect patients under section 3 of the Health and Safety at Work etc. Act 1974, are not normally uppermost in the corporate mind of health care organisations or of individual clinicians. However, there have now been a number of successful prosecutions following clinical incidents that have led to patients dying. The following cases brought under section 3 illustrate this development:

- Norfolk and Norwich NHS Trust prosecuted for the death of a patient during a cardiac angiogram: fine including costs £58,000[19]
- a university hospital prosecuted following the death of two patients in unrelated incidents during anaesthesia: fine including costs circa £30,000[19]
- a Scottish trust prosecuted in connection with a patient suicide: fine £10,000[19]
- a university hospital prosecuted following the death of a patient whose operation was not completed owing to poorly maintained equipment: fine including costs £50,000[20]

- Southampton University Hospitals NHS Trust prosecuted for failing to manage two doctors who failed to diagnose toxic shock syndrome resulting in a patient's death: fine including costs £110,000.[21]

The last case was preceded by the conviction of the two junior doctors involved in the care of the deceased patient for gross negligence manslaughter. Each doctor received an 18-month prison sentence suspended for two years. The criminal case against the trust under health and safety legislation concerned their failure to adequately supervise the junior doctors, and it was alleged that this led to the patient's death. The trust pleaded guilty and was fined accordingly. Ineffective clinical governance arrangements can therefore lead to legal sanction against both health care organisations and individuals.

11.7   Clinical governance in practice: a summary

It will be clear from this chapter that the clinical governance arena is crowded, fairly complex and constantly evolving. Governance in health care is addressed by a number of organisations allied to health care having remits to set standards, to guide, to check working practice and to penalise both organisations and individuals when arrangements do not match up to current requirements and standards.

For clinical governance to be taken forward appropriately in a health care organisation there has to be demonstrable commitment from the top of the organisation. This means at board and senior executive levels. The board of any organisation should concern itself with the arrangements for managing risk and for effective governance. Organisations normally do this by ensuring that an appropriately constituted committee reporting to the board has responsibility for governance and risk management. Health care organisations may therefore choose to take forward clinical governance within a broad governance and quality agenda, or to establish a separate committee to deal specifically with clinical governance. In either case, these high-level committees will be responsible for determining strategy and the necessary organisational arrangements and reporting regularly on progress to the board. Verification of how well clinical governance arrangements are working in practice is normally addressed within the organisation by its audit committee and externally by CQC and other bodies.

Supporting the high-level committees, clinical governance needs to be a part of the responsibility of all those who impact upon patients. This includes not just doctors and nurses, but also allied health care providers, pharmacists and clinical support services. To practise good clinical governance, these individuals and teams will need to be actively engaged in the following activities:

- CPD
- performance appraisal
- clinical audit
- incident and adverse-event reporting
- learning lessons from mistakes

- implementing best clinical practice
- commitment to high-quality health care provision.

Health care organisations benefit from having in place good arrangements for clinical governance by:

- reduced CNST contributions
- positive CQC and Monitor reviews
- enhanced quality of patient care
- reduced levels of clinical risk
- better outcomes for patients
- trained and competent staff.

In contrast, in the worst-case scenarios health care organisations that do not have good arrangements in place for clinical governance can face adverse national and local media attention, missed targets, critical reports that are published, and financial penalty by way of the CNST and prosecution in the criminal courts. Patients pay the ultimate price for poor clinical governance by loss of life or poor quality of life following clinical intervention. This on its own should be a continuous driver for excellence in clinical governance.

11.8   Notes and references

1. The Combined Code and Cadbury, Greenbury and Hampel Reports can be accessed at: www.ecgi.org/codes/documents/combined_code.pdf
2. HM Treasury, the 'Orange Book', *Management of Risk Principles and Concepts* (London, The Stationery Office, 2004).
3. NHS Executive, *Clinical Governance in the New NHS*, HSC 1999/065 (Department of Health, 1999).
4. Clinical governance: assuming the sacred duty of trust to patients, Professor Aiden Halligan, 2005.
5. NHS Executive, *A First Class Service: Quality in the New NHS* HSC 1999/32 (London, Department of Health, 1998).
6. National Audit Office, *Achieving Improvements in Clinical Governance: A Progress Report on Implementation by NHS Trusts*, HC 1055, 2002–03 (London, The Stationery Office, 2003).
7. Department of Health, *Integrated Governance Handbook 2006: A Handbook for Executives and Non-Executives In Health Care Organisations* (London, Department of Health, 2006).
8. Department of Health, *Equity and Excellence: Liberating the NHS* (London, Department of Health, 2010).
9. National Quality Board, *Review of Early Warning Systems in the NHS*, 2010.
10. National Quality Board, *Quality Governance in the NHS – A Guide for Provider Boards*, 2011.
11. Department of Health, *High Quality Care for All: NHS Next Stage Review* (London, Department of Health, 2008).
12. NPSA Board statement, 18 January 2002.
13. Department of Health, An Organisation with a Memory: Report of an Expert Group on Learning from Adverse Events in the NHS, 2000.
14. www.nhsla.com.

15. Marsh, NHS Litigation Authority Industry Report, April 2011.
16. General Medical Council, The Policy Framework for Revalidation: A Position Paper, July 2004.
17. General Medical Council, *Maintaining Good Medical Practice*, 1998.
18. Gifford Phil, Fit to Practise? Effective professional regulation in the UK, *Health Care Risk Report*, **16** (2010/2011), p. 17.
19. Vanessa L. Mayatt (ed.), *Tolley's Managing Risk in Healthcare: Law and Practice*, 2nd edn, (London, Lexis Nexis, 2004).
20. http://news.bbc.co.uk/1/hi/england/staffordshire.
21. Vanessa L. Mayatt, Health and safety prosecutions following harm to patients, *Health Care Risk Report*, **12** (2006), p. 9.

Key websites

www.hm-treasury.gov.uk
www.dh.gov.uk
www.npsa.nhs.uk
www.cqc.org.uk
www.nice.org.uk
www.nhsla.com
www.gmc-uk.org
www.hse.gov.uk
www.nhs.uk

B   An Ethical Perspective

Lucy Frith

Senior Lecturer in Bioethics and Social Science, Department of Health Services Research, University of Liverpool, Liverpool

The main aim of clinical governance is to improve the quality of care provided by the NHS and other health care providers, and it has been a central part of health care policy since the mid-1990s. It was developed in the United Kingdom partly in response to high-profile cases of poor care (e.g. Bristol Royal Infirmary) that showed a perceived need for more robust procedures for ensuring health care quality.[1] The aim of this chapter is to draw out some of the underlying ethical themes and principles of clinical governance and associated quality improvement mechanisms.

11.9   Clinical and quality governance

'Clinical governance is the framework through which all the components of quality, including patient and public involvement, are brought together.'[2] Clinical governance procedures are overarching frameworks that affect all aspects of health care delivery. Some argue that these organisational elements are not generally reflected in definitions of clinical governance and propose the following definition: 'Clinical governance is defined as a governance system for healthcare organisations that promotes an integrated approach towards management of inputs, structures and process to improve the outcome of healthcare service delivery where health staff work in an environment of greater accountability for clinical quality'.[3]

Seeing clinical governance in this way reflects its development – there is now an increasing focus on the wider organisational aspects of 'quality'. Clinical governance was seen as the preserve of clinicians and clinical managers, but quality governance involves the whole organisation in providing high-quality care.[4] The term 'clinical governance' is becoming less used (the Department of Health's clinical governance pages are no longer active and have been archived) and is being replaced by 'quality governance'. In this chapter I shall still use 'clinical governance' as a blanket term to mean the general procedures and structures that health care organisations put in place to facilitate the provision of 'high-quality' care.

The main elements of clinical governance include the following:

1.   Patient focus and public involvement – the NHS Act 2006 updated the duty for NHS bodies to involve and consult the public. The Coalition Government's plans for the NHS set out in the White Paper *Equity and Excellence:*

Liberating the NHS[6] in 2010 furthered this trend by adopting the slogan, 'No decision about me without me.'

2.   Clinical effectiveness – this can involve setting standards, and bodies such as the National Institute for Health and Clinical Excellence (NICE) and the National Service Frameworks (NSF) set standards and aim to ensure equality of access and standardisation of health provision throughout the NHS.

3.   Patient safety and risk management – this focuses on considering how patients might be harmed, preventing such harm, reporting risks and incidents and learning from these events.

The structures and processes used in clinical governance are the subject of almost continual change and the Health and Social Care Act 2012 will bring in further, as yet, unanticipated changes. An important feature of the changing health care environment in England is the increasing use of other organisations to provide services on behalf of the NHS. These might be independent (private) or third-sector providers such as social enterprises. There are, currently, almost 2500 independent hospitals and clinics offering a wide variety of services.[5] The encouraging of organisations to provide care means that the NHS will become one health care provider among many, and therefore how these other bodies manage their governance programmes will be a developing area for consideration.

11.9.1   Definitions of quality

Underpinning the ideas and procedures of clinical governance is a notion of what good-quality health care *is*. In order to talk meaningfully about quality we need to have some notion of what we mean by quality in this context. Darzi in the *NHS Next Stage Review*[7] put forward a definition of quality that is now generally used in policy documents. Quality comprises of three elements, as follows:

- Effectiveness – this is measured both by clinical and patient-related outcomes.
- Safety – this is a key element and came to the fore with publications such as *An organisation with a memory*.[8]
- Patient experience – this is becoming increasingly important in policy. The experience the patient has of their care should be seen just as important as the medical aspects of their treatment.

These elements of quality map on to the elements of clinical governance.

How quality is defined and measured is changing from the previous concern with performance targets (cutting waiting lists and reducing infection levels, for example) to an increasing focus on outcome measures and patient satisfaction. The *NHS Outcomes Framework* sets out what the NHS should be aiming to achieve and provides accountability mechanisms for the new NHS Commissioning Board: 'This means ensuring that the accountabilities running throughout the system are focussed on the outcomes achieved for patients not the processes by which they are achieved'.[9] How these 'good' outcomes are determined has developed from medically defined outcomes to include 'patient reported outcome measures' that seek to consider what patients might see as effective care themselves and ensuring patients have a positive experience of their care. It could also be argued that people's expectations of health care have changed, and therefore good-quality care has to encompass elements such as respectful treatment, taking on board patients' views and concerns and offering a greater choice over where they will be treated. The Care Quality Commission has, as part of its quality measurements, for example, a focus on people's right to be treated with respect, compassion, kindness and dignity.[5] Thus, the previously hidden ethical aspects of care are finding their way into quality measures.

I shall now consider the three elements of clinical governance: patient experience; clinical effectiveness and standard setting; and patient safety and risk management.

11.10   Patient experience and involvement

There are two main ways that patients' views and opinions are being increasingly incorporated in health care planning and organisation: a focus on the patient experience of health care as an important outcome and involving patients in health care policy decision-making.

11.10.1   Patient experience

The greater focus on patient experience as an indicator of quality builds on previous initiatives to involve patients in service design and improvement. The NHS Operating Framework 2012/13 says, 'NHS organisations must actively seek out, respond positively and improve services in line with patient feedback. This includes acting on complaints, patient comments, local and national surveys and results from "real time" data techniques.'[10] In 2012 the National Quality Board (NQB) published the NHS Patient Experience Framework, which sets out the important elements that affect a patient's journey through their care.

NHS patient experience framework:

1.   **Respect of patient-centred values, preferences, and expressed needs**, including: cultural issues; the dignity, privacy and independence of patients and service users; an awareness of quality-of-life issues; and shared decision making;
2.   Coordination and integration of care across health and social care system;
3.   **Information, communication, and education** on clinical status, progress, prognosis, and processes of care in order to facilitate autonomy, self-care and health promotion;
4.   **Physical comfort** including pain management, help with activities of daily living, and clean and comfortable surroundings;
5.   **Emotional support** and alleviation of fear and anxiety about such issues as clinical status, prognosis, and the impact of illness on patients, their families and their finances;

6. **Welcoming the involvement of family and friends**, on whom patients and service users rely, in decision-making and demonstrating awareness and accommodation of their needs as care-givers;

7. **Transition and continuity** as regards information that will help patients care for themselves away from a clinical setting, and coordination, planning, and support to ease transitions;

8. **Access to care** with attention for example, to time spent waiting for admission or time between admission and placement in a room in an in-patient setting, and waiting time for an appointment or visit in the out-patient, primary care or social care setting.[11]

NICE have recently issued guidance on the patient experience in adult care. 'This guidance provides the evidence and the direction for creating sustainable change that will result in an "NHS cultural shift" towards a truly patient-centred service.'[12] This sets out quality standards for patient experience such as: 'Patients are treated with dignity, kindness, compassion, courtesy, respect, understanding and honesty.'

The Darzi Report set the scene for this greater consideration of the ethical aspects of health care delivery by arguing that a constitution was needed to set out the core values and principles of the NHS, and this would be a 'powerful way' to ensure that these values 'are enshrined and protected'.[7] The first NHS Constitution was published in 2009, and the Health Act 2009 stipulated that all bodies providing NHS services (NHS, private and third-sector providers) must 'have regard' to the Constitution in all their actions and decisions. 'As our health care system becomes increasingly devolved, autonomous and entrepreneurial, there is a need for system-wide values, which reaffirm the social purpose of the NHS, to staff, patients and the public and inspire behaviours that put the needs of patients, staff and the public foremost in people's minds.'[13]

Paying attention to elements such as the patient's values and how their family and friends might be welcomed connects with elements of health care that people think are very important and arguably gives a focus for providing a better environment for promoting ethical care. These 'softer' measures that move away from narrowly defined clinical outcomes capture previously neglected elements of health care and go some way to addressing previous problems raised by definitions of quality. As Professor Campbell noted, 'The term "quality enhancement" is used, as though its meaning were self-evident. But in the absence of specification, the term is as empty as "quantity" – it refers merely to a dimension for measurement.'[14] With the Darzi definition and an incorporation of more patient-centred definitions of quality, there is an attempt to recognise that 'quality' is a value judgement. Now that quality measures also include how the patient experiences their care, there is enhanced recognition of these more subjective elements. However, although the incorporation of 'softer' measures does bring in more evaluative aspects, we need to remember that there could be disagreement over the definition of quality and there will not be one 'right' way of defining or interpreting the term. Hence, questions of what should we be doing will require us to make important value judgements and these should be made explicit so that they can be justified rather than assumed.

11.10.2   Involving patients

There are various ways that patients are to be involved in commenting on and deciding what services should be provided. A number of patient surveys are conducted, ranging from the national surveys carried out by the Care Quality Commission, annual patient surveys conducted by local trusts and PCTs, to small scale surveys conducted at ward level. Patient surveys were always a part of clinical governance from its inception; there is now a greater focus on patient involvement in actual decision-making, with patients being consulted as to the range of options which should be offered in the NHS, rather than just what they think about existing services. This is, in principle, a positive move. Giving patients the opportunity to influence what range of options and how those options will be delivered extends the notion of informed consent.

However, the Patients Forum, a coalition of voluntary patient health organisations, in a discussion document highlight how, with the changes in the structure of NHS provision, it might be harder than before for patient groups to influence decisions:

> The lack of stability and coherence in policy on patient and public involvement has made it difficult to create a climate of constructive dialogue with the Government and Department of Health . . . The range of regulatory bodies and next step agencies have contributed to a highly complex environment for health policy . . . Radical policies emerge and by the time the implications are understood it is too late to influence them.[15]

This lack of stability in policies on patient involvement was addressed in a House of Commons Report[16] in 2007 and has continued, as illustrated by policy changes in the last ten years. The Commission for Patient and Public Involvement in Health was established in 2003; however, a year later a Department of Health review recommended that it should be abolished.[17] This body was responsible for appointing and supporting the Patient and Public Involvement Forums (PPIFs) that were established in every NHS trust and PCT area in 2004. In 2006 their abolition was announced. These were replaced by Local Involvement Networks in 2008. With the Health and Social Care Act 2012 these are to be replaced by local HealthWatch organizations, and HealthWatch England that will be a statutory committee of the CQC. The continual changes in policy and the disruption they have caused has been recognised in the preparations for HealthWatch.[18] The Government's policies on public/patient involvement need to be implemented in a way that really gives people an opportunity to affect change, otherwise public/patient involvement will simply be a meaningless bit of rhetoric designed to give the impression of an NHS governed by consensus.

11.11   Clinical effectiveness – setting standards

Various bodies have been established to set standards and policies for the NHS. NICE produces evidence-based clinical guidelines and information on good practice, and a key function of this body is the systematic appraisal of medical interventions. For example, in 2012 NICE approved the use of the drug dabigatran (Pradaxa) for patients with atrial fibrillation for stroke prevention. This can be offered as an alternative to warfarin in order to reduce the risk of stroke and blood clots. Taking warfarin can be difficult for some patients due to the need for frequent check-ups and monitoring, whereas the use of dabigatran does not require such frequent testing. This is the first change in stroke prevention treatments for patients with atrial fibrillation at risk of stroke for 50 years.[19] The National Service Frameworks (NSF) have the overall aim of ensuring equity of access and standardisation of care for all patients in the NHS and link related policies to formulate an integrated national policy. Under current health policy these frameworks are now termed 'outcome strategies' and are part of the NHS Outcomes Framework.[20] For example, the Cancer Strategy was launched in 2011, and includes aims such as: increase survival rates so that by 2012/15 an extra 5000 lives can be saved; promote lifestyle changes to reduce preventable cancers and increase early diagnosis; improving patient support and patient experience.[21] These frameworks bring together the best evidence of clinical and cost effectiveness, with the views of users, to determine the best ways of providing a particular service.

The aim of setting standards in clinical governance is to determine the 'best' treatment or approach to a condition and implement these findings across the whole of the NHS, thus improving the quality of health care provision. These standards will be set by considering the medical evidence and by employing a rigorous methodology to determine the best treatment scientifically – such as the technology appraisal of the drug dabigatran (Pradaxa) mentioned above. I want to consider the view that evidence-based medicine will tell us which treatments are 'better' scientifically and argue that although medical science can make an important contribution to treatment decisions, value judgements still come into quality assessments. This view is gaining ground with the involvement of patients in developing guidelines alongside professionals.[22]

To say a treatment is effective, and hence of better quality, incorporates non-objective value judgements, namely, a judgement of what is a good outcome. It is generally argued that clinical trials are designed to find out certain effects of a drug – for example, the lowering of plasma cholesterol levels; these effects are capable of being measured by a piece of laboratory equipment. The findings that this equipment produces will be independent of the experimenters' perceptions and hence can be said to objective. However, the significance given to the effect, whether that effect is to be termed a good outcome, is not factors inherent in the data but the values we ourselves impose on the data. Effectiveness, good outcomes, quality, a 'better' treatment are not pre-existing facts waiting to be discovered by medical science: they are value-laden assessments of the weight given to a particular effect of the treatment.[23] Thus, to say a treatment is effective is summing up one's opinion on the data.

11.11.1   How we employ data in cost-effectiveness decisions

If we agree that clinical trials produce generally accepted factual data about the interaction of particular drugs or therapies: 'The evidence itself will not automatically dictate patient care but will provide the factual basis on which decisions can be made'[24] The evidence of effectiveness may form the basis of a very good reason for pursuing a particular course of action, but value judgements are needed to tell us whether we *should* take that course of action. As Muir Gray says in *Evidence Based Health Care*, 'Decisions about groups of patients or populations are made by combining three factors: 1. evidence; 2. values; 3. resources.'[25]

A central area where values shape how we should use the data and scientific evidence is that of priority-setting.[26] When bodies such as NICE decide on which health care interventions to recommend, they have to balance two possibly competing claims: do we promote the interests of individual patients as paramount and focus on the effectiveness of the treatment? Or should this individual ethic make way for concerns over the collective good, a population-based ethic and focus on the cost effectiveness of the treatment?

Alan Maynard argues that evidence-based medicine (EBM) focuses on finding out which treatments are most effective and is therefore grounded in the individual ethic.[27] EBM is concerned with finding out what is the most effective treatment for a particular patient. However, the treatment that is the most effective might not also be the most cost- effective. A physician who adopted the population-based ethic would be more concerned with recommending a treatment that was cost-effective and in the interests of society as a whole, rather than just the interests of the individual patient. This is one of the key value judgements that has to be made by all health care systems, and it is not a dilemma that can be solved by appealing to scientific evidence: it can only be solved by deciding what kind of values we wish to see drive health care.

NICE has as its remit the appraisal of health care technologies not just on grounds of clinical effectiveness but cost effectiveness (see Hughes & Doheny[28] for a case study of such a decision). While the public are more accepting of the supposed objective nature of clinical effectiveness, a denial of a treatment on the grounds of cost-effectiveness is often seen to be a form of health care rationing – denying treatment options purely on the grounds of lack of funding. In a review of the decisions NICE made between 1999 and 2005, Raftery noted that a fifth of guidances rejected the use of the intervention and the remainder recommended use with restrictions.[29]

There have been a number of cases where NICE has come into conflict with patient groups over their decisions not to provide particular treatments on the NHS (such as the debates over the drug beta interferon for multiple sclerosis in the early 2000s). In 2005 NICE reviewed its guidance on drugs for Alzheimer's disease and published draft guidance that Aricept, Reminyl and Exelon should no longer be available to NHS patients as they were not cost-effective. This recommendation was highly contested by groups such as the Alzheimer's Society and led to the formation of the Action on Alzheimer's Drugs Alliance. This body campaigned against this restriction of medications provided on the NHS, and after various appeals and additional guidance from NICE in 2006 (that recommended that the three drugs only be prescribed to people with moderate stage Alzheimer's with a mini-mental state examination (MMSE) score of between 10 and 20), in 2011 NICE issued guidance that allowed the three drugs to be prescribed for people with early-to-moderate Alzheimer's and Ebixa prescribed for people in the later stages of the disease. As the Alzheimer's Society say: 'This is a momentous stage of the *Access to Drugs Campaign* and Alzheimer's Society particularly welcomes the removal of specific reference to MMSE score in the NICE guidance. Access to treatment will be based on a more holistic assessment of severity and response, rather than be bound by a score on one particular measure'.[30]

This example illustrates two important points. First, patients and patient groups, in this case the Alzheimer's Society, could have different definitions of an effective treatment than the standard-setting agency holds. Second, cost is a factor in weighing up what treatments should be recommended and in this case it was claimed that the outlay to the NHS was not justified by the benefit it produces for the recipients. Whereas, the Alzheimer's Society argued that NICE's cost-effectiveness assessment was too narrowly focused and did not take into account the fact that the cost of caring for suffers was largely born by their families. In such a deliberation there is no scientific way of answering the question of what this treatment is worth. It is a matter for society to decide what values and priorities are important.

11.11.2   Standards in practice

One of the main ways that quality is managed under clinical governance is through the employment of care-pathways and clinical guidelines. Part of the process of clinical governance is to systematically assess current practice and formulate clinical guidelines that represent best practice. Since April 1994 all trusts have to show that they have started to develop clinical guidelines. The rationale behind guidelines is an attempt to both increase the quality of care and reduce the inequalities in access to health care. As NICE state:

> Good clinical guidelines aim to improve the quality of healthcare. They can change the process of healthcare and improve people's chances of getting as well as possible. Clinical guidelines can:

- provide recommendations for the treatment and care of people by health professionals
- be used to develop standards to assess the clinical practice of individual health professionals
- be used in the education and training of health professionals
- help patients to make informed decisions
- improve communication between patient and health professional.[31]

The regional variations in service delivery and health outcomes have been seen as a central problem for the NHS. For example, the *NHS Atlas of Variation*[32] shows in great detail the variation between different regions over a range of indicators (for instance, prescribing, treatment, number of hospital admissions, numbers with specific conditions and length of hospital stay). Examples of variation between regions are: 'A 25-fold variation in anti-dementia drugs prescribing rates across England; Patients with Type 2 diabetes are twice as likely to receive the highest standard of care in some areas of England in comparison to others.'[32] It has been claimed that the 2004 NICE[33] guideline on infertility treatment provision for example, that was designed to end what was perceived as a 'postcode lottery', has gone some way to alleviating regional disparities in infertility treatment.[34]

When applying the guidelines to the treatment of individuals, ethical dilemmas can arise. Treatments which produce the desired effect can differ from person to person. Even patients with identical manifestations of a particular disease could give different weight to various outcomes depending on personal taste, social and family situations, life priorities and so on. Guidelines can incorporate an assessment of quality that is held to be the same for all patients. This could come into conflict with an individual's particular conception of desirable benefit and their own personal quality assessment. Many authors have drawn attention to the importance of recognising that good outcomes must be seen as relative to the patient. Hopkins and Solomon[35] illustrate this point with the example of the management of stroke patients. They say that the course of the treatment and the outcomes of rehabilitation cannot be predetermined because each person's disability is unique. Hence the therapist has to concentrate on the goals and needs of the particular patient.

Guidelines rely on patient homogeneity, that is patients being very similar. In stroke rehabilitation, where patient variation is high, it is difficult to write a precisely defined clinical guideline. There are, on the other hand, areas of health care where patient variation is much lower, the removal of wisdom teeth, for example. When this is the case, guidelines can be useful. 'In conditions such as day case surgery, a single patient record is easy to introduce. In an intensive care setting, where variations are more common, a pathway together with freehand documentation may be more suitable.'[36] There may be areas where guidelines are more applicable; however, this should not be extended to areas of health care provision where guidelines may be inappropriate. Even when patients are suffering from the same condition, guidelines should not be applied unthinkingly. Room should be made for the needs and wants of the patient to be accommodated. It could be argued that due to the individual nature of many treatment decisions, it could be difficult to produce guidelines that reflected each patient's treatment preferences.[37] This drive to write standardised care pathways for patients could conflict with the other drive of current health care policy to be more a patient-centred.

11.11.3   Formulating guidelines

Guidelines can be used in a positive way and could increase patients' autonomy by involving them in the very formulation of guidelines and setting standards. Patients often have very different perspectives from the health care professionals and soliciting their views on their health care provision could be invaluable. The National Service Frameworks are charged with bringing together the views of service users to determine the best way to provide particular services. NICE involves the public and patients in its guidelines by facilities for commenting on proposals, joining a NICE committee, and suggesting topics for guidance. Patient groups can also be involved in guideline development. The benefits of this are that patients and carer members can add insights into:

- the practical, physical and emotional challenges associated with living with, or supporting someone with, a particular medical condition
- the many different things individual patients may want from their treatment and care
- how acceptable different options for care and treatment are to people
- what factors might affect patients' preferences for different types of treatment and care
- whether different groups of patients may have different views or needs, for instance, with regard to age, ethnicity, sex or disability
- what information and support patients and carers need to help them understand and deal with their condition.[38]

Service users were involved in the writing of the mental health NICE guidelines, and this improved the guidance produced. It has been argued that this involvement:

> can lead to progress in three main areas of guideline development and service user involvement:
>
> - translating evidence to recommendations
> - optimizing the acceptability of recommendations
> - reconciling different types of knowledge.[39]

However, scepticism can be expressed about the utility of involving patients in guideline development. First, it is ironic that after the initial development of EBM, that was designed to eradicate personal opinion and limited case reports – experiential knowledge (albeit those of the professional) – patient involvement in guidelines seeks to bring this form of knowledge back into clinical practice. While such inclusion is not *prima facie* a problem (although there might be issues about combining the scientifically produced knowledge with this different form), there are possible difficulties. It might become rather tokenistic – one or two patients talking for all patients, and there might be doubts that they can 'represent' a full range of patient views, thus only giving a personal picture. Often in patient involvement a limited number of views are solicited in an unsystematic way. To better get patient views a properly designed study (such as in-depth qualitative interviews, for example) should be conducted. There are practical problems with this (time, money), but if patient involvement is as important a current health policy deems it is, then robust methodologies of eliciting views and involving patients in guideline production need to be developed.

It is also argued that patients do not have the skills to appraise evidence in the way professionals do. One way of improving patient involvement is to offer training so that patients can more actively participate in the process. However, by providing training and support for service users in how to appraise scientific evidence and guideline development, they can become 'expert' patients. This can lead to them becoming distanced from their experiential knowledge base and 'become a fellow academic'.[40]

A literature review by van de Bovenkamp and Trappenburg[40] found that there is little evidence that active patient participation increases the quality or legitimacy of guidelines and that most studies and commentaries simply state such participation is important or appeal to it on principled grounds. One of the dangers they highlight with this approach is that there is a temptation to think that if patients are involved in the guideline development itself, then there is no need to pay attention to patient preferences at an individual level – it is assumed these have already been incorporated at development level. As van der Weijden et al. state: 'Patient participation in CPG development, which is an important innovation in itself, is not substitute for involvement of patients or consumers in individual clinical decisions. Indeed, patient representatives cannot be expected to provide input on what "the patient" with a particular disease prefers and what "the patient" experiences'.[37] Van de Bovenkamp and Trappenburg[40] show that there is another conception of patient involvement in guidelines that has become rarer in the literature than the active conception outlined above, that is guidelines should make room for individual patient preference. This could be done, they suggest, by incorporating a section on patient–physician communication so that discussions and patient preference can be incorporated into the treatment plan. Thus, there is 'a need for flexible guidelines that enable and facilitate patient involvement in medical decision making'.[37]

Used in this way guidelines can enable patients to be better informed and facilitate greater shared decision-making between patient and professional. For example, when patients enter hospital, they could be given a copy of the clinical guidelines, and this can indicate what should be happening during the course of their treatment. It will give them an informed basis on which to question and challenge their treatment provision. This model has been adopted by a Liverpool hospital. The guideline is explained to the patient, and they usually have access to it during their stay in hospital.[41] The patients therefore have a document that they can refer back to at any stage and so do not have to take in all the information at the beginning of their treatment.

11.12   Patient safety and risk management

One of the main ways that quality of health care provision is overseen is through the adoption of clinical risk management programmes (CRM) (for instance the National Patient Safety Agency). It is the responsibility of the health care professional to promote the welfare of individual patients and ensure that they receive the best and safest care. In this section I examine how such schemes can be used to create an environment which makes it easier for professionals to carry out their ethical duties.

One aspect of CRM that can be used as an important measure for preventing harm to patients is near-miss reporting and notifying of adverse events. Such events are a common problem for the NHS: between April and June 2011 there were 333,654 incidents reported, and the most common single type of incident was a patient accident (27 per cent) taking place in general or acute hospitals (72 per cent).[42] In 2010–11 97,500 written complaints were received by hospital and community health services, of these 44.8 per cent were about medical staff and 22.1 per cent about nurses, midwives and health visitors.[42]

To rectify such problems: 'The NHS needs to develop: a unified mechanism for reporting and analysis when things go wrong [and] a more open culture, in which errors or service failures can be reported and discussed.'[8] The current themes are to promote patient safety through a culture of candour,[43] and this is reiterated in the Coalitions Government's White Paper, *Equity and Excellence: Liberating the NHS*,[6] 'we will require hospitals to be open about mistakes and always tell patients if something has gone wrong'. This notion of openness is based on two arguments: first that if professionals are open and honest, then patients cope better with a safety incident.[43] People appreciate honesty, and it is the deceit involved in covering up of mistakes that often causes a bigger problem than the mistake itself. Second, there is an ethical argument that one should be honest and tell patients what has happened – whatever the consequences of such a disclosure. 'It is important to remember that saying sorry is not an admission of liability and is the right thing to do.'[43]

An interesting ethical issue is whether patients should be told that there has been a mistake when nothing has actually gone wrong. Chamberlain et al.[44] argued that such errors should be disclosed even when there is no resulting harm. They argue that this can increase trust in the doctor–patient relationship; facilitates open discussion and informed consent; and is beneficial for the health care organisation. However, as they note, there may be downsides to this, that patients could lose trust in their doctors and become more worried about their medical care. Any disclosure of error or near-miss needs to be done in a sensitive way, and they give the following advice:

- Disclose the error in a timely manner. Do not wait to see if the patient or family member discovers the error.
- Do not use ambiguous language to mislead the patient. Be clear and concise using terms that the patient and the family can understand.
- Explain potential outcomes, including if the medical team does not foresee any long-term consequences.
- Invite questions from the patient or family members.
- Apologize for the error, and explain that the error will be reported to the medical institution.[44]

The NPSA guidance[43] also includes useful advice on approaching patients and dealing with disclosure.

Any reduction in processes leading to patient harm, incidents of staff incompetence and general bad practice are to be applauded. However, there are difficulties with this approach, when one considers the context in which it operates. Janet Lyon[45] has argued that, in order for an adequate system of near-miss reporting to operate, the staff must be able to trust their employer to use the information responsibly. Various cases demonstrate this might not be the case. Dr Stephen Bolin, a consultant anaesthetist at Bristol Royal Infirmary, spent five years trying to draw attention to the problems with the paediatric cardiac surgery delivery. In light of the concerns that staff were not reporting incidents, the Public Interest Disclosure Act 1998 was passed to enable employees to raise concerns about dangerous or poor practice without endangering their careers, protecting whistle-blowers from sacking or victimisation. Even with legal safeguards in place staff members could feel threatened by having to report mistakes and accidents to the risk manager (see Wu,[46] for a discussion of the practicalities of talking about mistakes). Later cases such as events at Mid Staffordshire Hospital Trust between 2005 and 2009 show that a trusting environment is not always created. The Trust was found to have a 'closed culture' with a lack of information sharing and a focus on processes rather than quality of care.

It has been argued that often staff are 'the second victim' of adverse incidents, and there needs to be a recognition of the needs of the staff involved in incidents and how to support them.[47] The NHS Executive[48] has stated that 'the results of the risk management process should not be used for punitive or disciplinary purposes.' It also states that the information given should be kept confidential and that the informant should remain anonymous. Such confidentiality could ensure that the near-miss reporting scheme could effectively carry out the stated aims. There is now greater guidance for provider boards on how to ensure adequate governance arrangements to ensure quality of care.[4] Thus, such governance arrangements could be used to create a working environment which helps the professional to practise ethically. Elements of such an environment are deemed to be creating: an open culture; a just culture; a reporting culture; a learning culture; and an informed culture.[49] This would be beneficial to both staff and patients and ensure that the ethical aims of risk management schemes could be realised. As long as the possible fears of the staff are borne in mind by employers, a culture of trust could be fostered and non-punitive mechanisms developed for addressing the concerns of employees.

That such a culture is developing could be evidenced by findings from a General Medical Council (GMC) research project on their fitness to practise reporting mechanisms. Recent figures show a rise in GMC investigations into doctors on fitness to practise issues: in 2010 there were more than 2000, an 18 per cent increase compared with 2009, and 92 doctors were removed from the register, the highest ever total in one year.[50] The GMC attributes this not to doctors becoming worse but to:

- changes in public attitudes, in part driven by some awareness of high profile cases
- changes in colleagues' attitudes, driven largely by the perceived improvement in systems for raising confidential concerns
- improved governance and management systems for detecting and dealing with performance concerns, and an increased focus on outcomes and maintaining high standards of patient safety.[51]

The GMC stipulates that it is a doctor's duty to inform the appropriate authority about a colleague whose performance is questionable,[52] and the Nursing and Midwifery Council also has such requirements in their code.[53] The appropriate response to an allegation of incompetence clearly depends on the type of accident or incompetence that is reported. Serious misconduct, or wilfully disregarding the welfare of the patient should merit disciplinary action. The issue that is of more concern here is a genuine accident or mistake that the practitioner did not wilfully cause. Whether the accident was caused by a lack of skill or an inadequate process, these factors should be able to be addressed without the practitioner facing any form of disciplinary procedure.

11.13   Conclusion

The imperative to improve the quality of health care can be seen as a positive move to ensure that both health care providers and individual practitioners are held to be more accountable and responsible for the quality of the care they deliver. However, although quality of health care provision is something we all want, the term 'quality' is very hard to define. Once it is recognised that questions of what we should be doing have important ethical dimensions, then these ethical and value judgements can be more thoroughly debated and held up to scrutiny.

11.14   References

1. G. Scally & L. Donaldson, Clinical governance and the drive for quality improvement in the new NHS in England. *British Medical Journal*, **317** (1998), pp. 61–5.
2. D. R. Steel, Foreword from Scotland. In: Royal College of Nursing, *Clinical Governance: A resource guide* (London, RCN, 2007) http://www.clinicalgovernance.scot.nhs.uk/index.asp (accessed May 2012).
3. C. Som, Clinical governance a fresh look at its definition. *Clinical Governance*, **9** (2) (2004), pp. 87–90.
4. National Quality Board, *Quality Governance in the NHS – A guide for provider boards* (NQB, 2011), https://www.gov.uk/government/uploads/system/uploads/attachment_data/file/152061/dh_125239.pdf.pdf.
5. Care Quality Commission, *The State of Health Care and Adult Social Care in England* (London, The Stationery Office, 2011).
6. Department of Health, *Equity and Excellence: Liberating the NHS* (London, The Stationery Office, 2010).
7. Department of Health, *High Quality Care for All (the Darzi Report)* (London, DoH, 2008).
8. Department of Health, *An organisation with a memory: Report of an expert group on learning from adverse events in the NHS* (London, DoH, 2000).
9. Department of Health, *The NHS Outcomes Framework* (London, DoH, 2011).
10. Department of Health, *The Operating Framework for the NHS in England 2012–13*, (Lonfon, DoH, 2011).
11. National Quality Board, *NHS Patient Experience Framework* (London, NQB, 2012), https://www.gov.uk/government/uploads/system/uploads/attachment_data/file/146831/dh_132788.pdf.pdf
12. NICE *Patient experience in adult NHS services: improving the experience of care for people using adult NHS services*, NICE clinical guideline 138 (London, NICE, 2012).
13. Institute for Innovation and Improvement. *Living our Local Values* (London, NHS, 2008).
14. A. Campbell, Clinical governance – Watchword or buzzword? *Journal of Medical Ethics*, **27** (suppl. I) (2001), pp. i54–6.
15. Patients Forum, Options for the future (London, The Patients Forum, 2006).

16. House of Commons, *Health Committee Patient and Public Involvement in the NHS Third Report of Session 2006–07* (London, The Stationery Office, 2007).
17. Department of Health, *Patient and public involvement: A brief overview* (London, DoH, 2004) www.dh.gov.uk/PolicyAndGuidance/OrganisationPolicy/PatientAndPublicInvolvement.
18. Department of Health (2011) HealthWatch Transition Plan.
19. NICE (2012) Dabigatran etexilate for the prevention of stroke and systemic embolism in atrial fibrillation, Technology appraisals, TA249 – Issued: March 2012.
20. Department of Health (2011) *NHS Outcomes Framework 2012/13* (London, DH, 2011).
21. Department of Health (2011) *Improving outcomes: A strategy for cancer*, DH.
22. A. Boivin *et al.*, Patient and public involvement in clinical guidelines: International experiences and future perspectives. *Quality and Safety in Health Care*, **19** (2010), p. e22. doi: 10.1136/qshc.2009.034835.
23. I. Kerridge, Ethics and EBM: Acknowledging bias, accepting difference and embracing politics. *Journal of Evaluation in Clinical Practice*, **16** (2010), pp. 365–73.
24. W. Rosenberg & A. Donald, Evidence Based Medicine: An approach to clinical problem solving. *BMJ (Clinical Research Ed.)*, **310** (1995), pp. 1122–6.
25. J. Muir Gray, *Evidence-Based Health Care: How to Make Health Policy and Management Decisions* (London, Churchill Livingstone, 1997).
26. A. Maynard, Rationing health care: An exploration. *Health Policy*, **49** (1999), pp. 5–11.
27. A. Maynard, Evidence-based medicine: An incomplete method for informing treatment choices. *The Lancet*, **349** (1997), pp. 126–8.
28. D. Hughes & S. Doheny, Deliberating Tarceva: A case study of how British NHS managers decide whether to purchase a high-cost drug in the shadow of NICE guidance. *Social Science and Medicine*, **73** (2011), pp. 1460–78.
29. J. Raftery, Review of NICE's recommendations 1999–2005. *British Medical Journal*, **332** (2006), pp. pp1266–8.
30. Alzheimer's Society (2012) The story so far http://alzheimers.org.uk/site/scripts/documents_info.php?documentID=489 (accessed May 2012).
31. NICE (2012) Clinical guidelines. http://www.nice.org.uk/aboutnice/whatwedo/aboutclinicalguidelines/about_clinical_guidelines.jsp (accessed May 2012).
32. NHS Right Care (2011) *The NHS Atlas of Variation 2.0.* http://mediacentre.dh.gov.uk/2011/12/12/atlas-maps-out-variation-in-nhs/ (accessed May 2012).
33. NICE (2004) Fertility: Assessment and treatment for people with fertility problems, http://www.nice.org.uk/page.aspx?o=CG011.
34. Department of Health (2009) Primary care trust survey: Provision of IVF in England 2008.
35. A Hopkins & JK Solomon, Can contracts drive clinical care? *BMJ (Clinical Research Ed.)*, **313** (1996), pp. 477–8.
36. D. Kitchiner & P. Bundred, Integrated care pathways. *Archives in Disease in Childhood*, **75** (1996), pp. 166–8.
37. T. van der Weijden *et al.*, How to integrate individual patient values and preferences in clinical practice guidelines? A research protocol. *Implementation Science*, **5** (2010), p. 10.
38. NICE (2009) Factsheet 1: How NICE develops clinical guidelines and what documents we publish.
39. E. Harding *et al.*, Service user involvement in clinical guideline development and implementation: Learning from mental health service users in the UK. *International Review of Psychiatry*, **22** (2011), pp. 352–7.

40. H. van de Bovenkamp & M. Trappenburg, Reconsidering patient participation in guideline development. *Health Care Analysis*, **17** (2009), pp. 198–216.
41. D. Kitchiner *et al.*, Integrated care pathways. *Journal of Evaluation in Clinical Practice*, **2** (1) (1996), pp. 65–9.
42. National Reporting and Learning System (2012) *Quarterly data workbook*, http://www.nrls.npsa.nhs.uk/resources/collections/quarterly-data-summaries/?entryid 45=133438 (accessed May 2012).
43. National Patient Safety Agency, (2009) Being Open, DH.
44. C.J. Chamberlain *et al.*, Disclosure of non-harmful errors and other events. *Archives of Surgery*, **147** (3) (2012), pp. 282–6.
45. J. Lyon (1996) *The Trojan Horse: Problems of CRM*, MSc Dissertation, University of Liverpool.
46. A. Wu, Medical error: The second victim. *BMJ (Clinical Research Ed.)*, **320** (2000), pp. 726–7.
47. A. Wu & R. Steckelberg, Medical error, incident investigation and the second victim: Doing better but feeling worse? *Quality and Safety*, **21** (2012), pp. 267–70.
48. NHS Executive, *Risk Management in the NHS* (London, HMSO, 1994).
49. Patient Safety First, (2010) Implementing human factors in health care, London.
50. GMC (2012) GMC Fitness to Practise Statistics, http://www.gmc-uk.org/news/10866.asp (accessed May 2012).
51. GfK NOP Social Research (2011) Research into Fitness to Practise referrals, JN 452511.
52. General Medical Council (2006) *Good Medical Practice* (London, The General Medical Council).
53. Nursing and Midwifery Council, *The NMC Professional Code of Conduct: Standards of Conduct, Performance and Ethics* (London, NMC, 2008).

12 Clinical Research and Patients

A The Legal Perspective*

Natasha Hammond-Browning

Lecturer in Law, Southampton Law School, University of Southampton, Southampton

The issue of clinical research on human patients poses complex bioethical and legal dilemmas for nurses. Over the last 25 years nurses have steadily assumed a greater role in the conduct of clinical research, largely because of the increasing emphasis on evidence-based medicine, but also because involvement in research may help to validate their professional status. Nevertheless, it has been argued that there are still too few nurse researchers and that most nurses in practice are not sufficiently research-aware.[1] In an attempt to remedy this, the national strategy for nursing, midwifery and health visiting is committed to developing 'a strategy to influence the research and development agenda, to strengthen the capacity to undertake nursing, midwifery and health visiting research, and to

*This chapter is a revised version of the chapter in the last edition of this book, which was written by Marie Fox, University of Birmingham.

Nursing Law and Ethics, Fourth Edition. Edited by John Tingle and Alan Cribb.
© 2014 by John Wiley & Sons, Ltd. Published 2014 by John Wiley & Sons, Ltd.

use research to support nursing, midwifery and health visiting practice'.[2] Such initiatives make it imperative for nurses to have a clear understanding of the ethical and legal implications of engaging in clinical research.

The fundamental ethico-legal issue raised by clinical research involves a balancing exercise, between on the one hand the interests of the health professional carrying out research and of medical science itself, and on the other the welfare of those human patients or volunteers who are the subject of research.[3] Against that backdrop, the aim of this chapter is to explore the legal framework within which clinical research may be conducted. It should be noted that nurses have the same ethical and legal obligations as any other health professional,[4] although the particular position of the nurse and her relationship to her patients may present specific problems in some cases. However, as previous Royal College of Nursing guidance has stressed, 'In ethical terms . . . nurses have no more right than any other health professional to hide behind notions of subordination, compliance and obedience to justify avoiding personal responsibility for what they do as part of a research study'.[5]

It is worth noting that there is a relative absence of clear legal rules regulating research, although legislative intervention in this area is now growing and there is a proliferation of professional guidance. Thus although the Animals (Scientific Procedures) Act 1986 and the Human Fertilisation and Embryology Act 1990 created statutory bodies to regulate and license research that may lawfully be carried out on animals[6] and human embryos,[7] there has never been a statutory regime that licenses research on human patients in a comparable way. Equally, the common law in this area is marked by the absence of case law pertaining specifically to medical research. Thus, historically, the legal framework governing research has drawn heavily upon the principles laid down in relation to consent to conventional medical treatment and upon guidance for health professionals derived mainly from international declarations, which in turn have influenced codes of practice promulgated by professional bodies. However, in the past ten years there have been significant legal developments in this area. In the first place, concerns about clinical trials prompted the Department of Health to introduce a framework for clinical governance, while the introduction of a European Union Directive on the conduct of clinical trials, designed to harmonise the regulation of such trials throughout the EU, required the United Kingdom to produce new regulations to govern certain types of clinical research, which have been in force since 2004. More recently, the UK Government, as part of its *Plan for Growth*, laid before Parliament new regulations to establish the Health Research Agency (HRA) which has the National Research Ethics Service (NRES) at its core.[8] The HRA was established on the 1 December 2011 upon enactment of *The Health Research Authority Regulations 2011* and its remit applies to England only.

12.1   Definition of clinical research

Clinical research is traditionally classified in a number of ways. It is first distinguished from conventional treatment that uses approved methods and

322 Nursing Law and Ethics

techniques for therapeutic purposes. It is then subdivided into two broad classes of research. The first consists of those that do not involve any direct interference with the subject – for example, those involving psychological observation,[9] and the use of personal medical records or tissue samples. It can be difficult to draw distinctions between this and the second category – invasive research – which gives rise to much greater concern, as it involves direct physical or psychological interference with the subject. The focus in this chapter is on the issue of invasive research on human beings, but in the light of concerns and consequent legislation the issue of research using personal information and tissue samples is discussed (briefly) below. Invasive research on human subjects is conventionally further divided into two types:

(1) Therapeutic research is performed on a patient, and the use of new methods and techniques carries prospects of direct benefit to the individual patient.

(2) Non-therapeutic research involves the use of new procedures or drugs for purely or mainly scientific purposes that are unlikely to benefit the individual participant. While it may herald some collective benefit, the aim of the trial is the acquisition of scientific knowledge, and it is often carried out on healthy volunteers.[10]

It is worth noting that this therapeutic/non-therapeutic dichotomy, which has generated much bioethical scholarship, has been subject to attack. Commentators have suggested that it is a problematic distinction for the following reasons. First, in some cases therapeutic research may be more hazardous than non-therapeutic research. Second, it is often difficult to distinguish between research and innovative therapy. For instance, it is unclear whether a new surgical technique, such as keyhole surgery, should be subject to special regulation, as the introduction of a new drug procedure would be.[11] Third, in response to the lobbying of organised health pressure groups, such as AIDS patients, high-quality clinical care and responsible research have come to be recognised as a continuum rather than a dichotomy.[12] Priscilla Alderson has argued that '"[t]herapeutic" is an oddly fuzzy, unscientific word; it expresses possibly unfounded hopes for the future as if they were present realities, it confuses the aim of research with the activity . . . scientific rigour would assess research in terms of outcome, effectiveness and efficiency'.[13]

Notwithstanding the validity of these points, there may be good reason to retain the therapeutic/non-therapeutic distinction, given that advances attributed to research that is clearly non-therapeutic have been obtained at the cost of many blighted lives. In this regard, it is significant that historically these costs have been disproportionately borne by members of oppressed groups in society.[14] A major advantage of the distinction is that it enables commentators to argue that there should be a greater obligation to disclose risks in the context of non-therapeutic research.[15] Consequently, considerable controversy has been generated by the revision of the Declaration of Helsinki – the pre-eminent international agreement governing research – which in 2000 abandoned the distinction between therapeutic and non-therapeutic research. As some commentators have noted, an implied distinction between therapeutic and non-therapeutic research continues to underpin much of the guidance on research ethics promulgated by national professional bodies.[16] Moreover, issues arising from the catastrophic collapse of six healthy volunteers who participated in a Phase I trial of a drug compound – TGN1412 – designed to mitigate auto-immune and immunodeficiency diseases at Northwick Park Hospital in London in 2006 has indicated that the therapeutic/non-therapeutic distinction may continue to have ethical purchase. Certainly, the Northwick Park trial poses questions regarding the efficacy of the regulatory framework in general, which will be addressed below. These pertain to the validity of information about risks disclosed to the participants, the amount of money offered as an inducement (each participant was paid £2000), the complex way in which newer drugs function compared with the simpler compounds on which trials have traditionally focused, the reliability of prior animal testing, the failure to seek expert information from overseas sources, the absence of 'staggered dosing' in administering the compound, and the decision to administer the drug to healthy volunteers rather than to cancer patients who would have been less susceptible to toxicity (but more difficult and time-consuming to recruit). Latterly, the adequacy of insurance cover has also been raised.[17]

12.2   Regulation of clinical research

12.2.1   International declarations

The Declaration of Helsinki was promulgated largely as a result of the involvement of health professionals in medical experimentation amounting to torture on stigmatised social and ethnic groups in Nazi Germany. Indeed many ethico-legal concerns raised by clinical research have their roots in the Nazi era. The aftermath of the Nuremberg trials of Nazi war criminals witnessed the promulgation of the Nuremberg Code, which in 1964 was revised and expanded by the World Health Organization's Helsinki Declaration. It has subsequently been amended in 1975, 1983, 1989, 1996, 2000 and 2008.[18]

While the Nazi-era experiments exemplify the most appalling abuses of research, numerous subsequent examples highlight the continuing need for international regulation.[19] Particular concern has been prompted by medical research on subjects in the economic South, where standards may be lower and subjects less likely to benefit from expensive drugs marketed in the 'developed' world. Trials of AIDS drugs and vaccines, in particular, have courted controversy.[20]

Domestically, all nursing research carried out in the United Kingdom should comply with the fundamental principles enshrined in the Helsinki Declaration. This stresses that the first responsibility of the health professional is to his or her patient, and that considerations related to the well-being of the individual research subject should take precedence over all other interests (paras 4 and 6). Risks and burdens to the patient should be carefully assessed and must be compared with foreseeable benefits to them and others affected by the condition under investigation (para. 18), and that subjects are fully informed of them (para. 24). Furthermore, biomedical research must conform to generally accepted scientific procedures and be approved by an appropriate ethical review committee, conducted only by individuals with appropriate training and qualifications and supervised by a clinically competent medical professional (paras 12,15–16). The 1975 revision of the Helsinki Declaration recommended codes of practice for researchers, and this has resulted in guidelines promulgated by national bodies, of which the most prominent are those produced by the Royal College of Physicians[21] and the Royal College of Nursing,[22] as well as the guidelines that the Department of Health has recently published. *Governance Arrangements for NHS Research Ethics Committees: a harmonised edition* (hereafter the GAfREC harmonised guidelines) replaces the previous guidelines issued by the Central Office for Research Ethics Committees (COREC) (the GAfREC guidance).[23] Each of these sets of guidelines is underpinned by principles similar to those contained in the Helsinki Declaration. The Council of Europe's Convention on Human Rights and Biomedicine (1997) and its additional protocol on Biomedical Research (2005) have reaffirmed these principles.[24]

Although such guidelines are useful in stipulating patient rights and stressing the ethical obligations of researchers, they are not directly enforceable in law, and indeed the United Kingdom has yet to sign the Convention on Human Rights and Biomedicine. Moreover, guidance is inevitably framed in broad terms that leave considerable discretion to the researcher, particularly in assessing physical, psychological and emotional harm.

12.2.2   The criminal law

Notwithstanding the discretion thus entrusted to the scientific researcher, it should be noted that all activities undertaken by health professionals are circumscribed by the criminal law. English criminal law provides that undue harm may not be inflicted on an individual even if they are prepared to consent to the infliction of such harm (*R v. Brown* (1993)). In a consultation paper, *Consent in the Criminal Law*, the Law Commission (the body that deals with law reform issues in England and Wales) addressed the issue of what harm a person may legitimately consent to. It provisionally suggested that:

> a person should not be guilty of an offence if she causes injury to another, of whatever degree of seriousness, if such injury is caused during the course of properly approved medical research (i.e. approved by a Local Research Ethics Committee) and with the consent of the other person.[25]

This is consistent with the Law Commission's general stance regarding medical treatment, which is that legitimate clinical procedures may be undertaken regardless of the degree of harm that may result. However, the Commission did not address the key question of how 'acceptable risk' may be defined. This leaves open the issue of whether a high-risk trial may be undertaken if the patient is prepared to accept that risk – a matter considered below in the context of xenotransplantation. Certainly, failure to obtain the consent of an individual before she is included in a clinical trial may give rise to a criminal prosecution for battery. There is a remote possibility that a prosecution could be brought for manslaughter if a research subject died while participating in a high-risk trial. For instance, given the ethical concerns voiced about the Northwick Park trial above, it is possible that such a trial could have given rise to homicide charges had any of the subjects died. In 2001 similar concerns about the adequacy of risk and safety analysis were raised by the death of Ellen Roche – a 25-year-old lab technician – who had been enrolled as a healthy volunteer in an asthma trial at Johns Hopkins University Baltimore. Critics claimed that subjects were exposed to unacceptable risks because of lax oversight at federal, institutional and investigative levels.[26]

12.2.3   The civil law

As well as potentially constituting a criminal offence, battery/trespass to the person is also a civil wrong entitling the patient to sue for compensation. Thus, where any research involves examining, operating on or injecting the patient, consent must be obtained in advance for it to be carried out lawfully; unauthorised contact entitles the patient to damages. Consequently, obtaining adequate consent to participation is the key legal requirement in relation to nursing research, since authority to carry out research on a competent adult human subject derives from that person's consent.[27] Effectively, English law imposes responsibility on the individual research subject to protect herself from abuse by giving or withholding consent.[28] The upshot, as Berg has noted, is that in the past virtually all documented cases of abusive medical experimentation have been those that failed to employ satisfactory informed consent procedures.[29] Therefore, it is not surprising that the key principle enshrined in the Helsinki Declaration is that:

> each potential subject must be adequately informed of the aims, methods, sources of funding, any possible conflicts of interest, institutional affiliations of the researcher, the anticipated benefits and potential risks of the study and the discomfort it may entail, and any other relevant aspects of the study. The potential subject must be informed of the right to refuse to participate in the study or to withdraw consent to participate at any time without reprisal. Special attention should be given to the specific information needs of individual potential subjects as well as the methods used to deliver the information. After ensuring that the potential subject has understood the information, the physician or another appropriately qualified individual must then seek the potential subject's freely-given consent, preferably in writing. If the consent cannot be expressed in writing, the non-written consent must be formally documented and witnessed. (para. 24)

Similarly, in a nursing context, the Nursing and Midwifery Council's Code of Professional Conduct provides, *inter alia*:

All nurses . . . must ensure that you gain consent before you begin treatment or care . . . must respect and support people's rights to accept or decline treatment or care . . . must uphold people's rights to be fully involved in decisions about their care.[30]

Hence, a major issue in relation to consent to nursing research is how to ensure that the consent is 'freely-given' and 'informed'. As we saw in Chapter 7A, in relation to medical treatment, the courts have stated that so long as a patient gives a very general consent to treatment, the health professional will not be liable in the tort of battery (*Chatterton* v. *Gerson* (1981)). Although in *Sidaway* v. *Bethlem* (1985) the House of Lords rejected the view that the doctrine of informed consent forms part of English law in the context of medical treatment, it is clear in the post-*Sidaway* case law that the courts are increasingly prepared to call doctors to account, and reject the view that a responsible body of medical opinion is decisive in determining what should be disclosed to the patient. Cases such as *Pearce* v. *United Bristol Healthcare NHS Trust* have highlighted the importance of disclosing risks that would have affected the reasonable person's decision as to whether to consent to treatment, in order to avoid a finding of negligence. Moreover, although there have been no decided English cases on the duty of disclosure pertaining to clinical research, it is generally accepted by legal commentators that, in the context of research, law would impose stronger duties of disclosure.[31] Thus someone who volunteers for research is entitled to a fuller explanation of the nature of the trial and the risks it carries than would be the case in relation to conventional medical treatment. It is highly probable that English law would follow Canadian law[32] in adopting an objective test requiring a researcher to disclose all relevant facts that a reasonable subject would wish to know, and to provide the opportunity for questions, to which full and honest answers would be given.[33] The General Medical Council (GMC) frames this requirement in the following terms:

> Seeking consent is fundamental in research involving people. Participants' consent is legally valid and professionally acceptable only if they have the capacity to decide whether to take part in the research, have been properly informed, and have agreed to participate without pressure or coercion . . . You must give people the information they want or need in order to decide whether to take part in research. How much information you share with them will depend on their individual circumstances. You must not make assumptions about the information a person might want or need, or their knowledge and understanding of the proposed research project . . . You must make sure that people are given information in a way that they can understand. You should check that people understand the terms that you use and any explanation given about the proposed research method.[34]

However, given that researchers themselves may lack adequate information about the risks of a proposed new drug or course of treatment, some commentators query whether informed consent is truly possible in the context of clinical research.[35] Certainly, it is questionable whether the intended experimental subject can validly consent to procedures the results of which are uncertain, of dubious benefit or clearly harmful[36] – issues that are canvassed below in relation to xenotransplantation. It is thus not surprising that in those few court cases where judges have addressed the issue of consent to research, they have tended to limit their role to ensuring that fully informed, voluntary consent has been given. Yet, as Tobias has pointed out, notwithstanding the legal emphasis on informed consent 'neither lawyers, ethicists, nor medical scientists have so far agreed precisely what this term actually means'.[37] In this regard, Jackson highlights the existence of various grey areas. For instance, should a researcher disclose details of the funding of the trial, including any personal or financial benefit that she hopes to obtain, or the fact that she has been paid to carry out the trial?[38] Furthermore, McNeil has contended that, notwithstanding the emphasis that courts have traditionally placed on obtaining consent, consent alone is an inadequate basis on which to regulate experimentation on human subjects. In his view, the focus on consent fails to fully address issues such as the weighting of the risks and benefits of experimentation for the subject and society, and enables courts to avoid issues such as whether they should endorse guidelines for researchers.[39]

Following the tragic consequences of thalidomide, which was marketed as a remedy for morning sickness during pregnancy and caused severe limb deformities in children, legislation was introduced to regulate the introduction of new pharmaceuticals. The Medicines Act 1968 introduced a new system for licensing and monitoring of new drugs overseen by the Medicines Control Agency, which in 2003 merged with the Medical Devices Agency to form the Medical and Healthcare Products Regulatory Agency (MHRA). In 2001 a Directive was issued by the European Parliament on the approximation of the laws regulating clinical trials of medicinal products, with the aim of ensuring that good clinical practice is observed in the design, conduct, recording and reporting of clinical trials on human subjects throughout the European Union.[40] The outcome in the United Kingdom has been the enactment of the Medicines for Human Use (Clinical Trials) Regulations 2004 (hereafter referred to as the Clinical Trials Regulations). Under this legislation, an authorisation must be sought from the MHRA before new medicines can be tested in clinical trials. The 1968 Act and 2004 regulations have established a complex reporting system to monitor the impact of the drug in question. Any unexpected or adverse outcomes during treatment with the drug must be reported to the MHRA.[41] The so-called 'yellow card' scheme enables nurses, midwives and health visitors, as well as GPs and patients themselves to report any adverse drug reactions, following research indicating that GPs were failing to report adequately.[42]

12.2.4   The relationship between the investigator and the research subject

A further factor that impacts on the process of obtaining consent is the sometimes problematic nature of the relationship between the research subject and the health care professional engaged in research. As McNeil argues, the history of human experimentation is one of imbalance in favour of the interests of the researcher.[43] It has been extensively documented how in the research context the role of the health care professional has changed from that of a physician (or more recently a nurse) to that of a scientific investigator, to become, in Jay Katz's term, a 'physician-investigator' (or 'nurse-investigator'). Not only does this entail a potential conflict of loyalties to patients, employers and research aims, as a result of her multiple priorities as teacher, researcher, health professional and administrator;[44] it also means that the researcher is likely to be seen in a more ambivalent light by the subject. Kennedy has suggested that a health professional's primary duty to care for her patient is inevitably compromised by her duty to carry out clinical trials with due scientific rigour.[45] The researcher's commitment to such rigour leaves the patient in an even more disempowered position than is normally the case in engagement with health professionals, since scientific ideology generally requires the researcher to view the subject with dispassion and detachment.[46] As Katz points out, it follows that 'the commitment to objectivity invites the investigator's thought processes to become objectified and, in turn, to transform the human beings who are the subjects of research into data points to be plotted on a chart that will prove or disprove a research hypothesis'.[47]

Such power imbalances are especially likely to arise where the research subject is differentiated from the investigator by factors such as gender, class, race and ethnicity, which may pose communication difficulties. Given these disparities in power, researchers should bear in mind Morehouse's claim that '[t]here are many ways of introducing a research project to a patient which fall short of pressurising the patients, but certainly do not conform to total objectivity'.[48] This may particularly apply in the case of vulnerable groups of patients, discussed below. The Declaration of Helsinki provides that:

> When seeking informed consent for participation in a research study the physician should be particularly cautious if the potential subject is in a dependent relationship with the physician or may consent under duress. In such situations the informed consent should be sought by an appropriately qualified individual who is completely independent of this relationship. (para. 26)

In common with many legal documents, the Helsinki Declaration focuses on the role of doctors. However, the tension between scientific objectivity and concern for the patient is likely to be particularly disconcerting for nurses. Not only can it be argued that nursing is more firmly grounded in notions of care and nurturance than other health professions,[49] but in practice nurses tend to have closer relationships with their patients than do doctors. It may follow that nurses are viewed as better placed to explain the consequences of enrolment in a trial to a patient and to obtain their consent. Certainly, if a nurse finds herself in the position of seeking consent, guidelines promulgated by bodies such as the Medical Research Council (MRC) and GMC stress the need for explanations to be given in clear and easily comprehensible language. Any special communication or language needs of the participants should be taken into account.

As highlighted by the Griffiths Review into the conduct of research trials involving children at North Staffordshire Hospital during the 1990s, it is important to appreciate the difficulty of understanding and giving a valid consent at a time of severe physical, psychological or emotional stress.[50] The GMC guidance states that honesty and integrity are key to obtaining valid consent and stresses that researchers '. . . must be open and honest with participants and members of the research team, including nonmedical staff, when sharing information about a research project. . . . answer questions honestly and as fully as possible.'[51] The MRC suggests that it is useful, as well as good practice, to seek advice from consumers or lay persons in drafting information for potential subjects.[52] As noted above, subjects should also be clearly informed of their right to withdraw from participation at any time without reprisal.[53] Additionally, they must be given an explanation of how personal information will be stored, transmitted and published. In terms of the form of consent, we saw in Chapter 7A that written consent is generally only evidence of consent, but the Clinical Trials Regulations 2004 require that the decision must be 'given freely after [the participant] is informed of the nature, significance, implications and risks of the trial' and either must be in writing or 'if the person is unable to sign or mark a document so as to indicate his consent, is given orally in the presence of at least one witness and recorded in writing' (para. 3(1), Part 1, Schedule 1).

12.2.5   Consent to randomised controlled trials

Particular problems arise in the context of consent to randomised controlled trials (RCTs). RCTs, which aim to compare treatments or approaches in two or more groups of subjects who are allocated randomly to those groups,[54] have been promoted as the most scientifically valid method of evaluating procedures.[55] Those who endorse randomisation (which aims to rule out a purely psychological reaction to new drugs) argue that if drugs are not investigated using randomisation and blinding of both researchers and subjects to the process, then there is a strong possibility that bias will enter the study and affect the results. However, other commentators have suggested that RCTs may adversely affect the health professional–patient relationship by harming the bond of trust and mutual respect that is the ideal of medical practice, and run counter to the health professional's duty to decide what treatment is best for the individual patient.[56]

Oakley suggests that RCTs are ethically problematic since chance allocation may be antithetical to good ethical practice. In particular, she expresses concern at how 'the tension between the scientific aims of research and the humane treatment of individuals . . . is expressed in the very strategy of designing an experiment so as to restrict people's freedom to discuss with one another the commonality of the process in which they are engaged'.[57] What is certain is that the weighing-up of risks and how they are presented to potential participants is crucial with RCTs. Fletcher *et al.* suggest that the fundamental issue is the purpose for which the research is being carried out, and that generally a trial should only proceed 'if the likely benefits to the individual taking part in the research and/or to society as a whole far outweigh the risks of participation'.[58] Additionally, the Declaration of Helsinki provides that 'Physicians must immediately stop a study when the risks are found to outweigh the potential benefits or when there is conclusive proof of positive and beneficial results' (para. 20).

Given the uncertainties until such a point is reached, RCTs pose considerable problems for the law on informed consent, since the technique of randomisation makes it more difficult for the researcher to fully explain the risks to an individual patient. As Oakley notes, 'What people understand may not be what researchers think they do; "informed consent" is a shifting, complex process, rather than a discrete cognitive event'.[59] Certainly, the crucial issue in obtaining consent will be how the risks and benefits of the proposed research are presented to the research subject. Tobias has pointed to the practical difficulties of gaining informed consent in such trials, especially given the potential for misconception and anxiety, if the consequences of randomisation are fully explained to the patient. He argues that, instead, we should trust health professionals to engage in randomisation without explicit consent.[60] However, the consensus among legal commentators endorses Kennedy's view that with RCTs it is particularly important that the materiality of risk should be defined according to what the particular patient would want to know.[61]

The Griffiths Review into events at North Staffordshire in the 1990s highlighted numerous problems with the process for obtaining such consent.[62] Nurses were centrally involved and the review panel found that the nursing sister assigned to a project focusing on the treatment of respiratory problems in premature new-born babies did not appear to have been provided with a protocol or system for ensuring adequate documentation for all patients. It concluded that, in general, the nursing staff lacked adequate research experience for the tasks that they were asked to do, yet were not offered any training. Inadequate supervision by the researchers, coupled with a lack of support from the trust nursing management, contributed to problems in documenting whether consent forms had been completed.[63] There were particular concerns about the adequacy of information given to parents who were asked to enter their children in a trial in which a new technique – continuous negative extrathoracic pressure (CNEP) – was compared with the conventional treatment of positive pressure ventilation, given that some of the children subsequently suffered brain damage or died. Hopefully, the introduction of more detailed guidance on research governance (see below) will obviate these problems. However, nurses who are concerned by the conduct of trials or their qualifications for conducting them should be prepared to 'whistle-blow' where necessary.[64] What is clear is that participants must be fully aware on enrolling in an RCT that they will have no choice as to which treatment is given, and will not know what treatment they have been given until the end of the trial.

Additional problems are posed by RCTs involving placebos. The Helsinki Declaration states that:

> The benefits, risks, burdens and effectiveness of a new intervention must be tested against those of the best current proven intervention, except in the following circumstances:
>
> - The use of placebo, or no treatment, is acceptable in studies where no current proven intervention exists; or
> - Where for compelling and scientifically sound methodological reasons the use of placebo is necessary to determine the efficacy or safety of an inter-

vention and the patients who receive placebo or no treatment will not be subject to any risk of serious or irreversible harm. Extreme care must be taken to avoid abuse of this option.[65]

However, it has been queried whether such caution is justified, given the scientific value of placebo trials. Miller and Brody argue that 'it can be ethical to use placebo controls in scientifically valuable RCTs that involve withholding proven effective medical treatment, provided that the risks are not excessive and participants give informed consent'.[66] Guideline 11 of the revised guidance issued by the Council for International Organizations of Medical Sciences[67] (CIOMS) provides that 'as a general rule, research subjects in the control group of a trial . . . should receive an established effective intervention'. However, the guidelines sanction the use of placebos where there is no established effective intervention, or when withholding an established effective intervention would expose subjects to, at most, temporary discomfort or delay in relief of symptoms or when such established intervention would not yield scientifically reliable results and using a placebo would not add any risk or serious or irreversible harm to the subjects.

12.2.6   Research using personal information or human tissue

Many significant medical advances have resulted not from research trials involving human subjects but from the use of personal health information or human tissue samples retained following post-mortem examinations. For instance, such research has improved understanding of suspected health hazards, facilitated recognition of the epidemiology of new diseases (such as new-variant Creutzfeldt–Jakob disease (CJD) and its relation to the bovine spongiform encephalopathy (BSE) epidemic) and led to advice on reducing cot deaths. For many years such research was seen as less ethically problematic than research on human subjects, especially as well-coordinated use of such material can reduce the research demands on patients and the need for animal research.

However, such research has become hugely contentious. In particular, public outcry over unauthorised retention of children's organs at both Bristol Royal Infirmary and Alder Hey Hospital in Liverpool led to the establishment of public inquiries in the late 1990s,[68] and subsequently to the passage of the Human Tissue Act 2004. This legislation introduces a new regime to regulate use of human tissue, and once again the concept of consent is enshrined as the cornerstone. When the Human Tissue Bill was originally promulgated it contained requirements for specific consent[69] but in the course of the passage of the legislation through Parliament this was watered down (though see below). Thus, although section 1 of the 2004 Act stipulates that 'appropriate consent' must have been obtained before human tissue or organs may be removed for the purposes of research, the notion of 'consent' is not further defined in the Act itself. Section 3 does, however, specify three ways in which consent may be obtained for the use of cadaveric organs or tissue. First, the donor can stipulate her consent or lack of consent prior to death, either in writing (or by joining the organ donor register) or making her views clear to friends or relatives. Second, under section 4 of the Act she may appoint a person to represent her wishes after death for the purposes of giving or withholding consent to the removal of tissue or organs. Third, where no wishes have been indicated and no representative appointed, the consent of a person in a 'qualifying relationship' to the donor must be sought. Section 27(4) of the Human Tissue Act defines and ranks qualifying relationships, providing that the consent of a spouse or partner should be sought first, followed by that of a parent or child, and so on to the consent of a friend of long standing. Section 2(7) provides that a competent minor can consent to organ or tissue donation for research; and that where the child is not competent, the person with parental responsibility for her is authorised to consent or, in cases where no person has parental responsibility immediately prior to death, consent may be given by a person in a qualifying relationship to the child.[70] Where a living person wants to donate human organs or tissue for research purposes, according to section 3(2) of the Human Tissue Act 'appropriate consent' simply means the donor's consent, which is not further defined.

However, one of the Codes of Practice promulgated under the Act by the Human Tissue Authority established by the Act provides detailed guidance on obtaining consent for activities covered by the Act, which includes research on tissues donated by the living and taken from the deceased.[71] The code stresses that consent should be viewed as a process in which individuals . . . may discuss the issue fully, ask questions and make an informed choice (para. 33), that consent should be sought by a health professional who has been suitably trained (paras 48,52) and that the person must understand what the activity involves and, where appropriate, what the risks are (para. 32) Although, as we have seen, this requirement was absent from the final Act, the Code of Practice does specify that patients should be asked whether the consent they give is 'generic' (i.e. for any future project approved by an REC) or specific (para. 35), and they should be told if any samples will be put to commercial use (para. 149). It is good practice for the consent to be in writing, although this is not a specific requirement for research under the HTA (para. 33).

12.3   Ethical review

12.3.1   Research ethics committees

For most other forms of clinical research aside from that on tissues, the regulatory focus has, to some extent, now shifted from an emphasis on obtaining consent to ensuring compliance with codes of research practice, following the introduction of ethical review. Since 1968 official NHS policy has been that local research ethics committees (LRECs) should be established to oversee clinical research within the NHS. Under the EU Clinical Trials Directive ethics committee approval is now mandatory before any clinical trial can commence. Research Ethics Committees (RECs) were governed by Department of Health guidelines issued in 1991, which were revised under the research governance arrangements of 2001 and recently replaced by a 2011 harmonised edition.[72]

RECs have traditionally been envisaged as independent bodies, comprising both health professionals and lay persons, who are charged with the responsibility of protecting the rights and well-being of human subjects involved in a trial and have traditionally been self-regulating. However, since 1 May 2004 RECs that oversee clinical trials that come within the remit of the EU Clinical Trials Directive and the Clinical Trials Regulations 2004 that implement them (see section 12.2.3 above) are legally accountable to a new government body – the UK Ethics Committee Authority – which essentially comprises the Secretaries of State for health for England, Wales, Scotland and Northern Ireland. Although in theory this new Authority should overcome lots of the problems inherent in self-regulation – such as lack of transparency and accountability, and inadequate provision for monitoring and sanctions[73] – concerns have been expressed about subjecting research ethics to direct political control.[74] Equally controversial has been the recommendation by the Department of Health's Ad Hoc Advisory Group on the Operation of NHS Research Ethics Committees that the United Kingdom should move towards a fully professionalised REC workforce.[75] The consequence would be a reduction in the number of RECs, from around 200 currently to as few as 30, on the grounds of efficiency and reducing variation in decision-making.[76]

According to GAREC Harmonised guidance, the key function of RECs is defined as to 'review research proposals to assess formally if research is ethical' (para. 1.1.1). The Department of Health's Ad Hoc Advisory Group confirmed in 2005 that the key question for RECs to address is the ethical acceptability of the protocol, with appropriate specialists judging the scientific merit prior to the REC assessment of whether it satisfies appropriate ethical standards,[77] although this view has been criticised for its failure to demarcate scientific and ethical review.[78] The GAREC Harmonised guidance stipulates that 'A REC need not reconsider the quality of the science, as this is the responsibility of the sponsor and will have been subject to review by one or more experts in the field . . .' (para 5.4.2(a)). It thus takes the view that it is not the task of a REC to undertake additional scientific review. However, the REC should satisfy itself that the review already undertaken is adequate for the nature of the proposal under consideration. Before giving a favourable opinion, the REC must be '. . . assured about the ethical issues presented by the proposed research. These issues may vary, depending on the research in question. REC members receive training and guidance . . . about the issues they should consider, both in general and in particular cases. The training and guidance reflect recognised standards for ethical research, such as the Declaration of Helsinki, and take account of applicable legal requirements'.[79] Article 6 of the Clinical Trials Regulations 2004 and Para 3.2.9 of GAREC Harmonised guidance requires RECs to notify the applicant of its opinion within 60 days of receipt of a valid application in most cases, prompting concerns that workload and time pressures may remove the space for negotiation between institutions and RECs and impact adversely on the quality of decision-making.[80]

12.3.2   The limitations of research ethics committees

Although the existence of ethics committees is clearly desirable, various concerns have in the past been voiced about their effectiveness as a mechanism for scrutinising and monitoring clinical research, and it remains to be seen how the regime under the 2011 guidance will work in practice. The limitations of the self-regulatory system became strikingly apparent during the investigation into research on children at North Staffordshire Hospital. The Griffiths Inquiry found that, although the North Staffordshire REC generally operated in accordance with Department of Health Guidelines then in force, the level of detail in their minutes compared unsatisfactorily with minutes provided by a selection of other RECs to the review. Additionally, the computer-held register of research projects failed to include all the details required by the guidelines. The Inquiry also noted a lack of clarity in respect of how and when variations to a research project were to be reported.[81] Moreover, the LREC was criticised for doing little to ascertain whether its opinion was well informed or bore any relation to what other ethical review committees did or might have done in similar circumstances – increasingly this is regarded as a component of good practice (para. 9.2.2). A further concern related to the lack of training for members, with the Griffiths Inquiry finding that many members of the ethics committee had never been offered training.

These criticisms highlight the increasingly onerous duties entailed by membership of such committees. Thus, providing appropriate training for the members of RECs is a central plank of the current research governance framework for RECs. Para. 4.3.11 of the GAREC Harmonised guidance states that 'As a condition of appointment, REC members must agree to take part in initial and continual training appropriate to their role'. The North Staffordshire Inquiry also stressed that appointment of members should be an open process, compatible with Nolan standards and requiring public advertisement in the media, as well as through professional networks, and the submission of CVs. On the composition of RECs, it proposed that among the recommended 12–18 members there should be a balanced age and gender distribution, while efforts should be made to recruit ethnic minorities and those with disabilities. Such proposals seek to address past criticism concerning the under-representation of lay people, and the fact that one British study found that women and ethnic minority groups were poorly represented.[82] The GAREC Harmonised guidance now stipulates that there should normally be a maximum of 18 members (para 4.2.10), of whom at least one third are lay members (para 4.2.7), but that it should have a 'sufficiently broad range of experience and expertise, so that the rationale, aims, objectives and designs of the research proposals that it reviews can be effectively reconciled with the dignity, rights, safety and well being of the people who are likely to take part' (para 4.2.1). It also specifies that the REC should be balanced to reflect the diversity of the adult population of society' (para 4.2.4). Each REC should also '. . . have expert members to ensure methodological and ethical expertise about research in care settings and in relevant fields of care, as well as professional expertise as care practitioners' (para 4.2.6).[83]

Nurses who are members of RECs should also be aware of the possibility of legal action being taken against the decisions of RECs. Decisions may be judicially reviewed by the courts, and if RECs are found to have acted *ultra vires* or to have reached decisions irrationally or contrary to the rules of natural justice, then decisions may be referred back to the committee or struck down.[84] No negligence action has been brought against an REC, and in the past they have been deemed not to have a legal personality distinct from their members (in the way a company has legal personality), so it was thought likely that any action would lie against individual members, who are under a legal duty to act with due care in decision-making (although strategic health authorities do offer indemnity when members are appointed to RECs provided they act in good faith).[85] McHale suggests that since RECs have been placed on a statutory footing under the Clinical Trials Regulations, there may now be the possibility of a finding in negligence against the REC itself.[86] However, as Jackson notes, in practice any persons harmed as a result of an REC decision are more likely to proceed against potential defendants with greater resources, such as the pharmaceutical company sponsoring the trial.[87]

Prior to the Griffiths Review and the new research governance framework, there had long been disquiet over variations in the practices of ethics committees, such as those exposed at North Staffordshire. Such variations resulted in part from the way in which trials tended to be scrutinised on a local rather than national basis. In 1996 the Department of Health recommended that regional bodies – multicentre research ethics committees (MRECs) – should be established to scrutinise research protocols that proposed to undertake a number of trials at different locations throughout the country. While this certainly has reduced variation in local rates of approval, since LRECs are required to state reasons if they reject a protocol approved by an MREC,[88] a cynical view is that they are a convenient way of enabling researchers and drug companies to gain approval for projects notwithstanding objections at a local level.[89] Conversely, some commentators have contended that the process for seeking MREC approval is overly complex, leading to costly delays in the process of marketing drugs.[90] It is also worth noting that with the growth of new biotechnologies, such as reproductive technologies, gene therapy and xenotransplantation, a proliferating number of committees have been established to oversee research, with consequent problems relating to the overlapping roles and functions of these various bodies.[91] In an effort to deal with this fragmentation, COREC was established in 2000 to coordinate the work of the various ethics committees, it was succeeded by a new National Research Ethics Service on 1 April 2007. The research governance framework aimed to eliminate variations and inconsistencies in practice. In December 2011 the National Research Ethics Service became part of the Health Research Authority (HRA), which is envisaged to be 'a new pathway for the regulation and governance of health research' with the aim 'to streamline regulation, create a unified approval process, and promote proportionate standards for compliance and inspection within a consistent national system of research governance'.[92] Whether this happens only time will tell.

A further concern about RECs relates to the inadequate resources they have to monitor research once the initial approval is granted. McNeil contends that RECs are typical of self-regulating groups in their failure to deal adequately with non-compliance,[93] especially if the researcher is not seeking overseas grants or publication in international journals.[94] Although the Declaration of Helsinki stresses the obligation on researchers to provide monitoring information to the ethical review committee and in particular to report adverse events (para. 15), there is generally no sanction for failure to do so. To address this, the MRC requires that applicants for funding include with their research protocol their plans to ensure independent supervision of the clinical trial. It recommends that a trial steering committee be set up, which should include at least one of the principal investigators conducting the research, and at least three independent members, one of whom would chair the committee. It would meet to approve the final protocol before the start of the trial, and thereafter at least annually to monitor the progress of the trial and to maximise the chances of its being completed within the agreed timescale.[95]

The Griffiths Inquiry also stressed the responsibility of research ethics committees to review past decisions and to ensure that good management processes are built into research proposals. In this regard, the Clinical Trials Directive highlights the importance of monitoring. If a Member State has objective grounds for considering that the conditions in the request for authorisation are no longer met, or has doubts about the safety or scientific validity of the clinical trial, it will have powers to suspend or prohibit the clinical trial, or inform those responsible for conducting the trial how to remedy the situation (Article 12). Member States are required to appoint investigators to inspect sites on which clinical trials are conducted (Article 15); they must report all serious adverse events (Article 16). These requirements are implemented in the Clinical Trials Regulations, which impose strict requirements for the prompt reporting of actual and suspected serious adverse events (regulations 32–5). In addition, the GAREC Harmonised Guidance states that the research sponsor and other relevant bodies are responsible for enforcement if research is unsafe or not carried out as agreed and that RECS must require an annual report from the researcher (paras 3.2.15 and 3.2.17 and Annex G). However, it is still unclear whether these measures constitute a meaningful form of monitoring, given Jackson's contention that '[w]hile progress reports must be submitted, the committee's role is largely confined to collecting information volunteered by the researchers, rather than investigating the extent to which there has been compliance with the original protocol'.[96] Moreover this absence of effective mechanisms for monitoring is coupled with a practice whereby RECs have approved over 90% of research proposals after asking the researchers to consider minor modifications.[97]

In the USA criticisms of the ethical review system led to the establishment of a National Bioethics Advisory Commission to provide advice and recommendations on the appropriateness of certain government policies and practices in bioethics, including principles for the ethical conduct of research.[98] Some commentators have called for a similar commission to be set up in the United Kingdom.[99] While such calls have to some extent been superseded at the supranational level by the requirement to implement the Clinical Trials Directive, it is worth noting that, notwithstanding its claims to enhance the protection of research subjects, the Directive has been criticised as industry-led and designed to promote Europe as a research location.[100] Moreover, other commentators have stressed the value of RECs having knowledge of local investigators, which is steadily being lost in the drive to centralise.[101]

12.3.3   Research fraud and deception

A further obstacle to ensuring accountability of researchers is that cases of deception and fraud have been reported with increasing frequency over the last 15 years.[102] A high-profile example is the scandal over stem cell scientist Woo Suk Hwang who faked data in cloning experiments in South Korea, which was exposed in 2005.[103] Since scarce funding leads to pressure to demonstrate results for money invested and to publish widely for career advancement, there is considerable temptation to falsify results in this way. Numerous prestigious journals have acknowledged the extent of research fraud.[104] Although the Royal College of Physicians has stressed the necessity of following good practice and indicated in 1991 the need for a body to investigate allegations of fraud, no such body has been established. In 1997 the Committee on Publication Ethics (COPE) was established by a small group of medical journal editors to '. . . provide advice to editors and publishers on all aspects of publication ethics and, in particular, how to handle cases of research and publication misconduct. It also provides a forum for its members to discuss individual cases . . . COPE does not investigate individual cases but encourages editors to ensure that cases are investigated by the appropriate authorities (usually a research institution or employer).' COPE has also written a code of conduct and best practice guidelines for journal editors.[105] In the meantime it is the threat of litigation that holds researchers accountable, although the establishment of COPE has led to increased pressure on editors of scientific journals to pursue allegations of research misconduct.[106] A more general problem with the system for publishing research is that articles are much more likely to secure publication if the conclusions are positive, so that published research provides only a very incomplete picture of research projects actually undertaken.[107]

12.4   Vulnerable groups of research subjects

Researchers must be sensitive to the fact that some groups of potential subjects may be particularly vulnerable to pressure to participate in clinical trials, either because of doubts regarding their competence to participate or because their situation means that vulnerability is exacerbated by institutional and attitudinal factors. Particular concerns have been raised regarding research on children or mentally incompetent adults, and it is widely recognised that these groups should be accorded special protection. A specific failing identified by the Griffiths Review at North Staffordshire was the lack of specific guidance to researchers on how valid consent is to be obtained in vulnerable groups. Too often it was simply assumed that researchers were aware of the useful guidance contained in the Royal College of Physicians' guidelines. Once again this highlights the need for researchers to be fully informed of their legal obligations and current professional guidance. However, research with vulnerable groups should not be avoided, in some cases it is considered to be '. . . essential to conduct research in these groups in order to increase and enhance our understanding of the illness and disabilities from which they suffer, as well as to develop new and existing therapies to better treat their effects.'[108]

12.4.1   Children

Most clinical research is undertaken on competent adults. Indeed, the Nuremberg Code of 1947 and other early ethical guidance stressed that research should be carried out *only* on competent volunteers. However, in recognition of the different developmental, physiological and psychological differences in children, which make age- and development-related research important for their benefit, it is now generally accepted that children can participate in research protocols, provided strict safeguards are observed.[109] Clinical research involving child patients is important in the case of conditions that only or predominantly affect children, such as Duchenne muscular dystrophy, a rare single-gene disorder, which affects boys and typically results in death by the patient's late teens. The importance of research involving children has been highlighted in the wake of reports that nine out of ten drugs given to newborn babies and 50% of drugs prescribed for children of all ages have never been clinically tested on child subjects to ensure that that they are appropriate.[110] In recognition of the importance of adequate testing of drugs on children, the European Commission has signalled its intention to promulgate legislation that would compel pharmaceutical companies to undertake appropriate research on children to ensure that their therapeutic needs are addressed.[111]

Guideline 14 of the CIOMS guidance provides that, prior to undertaking research involving children, the researcher must ensure that:

- the research might not equally well be carried out with adults;
- the purpose of the research is to obtain knowledge relevant to the health needs of children;
- a parent or legal representative of each child has given permission;
- the agreement (assent) of each child has been obtained to the extent of the child's capabilities; and
- a child's refusal to participate in research will be respected.[112]

Thus, it seems that lawful research must relate to a condition from which the child suffers, must be designed to benefit that group, and there must be no alternative to the use of minors. Yet, beyond this, as Jackson notes, ethico-legal guidance remains inherently unclear. She suggests that it is misplaced to emphasise risk evaluation, rather than the burdens of participation, and that an assessment of the burdens should be weighed against the social benefits that may derive from involvement in research.[113]

Researchers should note that 'childhood' is a heterogeneous category and that it is important to take account of the different capabilities of children. Thus, older children who are capable of understanding the process, and better able to tolerate pain, should be selected ahead of younger children, unless there are significant age-related scientific reasons to include younger children. The Clinical Trials Directive stresses that minors should receive, from staff with experience with minors, information pertaining to the trial and its risks and benefits (Article 4(b)) – a condition implemented in the Clinical Trials Regulations.[114] As we saw in Chapter 10, English law permits a minor to consent to medical *treatment* if she is over 16 or is Gillick-competent. For some time it was unclear in English law how far this rule applied to research. The position has now been clarified by the 2004 Regulations, which define a minor as 'a person under the age of 16 years' (regulation 14). Thus, for a person younger than 16 the consent of her parents or legal representative (as defined in regulation 15) is necessary for participation in research to be lawful, regardless of whether she is Gillick-competent. The parent or legal representative should act on the basis of the minor's 'presumed will' under Article 4(a) of the Clinical Trials Directive. Thus a 'substituted judgement' test effectively replaces the common-law test of best interests in this context. While the Directive prohibits anyone under 16 from consenting to involvement in research, it does provide that the explicit *refusal* of a minor to participate should be considered by the investigator, provided the minor is capable of assessing the information provided and refusing consent (Article 4(c)). The regulations explicitly rule out the offering of any financial inducement to the minor or those authorised to consent to her involvement.[114] Given the scope of these regulations, much will depend on how they are interpreted. Edwards and McNamee have suggested that professional guidance in the UK is generally too permissive of research.[115] For instance, they point out that the Royal College of Paediatrics and Child Health (RCPCH) guidance[116] seems to breach the requirement in the Declaration of Helsinki ruling out research that prioritises the interests of third parties over those of the research subject by stating that 'research in which children are submitted to more than minimal risk, with only slight, uncertain or no benefit to themselves deserves serious ethical consideration'. By contrast Haggar and Woods suggest that the Clinical Trials Directive and other guidance may be seen as unduly restrictive with regard to the participation of children.[117]

In practice, most research on young children and babies will involve routine interventions, such as taking blood samples. In such cases it is important that parents are informed clearly that the samples are for research purposes and can be refused without adverse consequences for the child's treatment.[118] In the case of more invasive interventions, the events at North Staffordshire indicated that particular obstacles to obtaining informed consent may be encountered in trials involving sick babies, given the emotional stress parents are likely to be under. Guidance issued as a result by the RCPCH suggests that in emergency situations (e.g. where a newborn needs to be ventilated urgently), a form of provisional consent or agreement in principle should be sought by health professionals. This would allow options to be evaluated more fully after parents or legal representatives had had adequate time to reflect.[119]

12.4.2   The mentally incapacitated adult

Although incompetent adults clearly differ from children in many ways, similar issues are raised by proposals to carry out research on both groups. Once again the competence of the incapacitated person will have to be assessed carefully in relation to the particular procedure. As discussed in Chapter 7A, a patient may be competent to consent to one form of treatment but not to another. This applies equally in the research context.

The GMC guidance requires that the following criteria are met before a group of incompetent adults may participate in research:

> if it is related to their incapacity or its treatment;
>   if the research is expected to provide a benefit to them that outweighs the risks;
>   if the research is not expected to provide a direct benefit to them but is expected to contribute to the understanding of their incapacity, leading to an indirect benefit to them or others with the same incapacity, and if the risks are minimal.

Moreover, researchers '. . . must make sure that a participant's right to withdraw from research is respected. You should consider any sign of objection, distress or indication of refusal, whether or not it is spoken, as implied refusal'.[120]

Guideline 15 of the CIOMS guidance stipulates that:

> Before undertaking research involving individuals who by reason of mental or behavioural disorders are not capable of giving adequately informed consent, the investigator must ensure that:
>
> - such persons will not be subjects of research that might equally well be carried out on persons whose capacity to give adequately informed consent is not impaired;
> - the purpose of the research is to obtain knowledge relevant to the particular health needs of persons with mental or behavioural disorders;
> - the consent of each subject has been obtained to the extent of that person's capabilities, and a prospective subject's refusal to participate in research is always respected, unless, in exceptional circumstances, there is no reasonable medical alternative and local law permits overriding the objection; and,
> - in cases where prospective subjects lack capacity to consent, permission is obtained from a responsible family member or a legally authorized representative in accordance with applicable law.

However, under English law, in contrast to the situation with children, there has until relatively recently been no available proxy consent-giver for the incompetent adult, although, as we saw in Chapter 7A, according to the case of *F* v. *West Berkshire*, medical treatment could be provided on the grounds of necessity if it is in the patient's best interests.[121] *F* suggested that 'best interests' was to be judged by the health professional according to the *Bolam* test. However, recent cases have paid greater attention to human rights arguments in assessing best interests, and there are now compelling arguments that the *Bolam* test is a wholly inappropriate basis on which to determine whether an incompetent adult may be enrolled in a research project.[122] In the case of *Simms* v. *Simms*[123] Dame Elizabeth Butler-Sloss was prepared to sanction the use of experimental treatment on two teenagers aged 16 and 18 who were suffering from CJD – a devastating brain disease, which had left them incapacitated. Clinical trials on animals suggested that the experimental drug had inhibited the progress of a similar disease in mice, but it was completely untested in humans. However, note the special conditions obtaining this case, where the disease was fatal, no cure or recognised treatment existed, and the parents wished the experimental regime to be instituted. The judge noted:

> Where there is no alternative treatment available and the disease is progressive and fatal, it seems to me to be reasonable to consider experimental treatment with unknown benefits and risk, but without significant risk of increased suffering to the patient, in cases where there is some chance of benefit to the patient.[124]

Concerns over the uncertain legal position and the vulnerability of mentally incompetent adults led the Law Commission to propose that non-therapeutic research may be undertaken in certain situations but subject to additional safeguards. In particular, it suggested that any such proposal should be referred to a new mental incapacity research committee.[125] This proposal has been superseded by the enactment of the Clinical Trials Regulations 2004, which provide that for research on an incompetent adult to be lawful there must be 'grounds for expecting that administering the medicinal product to be tested in the trial will produce a benefit to the subject outweighing the risks or produce no risk at all' and that the clinical trial must be directly related 'to a life-threatening or debilitating clinical condition from which the subject suffers'.[126]

Under Article 5(a) of the Clinical Trials Directive, inclusion of an incapacitated person in research is permitted only if the informed consent of the person's legal representative is obtained, and, as in the case of enrolling children in research, this must be done on the basis of the 'presumed will' of the incapacitated person. This is the first time that proxy decision-making has been allowed in respect of health-related decisions for adults in the United Kingdom. Under Article 18 of the Clinical Trials Regulations, the legal representative may be a person who is 'suitable to act as the legal representative by virtue of their relationship with the [incapacitated] adult', who is unconnected with the trial. If no suitable person is available then the doctor primarily responsible for the person's treatment or a person nominated by the health care provider can be appointed as the professional legal representative. Doubts, however, have been raised about the adequacy of the system of legal representatives in protecting patient interests, especially as it seems in practice to rely on a form of 'fictionalised consent'.[127]

Yet, in theory at least, the involvement of the incompetent person in clinical research is tightly circumscribed. As 'clinical trial' is defined very broadly in Article 2 of the Clinical Trials Regulations[128] these regulations will encompass most forms of clinical research. However, for any non-medical research that falls outside the 2004 regulations, such as psychological studies, sections 30–31 of the

Mental Capacity Act 2005 apply.[129] These also provide that a number of conditions must be satisfied. However, as Pattinson notes, the conditions imposed by the 2005 Act are slightly more permissive than those contained in the 2004 regulations. The Act stipulates that the research must have the potential to benefit the participant or others with her condition and must pose no more than minimal risk, whereas the 2004 regulations require the research to be therapeutic or to carry *no* risk.[130] The 2005 Act seems more in line with the Convention on Human Rights and Biomedicine, which stipulates that non-therapeutic research on the incapacitated may exceptionally be carried out, provided that it entails only minimal risks and burdens for the individual concerned and has the aim of contributing:

> through significant improvement in the scientific understanding of the individual's condition, disease or disorder to the ultimate attainment of results capable of conferring benefit on the person concerned or other persons in the same age category or afflicted with the same disease or disorder or having the same condition. (Article 17)

Thus, as in the case of children it can be debated whether the applicable regulations are too restrictive or too liberal.

12.4.3 Other vulnerable groups

Researchers should be conscious of the fact that other potential subject groups may feel under particular pressure to participate in research, not through doubts about their competence, but because their circumstances render them vulnerable. Nurses will typically carry out research on patients who may feel compelled to participate out of a sense of obligation to the health professionals treating them. Similar considerations apply to medical and nursing students. Great care must be taken to explain rights to refuse or withdraw consent when research is proposed for these groups.

Caution may also be necessary when enrolling pregnant women, or women of child-bearing age, in view of the possible effects on the fetus should the research subject be or become pregnant.[131] However, it is controversial to label these women as 'vulnerable', and it is equally important that women should not be excluded from research protocols, as discussed in section 12.4.5 below.

12.4.4 Inducements and conflicts of interest

When recruiting members of vulnerable groups for clinical research, it is important that RECs examine how far the subject may be influenced by financial inducements. The GMC guidance states that doctors must 'make sure that participants are not encouraged to volunteer more frequently than is advisable or against their best interests. [Doctors] should make sure that nobody takes part repeatedly in research projects if it might lead to a risk of significant harm to them' (para. 17). Yet, in media coverage of the Northwick Park trial discussed above, it has emerged that payments in the United Kingdom routinely breach this guideline, and that certain individuals repeatedly 'volunteer' for enrolment in clinical trials.

Aside from inducements for subjects to enter trials, health care professionals also need to ensure that inducements or perks from drug companies sponsoring trials do not influence how they present benefits to potential participants. In 2000 it was reported that the outgoing editor of the prestigious *Journal of the American Medical Association* had called for restrictions on stock ownership and other financial incentives for researchers, claiming that growing conflicts of interests were tainting scientific research.[132] That this is regarded as a pressing ethical concern is reflected in the revised Declaration of Helsinki, which hitherto had been silent on the need for transparency about economic incentives in research. It now provides that all possible conflicts of interest should be disclosed (paras 14, 24 and 30; see section 12.2.3 below). In its 2000 guidance, the MRC points to the potential conflicts of interest, where a researcher's scientific judgement could be unduly influenced by financial gain or personal, academic or political advancement. It recommends that researchers should automatically ask themselves, 'Would I feel comfortable if others learned about my secondary interest in this matter *or* perceived that I had one?' If the answer is negative, that signals that the interest must be disclosed and addressed according to the appropriate policies established by employers, peer review bodies or journals.[133]

12.4.5   The pool of available research subjects

Given the historical emphasis on protecting research subjects, the exclusion of potential subjects from consideration for clinical protocols has only lately been identified as a significant bioethical issue. Such concern signalled a paradigm shift in how enrolment in clinical trials had come to be viewed.[134] While research on human subjects was initially perceived as a necessary aspect of public health, and then as a transgression of individual rights, in some cases tantamount to torture, it has since the 1980s increasingly come to be regarded as an avenue of access to better medical care. This shift was largely prompted by the thalidomide and DES drug disasters, which led to criticisms of the policy of excluding pregnant women from trials given the catastrophic impact of these drugs on children born to women who took them during pregnancy.[135] As noted above, pregnant women have historically been categorised as a vulnerable group, and as a result, guidance issued to researchers has in the past explicitly excluded certain women from biomedical research, if they were pregnant or of child-bearing age. Such exclusions raise important questions pertaining to autonomy and justice. While the justifications for explicit exclusions are generally couched in the rhetoric of protecting women and their unborn children, it is more likely to be attributable to fears of legal liability for any teratogenic impact on the unborn child. However, Merton has argued convincingly that such fears are more apparent than real, since no successful claim has been brought and a proper warning of known and unknown risks would in all probability extinguish the strict liability claims of both subjects and their children for either pre-natal or pre-conceptual harm.[136]

Explicit exclusions are now rare, and in the United Kingdom the GAfREC Harmonised guidelines require ethics committees to have regard to the requirement that:

> [t]he benefits and risks of taking part in research, and the benefits of research evidence for improved health and social care, should be distributed fairly among all social groups and classes. Selection criteria in research protocols should not unjustifiably exclude potential participants, for instance on the basis of economic status, culture, age, disability, gender reassignment, marriage and civil partnership, pregnancy and maternity, race, religion or belief, sex or sexual orientation. RECs should take these considerations into account in reviewing the ethics of research proposals, particularly those involving under-researched groups.[137]

Certainly, excluding women from research may ultimately be a more dangerous legal stance; pharmaceutical researchers in particular leave themselves open to litigation by omitting women, given that their products are then aggressively marketed to women. The CIOMS guidance does advise, though, that 'a thorough discussion of risks to the pregnant woman and to her fetus is a prerequisite for the woman's ability to make a rational decision to enrol in a clinical study' (guideline 16).

The second factor responsible for changing the way in which clinical trials are viewed has been the HIV/AIDS pandemic, which has further politicised the field of clinical research. Patients with these conditions have campaigned for just allocation of access to research and have characterised clinical trials as treatment when there is no proven treatment for a medical condition (thereby further blurring the dichotomy between research and therapy, noted at the beginning of this chapter). Stimulated by these developments, patients with other diseases, notably breast cancer and Alzheimer's disease, and their advocates have become more vocal about access to experimental drugs and treatments and have asserted the right to participate in trials. Consequently, being a research subject is no longer viewed as an unqualified sacrifice – rather it is seen as a potentially risky opportunity. The upshot is that researchers, long sensitised to the need for protection of research subjects, must now also focus on the need to include individuals and groups. In recognition of this, guideline 12 of the CIOMS guidance states that 'groups or communities should be selected in such a way that the burdens and benefits of the research will be equally distributed. The exclusion of groups or communities that might benefit from study participation must be justified'. The commentary on this guideline stresses the injustice involved in overusing certain populations, such as the poor or the administratively convenient.

All researchers should thus bear in mind the need for increased efforts to recruit certain populations, including patients with AIDS, minorities, the elderly[138] and women. This constitutes one aspect of good experimental design of a research protocol, as well as fulfilling the general ethical obligation of fairness or justice.

12.4.6   Review of research and compensation

Until 2004 if a clinical trial was approved by a REC, then the conduct of that research was largely left up to the research team and there were limited possibilities for review. A research subject injured as a result of defective drugs or surgical appliances can theoretically bring an action under the Consumer Protection Act 1987, arguing that a defective product was supplied. However, it is likely that researchers could successfully invoke the 'state of the art' defence, that is, that any defects in the product were not ascertainable given the state of scientific knowledge when it was marketed. Prospects of a successful negligence claim are also low, since negligence actions will probably fail, if a properly conducted research programme had been approved by a REC and carried out in accordance with a responsible body of professional opinion, although in exceptional circumstances negligence claims have succeeded.[139]

Although we have seen that the 2004 Clinical Trials Regulations offer greater scope for monitoring and oversight once projects are approved, the difficulties in pursuing a legal remedy for harm suffered as a result of participation in clinical trials has focused attention on mechanisms for compensating those who suffer harm. There is no formal legal requirement that participants in research should be indemnified. Association of British Pharmaceutical Industry guidelines do provide that where commercial companies sponsor research, they should give contractually binding guarantees to healthy volunteers if they should be injured, but these guidelines are not mandatory.[140] In recognition of the inadequate protection given to volunteers in clinical research, the Pearson Commission recommended years ago that 'any volunteer for medical research who suffers severe damage as a result should have a cause of action, on the basis of strict liability, against the authority to whom he has consented to make himself available'.[141] Unfortunately no Government has implemented this proposal.[142] The possibility of a major claim for compensation is particularly likely in the case of new chemical compounds such as those used in the Northwick Park case described above. The interim findings of the Medicines and Healthcare products Regulatory Agency (MHRA) suggested that the severe immune reaction in this case was occasioned not by human error but the way in which genetically engineered monoclonal antibodies in TGN1412 acted on the immune cells of the human body – something that could not have been predicted in prior animal studies.[143] Like various biotechnologies, these 'super-antibodies' may pose serious safety concerns. The issue of how very hazardous risks, which are difficult to estimate with any degree of certainty, should be presented to research subjects is also raised in the following case study on xenotransplantation. While the EU Clinical Trials Directive now requires that ethics committees take into account the provision for indemnity or compensation in the event of injury or death when deciding whether to approve a clinical trial (Article 6(h)), concerns have been expressed about how adequate the insurance of the German pharmaceutical company – TeGenero – that created TGN1412 is.[144]

A further related source of controversy relates to health care provided in the aftermath of clinical trials. As noted above, one incentive to enrol in a clinical trial is its perception as an avenue to high-quality medical care, but this raises ethical issues about the care of patients once their involvement in research is complete. Such concerns have been particularly acute where pharmaceutical companies withdraw from developing countries after the completion of a clinical trial.[145]

12.5   Case study: participating in biotechnological research projects – xenotransplantation trials

As new biotechnologies are developed, new ethical and legal dilemmas are raised for researchers. An example is offered by xenotransplantation, which potentially gives rise to incalculable risks.[146] Xenotransplantation may be defined simply as the transplant of tissue between species. Most attention to date has centred on the transplant of whole animal organs (such as hearts, kidneys and livers) into humans. Biotechnology companies are currently breeding genetically engineered pigs, which are viewed as a likely source of these organs. The ethics and safety of xenotransplantation was considered in two major reports in the mid-1990s.[147] Both concluded that xenotransplantation, using pigs as source animals, was an ethically acceptable solution to the chronic human organ shortage, although it was not deemed safe at that point to proceed to clinical trials involving humans given the huge risks the technology posed. Instead, the use of primates (effectively as 'surrogate' humans) was endorsed.

The major risk identified is that diseases will spread from the pig source to the recipient and possibly the wider population. Until December 2006, any decision to proceed to human trials had to be approved by the Xenotransplantation Interim Regulatory Authority (UKXIRA) established on the recommendation of the Department of Health review of this technology (the Kennedy Report). However, in December 2006 UKXIRA was disbanded and clinical trials of xenotransplants will now be overseen by RECs.

Even if REC approval were to be granted, questions remain concerning the role of health professionals involved in such trials. As with enrolment in most clinical trials, the crucial issue will be obtaining valid consent. However, xenotransplantation raises particular problems over and above the general difficulties of obtaining informed consent. In the first place, potential recipients of pig tissue are in an especially difficult situation, where it is questionable whether their decision to enter clinical trials actually represents an informed choice. If a particular class of patients realises that the only alternatives to enrolling in a potentially hazardous clinical trial are the slim chance of obtaining a suitable organ, or death, the likelihood is that they will be willing to take that risk regardless of the hazards it creates for them or others.

Second, as this is an entirely new procedure, it is arguably not possible to assess the inherent risks with any degree of accuracy. In general, little is known about pig diseases, but the history of animal–human viruses lends plausibility to the view that xenotransplantation offers a unique opportunity for prion-type diseases to jump the species barrier. This is particularly so given that, in the case of xenotransplantation, source animals are genetically engineered with human genes. Two problems arise. The first is the practical difficulty posed by the

Kennedy Report's suggestion that huge amounts of information would have to be given to research subjects. It proposes that for an informed decision to be given, potential recipients should be given information regarding the psychological and social effects of xenotransplantation, the source of tissue, breeding conditions and animal suffering, as well as genetic implications.[148] It is highly questionable that many patients are equipped to fully assimilate and evaluate such quantities of information.

A still more fundamental problem is whether individual recipients should be able to consent to a procedure that has the potential to unleash unsuspected hazards on the broader population. How should this sort of risk be explained to a potential participant in a clinical trial? Additionally, given these risks, those who enrol in the first trials to be authorised must submit to surveillance and monitoring of their movements.[149] This gives rise to problems about how to present potentially very intrusive interferences with civil liberties (including the right to reproduce) to potential research subjects.

Xenotransplantation thus highlights the need for fuller consideration to be given to the adequacy of counselling and information provision when subjects are enrolled in clinical trials, especially where the research concerns new technologies or genetically engineered compounds like TGN 1421 and there is no existing or adequate way of treating the disease.[150]

This case study also raises concerns over how an effective system of scrutiny and accountability may be implemented, especially when a number of committees with potentially overlapping remits exist to regulate this procedure.[151] It is somewhat unclear whether xenotransplant trials would fall within the scope of the Clinical Trials Regulations, but Beyleveld, Finnegan and Pattinson suggest that these would probably apply only to trials that involve the use of a new pharmaceutical and/or gene therapy/somatic cell therapy in addition to the transfer of organs or tissue.[152] A final issue raised by xenotransplantation is that, should the worst fears of its opponents be realised, a crucial factor is who should bear the costs of compensating victims and paying for their health care, particularly if a major new disease is unleashed on the broader population.

12.6   Conclusions

As will be apparent from the above review, the law regulating nursing research has traditionally been somewhat vague and, in the view of many commentators, loaded in favour of a pro-research agenda. In the early years of the 21st century, however, public concerns about many forms of research and the growing role of the European Union in regulating clinical trials,[153] combined with a political agenda that promotes research governance, has begun to impact significantly on this field. Nevertheless, it is somewhat early to judge what effect this will have on the practice of clinical research. As we have seen, some commentators see the main objective of European legislation as establishing Europe as a competitive research site, rather than improving the protection of research subjects. Others point to bureaucratic inconvenience, associated costs and lengthy delays in the process of approving new treatments, which makes the conduct of trials especially difficult where they are not backed by large pharmaceutical companies.[154]

Concerns continue to be expressed about the adequacy of monitoring arrangements and the heavy reliance on concepts such as consent and risk, which are difficult to define or judge with precision. Moreover, new arrangements aimed at protecting the interests of the incompetent and children rely on an assumption that legal representatives can second-guess what individuals would have wanted. The Griffiths Report has highlighted how, in the past, considerable disparity existed between best practice and the formal guidance available, which left considerable scope for individual latitude in how particular projects were managed. Even with more robust research governance arrangements, it will be difficult to ensure that guidance is always observed. The remit and workload of RECs is steadily increasing, leading to concerns about a loss of quality in decision-making and increased bureaucracy.

Additionally, regulation in this area remains in a state of flux. The Department of Health has recently revised its governance arrangements for RECs, barely ten years after the original arrangements were put in place. It remains to be seen how long it takes for the new harmonised arrangements to be reviewed and replaced.

Another important and problematic aspect of the current regulatory framework is the proliferation of various forms of guidance governing a range of clinical research practices on different subjects. As demonstrated above, the tensions that exist between the numerous legal, professional and international guidelines mean that, against a backdrop of growing public scepticism about clinical research, the researcher has to negotiate a complex web of regulations, which are often vague and in some cases contradictory.

As we have seen, the development of new technologies and synthetic compounds, coupled with the manner in which clinical research is increasingly dependent on private funding by pharmaceutical firms rather than government and academia, has raised new safety concerns and prompted calls for tighter regulation.[155] However, notwithstanding various doubts about the new regulatory mechanisms, and the changing nature of the research they seek to control, it is certainly the case that there is now considerable impetus (regardless of the motivations for it) to ensure that good clinical practice is observed in the conduct of research. In the meantime, the onus, as ever, is on researchers to be as truthful and clear as possible in their communications with participants about the risks and benefits of proposed research programmes, and to ensure that participants' interests are prioritised over those of society, medicine or professional advancement.

12.7   Acknowledgement

Natasha Hammond-Browning would like to thank Bob Lee for suggesting that she update this chapter and John Tingle for his patience during the process.

12.8   Notes and references

1. Department of Health, *Towards a Strategy for Nursing Research and Development: Proposals for Action, Department of Health* (London, Department of Health, 2000), p. 2; A. Kitson, A. McMahon, A. Rafferty & E. Scott, On developing an agenda to influence policy in health related research for effective nursing: a description of a national R&D priority setting exercise. *Nursing Times Research*, **2** (1997), p. 323.

2. Department of Health, *Making a Difference: Strengthening the Nursing, Midwifery and Health Visiting Contribution to Health and Health Care* (London, Department of Health, 1999).

3. N. Fletcher, J. Holt, M. Brazier & J. Harris, *Ethics, Law and Nursing,* (Manchester, Manchester University Press, 1995), p. 185.

4. Ferguson's research has highlighted the paucity of relevant legal knowledge on the part of clinical researchers – see P. Ferguson, Legal and ethical aspects of clinical trials: the views of researchers. *Medical Law Review*, **11** (2003), pp. 48–69.

5. Royal College of Nursing, *Research Ethics: RCN Guidance for Nurses* (London, RCN, 2004). Note that the RCN released a revised version in 2009, Royal College of Nursing, *Research Ethics: RCN Guidance for Nurses* (London, RCN, 2009).

6. M. Fox, Animal rights and wrongs: medical ethics and the killing of non-human animals, In R. Lee & D. Morgan (eds), *Death Rites: Law and Ethics at the End of Life* (London, Routledge, 1994).

7. See J. McHale & M. Fox, *Health Care Law: Text and Materials,* 2nd edn (London, Sweet & Maxwell, 2006), p. 725.

8. *The Plan for Growth* March 2011 http://cdn.hm-treasury.gov.uk/2011budget_growth.pdf *The Health Research Authority Regulations 2011* http://www.legislation.gov.uk/uksi/2011/2341/contents/made last accessed 18 December 2011.

9. This has proven controversial in the context of suspected abuse of child patients by parents. For instance, in a review of research practices at North Staffordshire Hospital in the 1990s, considerable controversy was generated by covert video surveillance of parents suspected of abuse and the question of whether this constituted a research programme. A Review Group set up to inquire into the events recommended that the Department of Health should issue guidance to aid professionals in the identification of such abuse. See NHS Executive West Midlands Regional Office, *Report of a Review of the Research Framework in North Staffordshire Hospital NHS Trust (The Griffiths Review)*, para. 12.4.1. In this regard, Guideline 6 of the Council for International Organisations of Medical Sciences (CIOMS) *International Guidelines for Biomedical Research Involving Human Subjects* (2002) proposes that an ethical review committee must approve all research where there is an intention to deceive, and specify that the researcher must demonstrate that no other research method would suffice – see commentary on Guideline 6, http://www.cioms.ch/publications/guidelines/guidelines_nov_2002_blurb.htm (accessed 19 November 2011). The CIOMS was formed in 1949 under the auspices of the WGO and UNESCO to promote biomedical research and offer international guidance.

10. This distinction was derived from earlier formulations of the Declaration of Helsinki – see J. Montgomery, Law and ethics in international trials, In C. Williams (ed.), *Introducing New Treatments for Cancer* (Chichester, Wiley, 1992).

11. British Medical Association, *Consent, Rights and Choices in Health Care for Children and Young People* (London, BMJ Books, 2001), p. 207.

12. R. Whyte, Clinical trials, consent and the doctor–patient contract. *Health Law in Canada*, **15** (1994), p. 50; C. Grady, *Review of the Search for An AIDS Vaccine: Ethical Issues in the Development and Testing of a Preventive HIV Vaccine* (Indiana, Indiana University Press, 1995).

13. P. Alderson, Did children change or the guidelines? *Bulletin of Medical Ethics*, **150** (1999), pp. 38–44 at p. 40, cited in BMA, *Consent, Rights and Choices in Health Care for Children and Young People* (London, BMJ Books, 2001), p. 185.

14. See note 19 below.

15. H. Brody & F.G. Miller, The clinical-investigator: unavoidable but manageable tension. *Kennedy Institute of Ethics Journal*, **13** (2003), pp. 329–46.

16. S.D. Edwards & J. McNamee, Ethical concerns regarding guidelines on the conduct of clinical research on children. *Journal of Medical Ethics*, **31** (2005), pp. 351–4 at p. 354.

17. I. Oakeshott & L. Rogers, Earlier trials had shown that drug group was highly toxic, *Sunday Times*, 19 March 2006; M. Goodyear, Learning from the TGN1412 trial, *British Medical Journal*, **332** (2006), pp. 677–8; J. Revill, Drug trial firm knew of risk, *The Observer*, 9 April 2006; C. Dyer, J. Carvel & P. Curtis, Victims could lose out after doubts about insurance cover, *Guardian*, 17 April 2006.

18. Declaration of Helsinki, latest amendment was made 2008, with clarification 2002 and 2004, http://www.wma.net/en/30publications/10policies/b3/.

19. Although the Nazi and Japanese experiments during World War II overshadow all subsequent abusive medical research on humans, other infamous examples include the Tuskegee experiments in 1932–72, which used Black males to determine the natural course of syphilis, even though the treatment had existed for centuries (see J. Jones, *Bad blood: The Tuskegee Syphilis Experiment* (New York, The Free Press, 1981)); experiments to test radiation as a therapy carried out in the USA until the early 1970s (see P. McNeil, *The Ethics and Politics of Human Experimentation* (Cambridge, Cambridge University Press), Chapter 1); and HIV research on prostitute women in the Philipines in the 1980s (see L. Laurence & B. Weinhouse, *Outrageous Practices: How Gender Bias Threatens Women's Health* (New Brunswick, Rutgers University Press, 1994/7), p. 23–4. For other examples, see BMA, *The Medical Profession and Human Rights: Handbook for a Changing Agenda* (London, Zed Books, 2001), Chapter 9.

20. J. Harris, Research on human subjects, exploitation, and global principles of ethics, In M. Freeman & A. Lewis (eds), *Law and Medicine: Current Issues*, vol. 3 (Oxford, Oxford University Press, 2000); E. Jackson, *Medical Law: Text, Cases and Materials*, 2nd edn (Oxford, Oxford University Press, 2010), p. 486.

21. Royal College of Physicians (RCP), *Guidelines on the Practice of Ethics Committees in Medical Research Involving Human Subjects*, 4th edn (London, RCP, 2007).

22. Royal College of Nursing, *Research Ethics: RCN Guidance for Nurses* (London, RCN, 2009).

23. Central Office for Research Ethics Committees (COREC), *Governance Arrangements for NHS Research Ethics Committees* (London, Department of Health, 2001) superseded on 1 September 2011 by *Governance Arrangements for NHS Research Ethics Committees: a Harmonised Edition* (London, Department of Health, 2011).

24. See Chapter 5 of the Convention for the articles governing scientific research. The full text of the Convention, and additional protocols is available at http://conventions.coe.int/Treaty/en/Treaties/Html/164.htm (last accessed 30 July 2013).

25. *Consent in the Criminal Law*, Law Commission Consultation Paper No. 139, paras 8.38–8.52 (London, The Stationery Office).

26. S. Graham, Johns Hopkins leads changes in human studies process, *Baltimore Business Journal*, 19 July 2002. Various criticisms were made of the ethical review

process by an internal investigation, although no major flaws in the trial design were found. Similar concerns were raised by a clinical trial into an experimental drug to treat hepatitis B conducted by the National Institutes for Health in 1993, where five patient volunteers died after the drug proved toxic in humans – S. Levine, Five patients die of liver failure in NIH Hepatitis B drug trial, *Washington Post*, 31 July 2001.

27. M. Brazier, *Medicine, Patients and the Law*, 4th edn (Harmondsworth, Penguin, 2007), p. 410.

28. C. Miller, Protection of human subjects of research in Canada. *Health Law Review*, **4** (1995), p. 8.

29. J.W. Berg, Legal and ethical complexities of consent with cognitively impaired research subjects: proposed guidelines. *Journal of Law, Medicine and Ethics*, **24** (1996), p. 18.

30. Nursing & Midwifery Council, *Code of Professional Conduct: Standards of Conduct, Performance and Ethics for Nurses and Midwives* (2008), paras 13–15.

31. P. McNeil, *The Ethics and Politics of Human Experimentation* (Cambridge, CUP, 1993), Chapter 1.

32. See I. Kennedy, The law and ethics of informed consent and randomized controlled trials, In I. Kennedy (ed.), *Treat Me Right* (Oxford, OUP, 1989). Moreover, as discussed in Chapter 7A of this book, even in the context of medical treatment the *Sidaway* standard of disclosure seems to have been modified by subsequent cases to require much fuller answers to questions.

33. In 1965 the Saskatchewan Court of Appeal held that the subject should be informed of 'all the facts, probabilities and opinions that a reasonable man might be expected to consider before giving his consent'. See *Haluska* v. *University of Saskatchewan* (1965) 53 DLR 2d, 436, 444 per Mr Justice Hall.

34. General Medical Council, *Good Practice in Research and Consent to Research* (London, GMC, 2010) paras 1, 4 and 7. available at: http://www.gmc-uk.org/static/documents/content/Research_guidance_FINAL.pdf (accessed 19 November 2011).

35. M. Bassiouni, T. Baffes & J. Evrard, An appraisal of human experimentation in international law and practice: the need for international regulation of human experimentation. *Journal of Criminal Law and Criminology*, **72** (1597) (1981), pp. 1611–2.

36. H. Beecher, Research and the individual. *Human Studies*, **5** (1970).

37. J.S. Tobias, BMJ's present policy (sometimes approving research in which patients have not given fully informed consent) is wholly correct. *British Medical Journal*, **314** (1997), p. 1111.

38. E. Jackson, *Medical Law: Text, Cases and Materials*, 2nd edn (Oxford, Oxford University Press, 2010), p. 470.

39. P. McNeil, *The Ethics and Politics of Human Experimentation* (Cambridge, Cambridge University Press, 1993), p. 135.

40. Directive 2001/20/EC of the European Parliament and of the Council of 4 April 2001.

41. For more detail on the regulatory system for licensing medicines, see E. Jackson, *Medical Law: Text, Cases and Materials*, 2nd edn (Oxford, Oxford University Press, 2010), Chapter 10; H. Teff, Products liability, In A. Grubb (ed.), *Principles of Medical Law*, 4th edn (London, Blackstone Press, 2004), pp. 985–1024; K. Mullan, *Pharmacy Law and Practice* (London, Blackstone Press, 2000), Chapter 4.

42. R. Mendick, GPs failing to report drug side-effects, *Independent on Sunday*, 15 April 2001; see also S. Bosley, Doctors urged to be more vigilant over drugs' side-effects, *Guardian*, 12 May 2006.

43. P. McNeil, *The Ethics and Politics of Human Experimentation* (Cambridge, Cambridge University Press, 1993), p. 13.

44. R. Morehouse, Dilemmas of the clinical researcher: a view from the inside. *Health Law in Canada*, **15** (1994), pp. 52–3.

45. I. Kennedy, The law and ethics of informed consent and randomized controlled trials, In I. Kennedy (ed.), *Treat Me Right* (Oxford, Oxford University Press, 1989).

46. See M. Fox, Research bodies: feminist perspectives on clinical research, In S. Sheldon & M. Thomson (eds), *Feminist Perspectives in Health Care Law* (London, Cavendish, 1998).

47. J. Katz, Human experimentation and human rights. *Saint Louis University Law Journal*, **38** (7) (1993), p. 35.

48. R. Morehouse, Dilemmas of the clinical researcher: a view from the inside, *Health Law in Canada*, **15** (1994), p. 52. Royal College of Physicians guidelines suggest that the subject should be sufficiently informed, told that participation is voluntary but should not be invited to take unacceptable additional risks, informed that she may decline to participate or withdraw at any time, and be informed of the progress and outcome unless justified otherwise. *Guidelines on the Practice of Ethics Committees in Medical Research Involving Human Subjects*, 4th edn (London, RCP, 2007).

49. See, for example, P. Bowden, *Caring: Gender-Sensitive Ethics* (London, Routledge, 1997), Chapter 4.

50. See note 9 above.

51. General Medical Council, para 22; see note 34 above.

52. Medical Research Council, *Guidelines for Good Practice in Clinical Trials* (London, Medical Research Council, 1998), para. 5.4.6.

53. See Helsinki Declaration, para. 24 – see note 10 above.

54. J. McHale, Guidelines for medical research: some ethical and legal problems. *Medical Law Review*, **1** (1993), p. 167.

55. See, for instance, MRC, *Guidelines for Good Practice in Clinical Trials* (London, Medical Research Council, 1998), p. 3.

56. G. Rawlings, Ethics and regulation in randomised controlled trials of therapy, In A. Grubb (ed.), *Challenges in Medical Care* (Chichester, Wiley, 1992), pp. 41–2.

57. A. Oakley, Who's afraid of the randomized controlled trial, In H. Roberts (ed.), *Women's Health Counts* (London, Routledge, 1990).

58. N. Fletcher, J. Holt, M. Brazier & J. Harris, *Ethics, Law and Nursing* (Manchester, Manchester University Press, 1995), p. 187.

59. A. Oakley, *Experiments in Knowing: Gender and Method in the Social Sciences* (New York, The Free Press, 2000), p. 287.

60. J.S. Tobias, BMJ's present policy (sometimes approving research in which patients have not given fully informed consent) is wholly correct. *British Medical Journal*, **314** (1997), p. 1111.

61. I. Kennedy, The law and ethics of informed consent and randomized controlled trials, In I. Kennedy (ed.), *Treat Me Right* (Oxford, Oxford University Press, 1989).

62. See note 9 above.

63. Griffiths Review, para. 9.3.5 (see note 9 above).

64. See further the discussion of whistle-blowing in Chapter 8A of this volume.

65. See note 9 above.

66. F.G. Miller & H. Brody, What makes placebo-controlled trials unethical? *American Journal of Bioethics*, **2** (2002), pp. 3–7.

67. Council for International Organizations of Medical Sciences, *International Ethical Guidelines for Biomedical Research Involving Human Subjects* (Geneva, CIOMS, 2002).

http://www.cioms.ch/publications/guidelines/guidelines_nov_2002_blurb.htm (accessed 18 December 2011).

68. Bristol Royal Infirmary Inquiry, the Inquiry into the management of care of children receiving heart surgery at the Bristol Royal Infirmary, *Interim Report: Removal and Retention of Human Material*, May 2000; The Royal Liverpool Children's Inquiry, 30 January 2001. See M. Brazier, Human tissue retention. *Medico-legal Journal*, **72** (2004), p. 39.

69. O. O'Neill, Some limits of informed consent. *Journal of Medical Ethics*, **29** (2003), pp. 4–7.

70. D. Price, The Human Tissue Act 2004. *Modern Law Review*, **68** (2005), pp. 798–821.

71. Human Tissue Authority, *Code of Practice 1: Consent* (London, HTA, 2009).

72. Central Office for Research Ethics Committees (COREC) (now NRES), *Governance Arrangements for Research Ethics Committees* (London, Department of Health, 2001) [hereafter GAfREC guidance], now superseded by the *Governance arrangements for research ethics committees: a harmonised edition* (London, Department of Health, 2011) [hereafter GAREC Harmonised).

73. J. Black, Constitutionalising self regulation. *Modern Law Review*, **59** (1996), pp. 24–56.

74. S. Kerrison & A.M. Pollock, The reform of UK research ethics committees: throwing the baby out with the bath water? *Journal of Medical Ethics*, **31** (2005), pp. 487–9.

75. Department of Health, *Report of the Ad Hoc Advisory Group on the Operation of NHS Research Ethics Committees* (2005) [hereafter Ad Hoc Advisory Group report]. Available from COREC at http://www.corec.org.uk (accessed 12 April 2006). For a critique of these proposals, see A.J. Dawson, The Ad Hoc Advisory Group's proposals for research ethics committees: a mixture of the timid, the revolutionary and the bizarre. *Journal of Medical Ethics*, **31** (2005), pp. 435–6.

76. See Association of Research Ethics Committees (AREC), *AREC Council Response to Implementing the Recommendation of the AD Hoc Advisory Group on the Operation of NHS Research Ethics Committees: A Consultation* (London, AREC, 2006).

77. Ad Hoc Advisory Group Report – see note 75 above.

78. A.J. Dawson, The Ad Hoc Advisory Group's proposals for research ethics committees: a mixture of the timid, the revolutionary and the bizarre. *Journal of Medical Ethics*, **31** (2005), pp. 435–6.

79. Department of Health, *Governance Arrangements for Research Ethics Committees: A Harmonised Edition* (London, Department of Health, 2011) at para. 5.3.1.

80. S. Kerrison & A.M. Pollock, The reform of UK research ethics committees: throwing the baby out with the bath water? *Journal of Medical Ethics*, **31** (2005), pp. 487–9.

81. See note 9 above.

82. J. Neuberger, *Ethics and Health Care: The Role of Research Ethics Committees in the United Kingdom* (London, King's Fund Institute, 1992).

83. See note 72 above. For more detailed discussion of the role of and decision-making processes employed by RECS, see E. Gerrard & A. Dawson, What is the role of the research ethics committee? Paternalism, inducements, and harm in research ethics. *Journal of Medical Ethics*, **3** (2005), pp. 419–23.

84. J.V. McHale, Guidelines for medical research: some ethical and legal problems. *Medical Law Review*, **1** (1993), pp. 160–86.

85. M. Brazier, Liability of ethics committees and their members. *Professional Negligence*, **6** (1990), p. 186.

86. J. McHale, Clinical research. A. Grubb, *Principles of Medical Law*, 3rd edn (Oxford, Oxford University Press, 2010), pp. 761–2; see also the discussion in the letters page

of the *Guardian* – D. Laurence, Ethics committees and drugs trials, 2 May 2006, and M. Levis, Limits of liability, 12 May 2006.

87. E. Jackson, *Medical Law: Text, Cases and Materials*, 2nd edn (Oxford, Oxford University Press, 2010), p. 494.

88. P. Glasziou & I. Chambers, Ethics review roulette: what can we learn? *British Medical Journal*, **328** (2004), p. 121.

89. K. Alberti, Multi-centre research ethics committees: has the cure been worse than the disease? *British Medical Journal*, **320** (2000), p. 1157.

90. N.R. Dunn, A. Arscott & R.D. Mann, Costs of seeking ethics committee approval before and after the introduction of multicentre research ethics committee. *Journal of the Royal Society of Medicine*, **93** (2000), pp. 511–2; K. Jamrozik, Research ethics paperwork: what is the plot we seem to have lost? *British Medical Journal*, **329** (2004), pp. 286–7.

91. M. Fox & J. McHale, Xenotransplantation: The Ethical and Legal Ramifications. *Medical Law Review*, **6** (1998), pp. 42–61.

92. *New Health Research Authority Comes a Step Closer* 27 September 2011 Department of Health http://www.dh.gov.uk/health/2011/09/health-research-authority (accessed 19 November 2011).

93. P. McNeil, *The Ethics and Politics of Human Experimentation* (Cambridge, Cambridge University Press, 1993), p. 10.

94. P. McNeil, *The Ethics and Politics of Human Experimentation* (Cambridge, Cambridge University Press, 1993), p. 110.

95. Medical Research Council, *Guidelines for Good Practice in Clinical Trials* (London, MRC, 1998), Chapter 6 and Appendix 3.

96. E. Jackson, *Medical Law: Text, Cases and Materials*, 2nd edn (Oxford, Oxford University Press, 2010), p. 461.

97. C. Miller, Protection of human subjects of research in Canada. *Health Law Review*, **4** (1995), p. 9.

98. *Protection of Human Research Subjects and Creation of NBAC*, Exec. Order No. 12,975, 60 Fed. Reg. 52,063 (1995). See A. Mastroianni & J. Kahn, Remedies for human subjects of Cold War research: recommendations of the Advisory Committee. *Journal of Law, Medicine and Ethics*, **24** (1996), pp. 118–26.

99. J. McHale, Guidelines for medical research: some ethical and legal problems. *Medical Law Review*, **1** (1993), pp. 184–5.

100. E. Cave & S. Holm, New governance arrangements for research ethics committees: is facilitating research achieved at the cost of participants' interest. *Journal of Medical Ethics*, **28** (2002), pp. 318–21.

101. S. Kerrison & A.M. Pollock, The reform of UK research ethics committees: throwing the baby out with the bath water? *Journal of Medical Ethics*, **31** (2005), pp. 487–9.

102. P.J. Friedman, Mistakes and fraud in medical research. *Law, Medicine and Health Care*, **20** (1992), p. 17; D.M. Parrish, Falsification of credentials in the research setting: scientific misconduct? *Journal of Law, Medicine & Ethics*, **24** (1996), p. 260.

103. See J. Watts & I. Sample, Cloning fraud hits search for stem cell cures, *Guardian*, 24 December 2005; I. Sample, Stem cell pioneer accused of faking all his research, *Guardian*, 11 January 2006; E. Check & D. Cyranoski, Korean scandal will have global fallout, *Nature*, **438** (2005), pp. 1056–7; Summary of the final report on Professor Woo Suk Hwang's research allegations by Seoul National University Investigation Committee, *New York Times*, 9 January 2006.

104. S. Lock, F. Wells & M. Farthing, *Fraud and Misconduct in Medical Research*, 3rd edn (London, BMJ Publishing Group, 2001).

105. Committee on Publication Ethics, *Code of Conduct and Good Practice for Journal Editors* http://publicationethics.org/files/Code_of_conduct_for_journal_editors_ Mar11.pdf (COPE, 2011) (accessed 18 December 2011).

106. F. Godlee, Dealing with editorial misconduct. *British Medical Journal*, **329** (2004), pp. 1301–2 (2002).

107. I. Chalmers, Unbiased, relevant and reliable assessments in health care. *British Medical Journal*, **318** (1999), p. 1167.

108. H. Biggs, *Healthcare Research Ethics and Law: Regulation, Review and Responsibility* (London, Routledge-Cavendish, 2010), p. 128.

109. BMA, *Consent, Rights and Choices in Health Care for Children and Young People* (London, BMJ Books, 2001), Chapter 9; P.B. Miller & N.P. Kenny, Walking the moral tightrope: respecting and protecting children in health-related research. *Cambridge Quarterly of Healthcare Ethics*, **11** (2002), pp. 217–29.

110. M. Henderson, How drugs for adults harm children, *The Times*, 18 February 2006; N. Fleming, Scaled down drugs 'risk to the young', *Daily Telegraph*, 18 February 2006; E. Webb, Discrimination against children. *Archives of Disease in Childhood*, **89** (2004), pp. 804–8.

111. L. Haggar & S. Woods, Children and research: a risk of double jeopardy? *International Journal of Children's Rights*, **13** (2005), pp. 51–72 at pp. 52–3.

112. CIOMS Guideline 14 – see note 9 above.

113. E. Jackson, *Medical Law: Text, Cases and Materials* (Oxford, Oxford University Press, 2006), p. 497.

114. Medicines for Human Use (Clinical Trials) Regulations 2004, Schedule 1, Part 4.

115. S. Edward & M.J. McNamee, The ethical concerns regarding guidelines for the conduct of clinical research on children. *Journal of Medical Ethics*, **31** (2005), pp. 351–4. See also V. Hasner Sharav, Children in clinical research: a conflict of moral values. *American Journal of Bioethics*, **W12–59** (2003).

116. Royal College of Paediatrics and Child Health (RCPCH), Guidelines of the ethical conduct of medical research involving children. *Archives of Disease in Childhood*, **82** (2000), pp. 177–82 at p. 179.

117. L. Haggar & S. Woods, Children and research: a risk of double jeopardy? *International Journal of Children's Rights*, **13** (2005), pp. 51–72.

118. J. McHale & M. Fox, *Health Care Law: Text and Materials*, 2nd edn (London, Sweet and Maxwell, 2006), p. 709.

119. Royal College of Paediatrics and Child Health, *Safeguarding Informed Parental Involvement in Clinical Research Involving Newborn Babies and Infants* (London, RCPCH, 1999).

120. General Medical Council, *Good Practice in Research and Consent to Research* (London, GMC, 2010), paras 25, 26 and 30.

121. *F v. West Berkshire Area Health Authority* [1989] 3 All ER 545; for the position in Scotland, see the Adults with Incapacity (Scotland) Act 2000. See further Chapter 7A.

122. J. McHale & M. Fox, *Health Care Law: Text and Materials*, 2nd edn (London, Sweet & Maxwell, 2006), p. 692.

123. *Simms v. Simms* [2003] 1 All ER 669.

124. J. Harrington, Deciding best interests: medical progress, clinical judgment and the 'good family'. *Web Journal of Current Legal Issues*, **2** (2003). available at: http://webjcli.ncl.ac.uk (accessed 7 April 2006).

125. Law Commission, Mental incapacity. *Law Commission*, **231** (1995), paras 6.29–6.36.

126. Medicines for Human Use (Clinical Trials) Regulations 2004, Schedule 1, Part 4.

127. J. McHale, Clinical research, In A. Grubb (ed.), *Principles of Medical Law*, 3rd edn (Oxford, Oxford University Press, 2010), pp. 748–9; S. Pattinson, *Medical Law and Ethics*, 3rd edn (London, Sweet & Maxwell, 2011), p. 416.

128. Article 2a of the Clinical Trials Directive defines 'clinical trial' as 'any investigation in human subjects intended to discover or verify the clinical, pharmacological and/or other pharmacodynamic effects of one or more investigational medicinal product(s), and/or to identify any adverse reactions to one or more investigational medicinal product(s) and/or to study absorption, distribution, metabolism and excretion of one or more investigational medicinal product(s) with the object of ascertaining its (their) safety and/or efficacy'.

129. Section 30(3) of the Mental Capacity Act 2005 excludes from that Act any clinical trials regulated under the Clinical Trials Regulations, so the application of the MCA to clinical research is very limited.

130. S. Pattinson, *Medical Law and Ethics*, 3rd edn (London, Sweet & Maxwell, 2006), p. 416.

131. Guideline 17, CIOMS guidance (see note 9 above) provides that '[i]nvestigators and ethical review committees should ensure that prospective subjects who are pregnant are adequately informed about the risks and benefits to themselves, their pregnancies, the fetus and their subsequent offspring and to their fertility'. However, it stresses that pregnant women should be presumed to be eligible to participate in biomedical research, although such research should be relevant to the health needs of pregnant women.

132. Reported by The Associated Press, May 17, 2000; available on www.my.aol.com/news.

133. Medical Research Council, *Good Research Practice* (London, MRC, 2000).

134. M. Fox, Research bodies: feminist perspectives on clinical research, In *Feminist Perspectives in Health Care Law* (eds S. Sheldon & M. Thomson), (London, Cavendish, 1998), pp. 122–3.

135. DES was a drug first prescribed in the USA in 1943, in the hope that it would avert miscarriages. Its efficacy was challenged as early as 1953, and by 1971 the FDA had banned its use during pregnancy after substantial evidence that it was associated with high rates of cervical cancer in the daughters of DES users.

136. V. Merton, The exclusion of pregnant, pregnable, and once-pregnable patients (aka women) from biomedical research. *American Journal of Law and Medicine*, **12** (1993), p. 369.

137. GAfREC Harmonised guidance para. 3.2.3 (see note 72 above).

138. F. Ross, Involving older people in research: methodological issues. *Health & Social Care in the Community*, **13** (2005), pp. 268–81.

139. A. Boggio, The compensation of the victims of the Creutzfeldt-Jacob Disease in the United Kingdom. *Medical Law International*, **7** (2005), pp. 149–67.

140. J.M. Barton *et al.*, The compensation of patients injured in clinical trials. *Journal of Medical Ethics*, **21** (1995), p. 166.

141. *Royal Commission on Civil Liability and Compensation for Personal Injury*, Cmnd 7054 (1978), para. 1341.

142. R. Gillon, No-fault compensation for victims of non-therapeutic research: should government continue to be exempt? *Journal of Medical Ethics*, **18** (1992), p. 59.

143. G. Vince, Drug trial horror: the official interim report, *New Scientist*, 5 April 2006; K. Archibald, It's time to test the testers, *Guardian*, 6 May 2006.

144. C. Dyer, J. Carvel & P. Curtis, Victims could lose out after doubts over insurance cover, *Guardian*, 17 April 2006.

145. E. Jackson, *Medical Law: Text, Cases and Materials*, 2nd edn (Oxford, Oxford University Press, 2010), p. 486.

146. M. Fox, Reconfiguring the animal/human boundary: the impact of xenotechnologies. *Liverpool Law Review*, **26** (2005), pp. 149–67.

147. Nuffield Council on Bioethics, *Animal-to-Human Transplants: The Ethics of Xenotransplantation* (London, Nuffield Council on Bioethics, 1996); *A Report by the Advisory Group on the Ethics of Xenotransplantation* (London, Department of Health, 1997) [hereafter 'the Kennedy Report'].

148. Kennedy Report, para. 7.11.

149. United Kingdom Interim Xenotransplantation Regulatory Authority, *Draft Report of the Infection Surveillance Steering Group of the UKIXRA* (1999).

150. S. Fovargue, Consenting to bio-risk. *Legal Studies*, **26** (2005), pp. 404–18.

151. M. Fox & J. McHale, Xenotransplantation: the ethical and legal ramifications. *Medical Law Review*, **6** (1998), pp. 42–61; S. McLean & L. Williamson, *Xenotransplantation: Law and Ethics* (Aldershot, Ashgate, 2005).

152. D. Beyleveld, T. Finnegan & S. Pattinson (2006) The Regulation of Hybrids and Chimeras in the UK. Report produced for CHIMBRIDS (Chimera and Hybrids in Comparative European and International Research), University of Mannheim.

153. J. McHale & T. Hervey, *Health Law and the European Union* (Cambridge, Cambridge University Press, 2004), Chapter 4.

154. A. Hemminki & P.K. Kellokumpu-Lehtinen, Harmful impact of EU clinical trials directive. *British Medical Journal*, **332** (2006), pp. 501–2.

155. A. Caplan & E. Rosenthal, Risky Business: Human testing for a profit: new scrutiny needed after two commercial clinical trials go wrong, *MSNBC Interactive*, 24 March 2006, www.msnbc.msn.com/id/11927387/ (accessed 25 April, 2006); E. Rosenthal, When drug trials go horribly wrong, *International Herald Tribune*, 9 April 2006.

B   An Ethical Perspective –
Nursing Research

Richard Ashcroft

Professor of Bioethics, School of Law, Queen Mary, University of London, London

Research is an essential element of innovation and quality improvement in health care. As such, it aims at something of great collective value. It can also be enormously personally rewarding to the researcher him- or herself. For the 'subjects' or 'participants' in research, the research process can be beneficial for their health or their well-being, both through the intervention they receive as part of the research process, and through the fact of participating in the research process itself.

Research can, however, be pursued selfishly; it can cause harm or distress to subjects; it can be irrelevant or unoriginal, and incompetently or fraudulently performed; and it can be exploitative. There is therefore no question that research is an ethically significant activity, and that any research project must be pursued in an ethically reflective way. Merely to say this is to skate over the complexities of doing so: the diversity of research methods, settings in which research can be pursued, purposes to which the results of research are put, people who do research and relationships between them. This chapter will present the elements of the ethics of research, illustrating these with examples. It will concentrate on two kinds of nurse (and midwife and health visitor) research activity: nursing research (research into the health care work and types of care and treatment that nurses do) and the work of research nurses (the role of the research nurse in clinical trials and other kinds of biomedical research). The nurses will also care for patients in clinical trials and other studies in which the nurse has no direct involvement, but for most purposes the ethical principles will be similar, since in all circumstances the nurse's primary responsibility is for the patient. What varies between the roles of nurses with care of patients in research, research nurses and nursing researchers is the degree of responsibility for the research and control over it and the kinds of dilemma that may arise.

12.9   The sources of nursing ethics

Ethical principles for professionals have a number of sources. These include:

- the law
- professional codes of conduct
- fundamental moral principles

- the core values of
  - the individual
  - the institution
  - the profession
  - society.

This list has no special order, as it is a matter of controversy which source of ethics is most reliable, and which takes priority. However, most of us would agree that nurses have a strong obligation to abide by, and work within, the law. The law does not determine precisely what is ethical: for instance, many actions are lawful but possibly unethical, and some actions may be ethical without being lawful. Examples might include abortion and euthanasia – many people who think abortion ethical also think euthanasia ethical, while in law abortion is legal in many circumstances and active euthanasia is unlawful. Conversely, many people who think euthanasia is unethical also think that abortion is unethical.

The role of professional codes of ethics and conduct is in part to define the nature of the profession they regulate. They identify certain actions that might be permitted for lay people but are not permissible in nurses, and other actions that are permissible in nurses but not permitted for lay people. Codes set out the higher standards of competence, rights and duties that go along with being a nurse. Many of these rights and duties have an ethical character, but many are more in the nature of the requirements of professional etiquette. In identifying the roles that the law, ethics and professional codes have for nurses and others, we must turn eventually to the ethical foundations of these codes – the fundamental principles and values that are meant to underlie these codes.

An example of a fundamental moral principle is the principle of non-maleficence: individuals have a duty to refrain from harming others. This principle is particularly associated with the caring professions, but it is not specific to them alone. Rather, it has special importance for the caring professions simply because their patients or clients are particularly vulnerable, and thus at greater risk of being harmed, and because the skills and tools of the caring professions are particularly liable to being turned to harmful ends. However, saying that this principle is fundamental is not to say that it is absolute. Thus, certain actions do cause harm (e.g. venepuncture) but are justified by their being carried out with beneficent intentions (e.g. to provide pain relief). Hence, fundamental principles must be balanced against each other; in this case, non-maleficence is balanced with beneficence and with respect for autonomy (the individual must be asked for his or her consent).

The question of epistemology of values (how we know them) has exercised philosophers for generations. It appears in an interesting way in research ethics. First, research ethics, like health care ethics generally, is a field that has experienced considerable historical evolution, as its principles have become more clearly articulated and ramified over time. The key scandals in the ethics of research always raise questions of whether the responsible agents knew that they were acting wrongly, and whether it was possible for them to know. Even if we can show that they did not and could not have known that they were in the wrong, we may perhaps argue that they are nonetheless culpable. Relatedly, the guilty individuals or institutions may insist that their critics and colleagues were just as guilty, and that they are unjustly escaping censure, or are being judged hypocritically. Exactly these arguments were used in their defence by the Nazi doctors at the Nuremberg Trial, for instance.

The epistemology of values and the difficulty of balancing principles lead us to consider a problem that is much discussed in the nursing ethics literature: whether any principles exist, whether they are in any sense universal or objective, and whether the 'principles' approach is consistent with the orientation of caring, which many argue is what typifies the nursing relationship. This is a large topic, which is beyond the scope of this chapter. However, for present purposes it is important to distinguish between the genuine problems of knowledge and application of principles, and the relativist proposal that ethical principles are merely matters of stance and subjective attitude.

I suggest that moral relativism is neither a practical possibility – since in fact all nurses are regulated by a framework of law and by professional codes of conduct – nor a viable intellectual stance. Even 'situational' approaches, such as the 'ethics of care' approach, turn on judgements that certain values are non-negotiable. Where ethical approaches differ is generally in relation to how we know and apply values and principles to situations. Epistemological questions arise in another context in research ethics, as we will consider in the next section.

12.10   Ethics and the design of research

It is commonly said that 'bad science is bad ethics'. Before we consider why this is so, we must understand better what is meant by 'bad science'. I propose the following definition as a description of science: science is the activity of the disciplined, collective acquisition of reliable, generalisable knowledge; science is also the evolving set of outcomes of that activity.

The scientific activity includes a great range of methods, styles, techniques and practices, such that 'good' science is hard to define and perhaps amounts to nothing more than 'successful' science. Nevertheless, bad science is easier to define. Bad science is 'science' that contradicts the very idea of science as defined above. Hence, science that is methodologically ill-defined or likely to result in meaningless or unreliable data, unjustified knowledge claims or no significant contribution to generalisable knowledge at all is bad science. What is meant by 'generalisable' is somewhat controversial, but at least it requires the scientific experience to be communicable, that is, understandable by others and in some way usable by others. Science is about public knowledge rather than some essentially private experience. This view applies as much to qualitative or action research as to quantitative research or other 'natural science' inquiry. Likewise, scientific research that is kept secret or is unreported breaches the requirement that science be a collective enterprise.

This account of bad science is meant to cover the whole range of scientific methods, from statistical analysis of large numerical data sets to qualitative research interviews. Translated into practical terms, some obvious recommendations come out:

- The study should start with a satisfactory literature review that permits the definition of the research question in such way as to show that the question is important, that it has practical relevance and that we don't already know the answer to the question. No inquiry is so 'naive' or 'novel' that it does not build in some way on previous work or on previously developed methods, and these debts need to be brought into view and analysed, so far as this is possible.
- The design of the study must be reliable and likely to answer the research question in such a way that the validity of the answer is determinate and the findings of the study are interpretable and applicable by other practitioners and researchers.
- The results of the study must be publishable and, even if negative, must actually be published within a reasonable time from the completion of the study to permit other researchers and the public to learn from the study (its weaknesses no less than its strengths). The publication should be a fair and accurate account of the research design and results. There is an equivalent duty on the editor of the journal or book and reviewers for the journal or book to give a fair and competent assessment of the article or chapter submitted for publication.

All of these recommendations are now included in the Declaration of Helsinki, which is the most important international ethical guideline regulating biomedical research. However, they are here restated in language that shows their applicability as widely as possible to the diversity of research methods used in nursing today, including qualitative and health services research methods. With bad science defined, it should be clear why 'bad science is bad ethics'. In the first place, research involves exposing patients or colleagues or other research subjects to the risks of the research. Hence if this research is unlikely to produce reliable results, it is arguable that the subjects are exposed to risk without this in any way being balanced by the prospect of benefit to society. To the extent that participants are taking part with altruistic motives, bad research misrepresents itself as an opportunity to benefit others, when it has no prospect of doing so. As such, it could be seen both as an insult to the altruism of the participants, and their deception. To the extent that the research offers some benefit to the participants in terms of access to new treatment, increased access to nursing or other health care services, or financial or other inducements, there is still an issue about the waste of resources bad research involves. Research always involves staff time and use of basic resources, even where there is no additional grant funding component. Hence there is always an 'opportunity cost', as the economists say, involved in doing research. The opportunity cost of bad research is at least the opportunity of using staff and other resources more effectively, in either caring for patients or carrying out bona fide research, for instance. Research ethics typically ignores the ethical issues involved in resources and facilities management in the health services, but this is morally short-sighted.

12.11   The competence of the research staff and research governance

One important exception to the requirement that the research design be 'good' science appears to be research carried out as part of the researcher's own education or training. Does 'student research' have to be judged by standards as high as those by which 'real' research is judged? There are different schools of thought here, but in essence it comes down to how the researcher (student) wishes the research to be considered. Is it an educational project, designed to instruct the student in research methods and management? Or is it primarily intended as research, that is, an attempt to add to collective knowledge? If the latter, then the research standard applies. The project must be assessed as objectively as possible in the light of existing knowledge and standards of research method. If the former, then the project must meet a different, not necessarily lower, standard.

The educational project must be evaluated as a project that aims to teach the student something about research method and management. As such, it must be evaluated in the same way that any educational intervention is – according to the aims and objectives of the teaching and the capacity this work has for permitting fulfilment of those aims and objectives. To some extent, these overlap with the aims and objectives of research; the best student research is often publishable in its own right. Moreover, at a certain standard the appropriate educational aim is to produce work that can stand the rigours of objective peer review. This is certainly the case of work produced for master's degrees by research, and for doctoral research.

The moral issues involved in educational projects are not, finally, different from those involved in research projects: the subjects must be told of the aims of the research and what it is hoped to achieve. In educational projects, they must be told that this is to help the student learn – as when a student nurse takes part in ward rounds and clinical care of patients. In research projects, they must be told that this research will aim to add to knowledge. In either case, the patient's consent should be sought (where possible) and the risks and benefits of the research explained, and so on. What differs between the educational project and the research project is simply the explicit non-clinical aim of the activity over and above its clinical aim, if any.

Just as the standard of the design may vary in the research and educational contexts, so too may the standard of competence expected of the principal investigator. However, there are limits. In research projects, there is a clear obligation for the research undertaken to lie within the competence of the investigator (or investigating team together) to carry out the work. This is clearly true in clinical negligence terms, but even where the possible incompetence has no clinical consequences for the subject, the general obligation not to do 'bad science' entails the duty to carry out only such research as can be done competently.

When the investigator is carrying out an educational project, the competence requirement obviously varies somewhat. Additionally, innovative research may well involve pushing the boundaries of the investigator's competence. What these situations illustrate is that 'competence' is as much an institutional as an individual affair. In the cases of the student or inexperienced or methodologically innovative researcher, competence must be secured by appropriate supervision and support, clear lines of accountability and, where necessary, physical oversight of the research activity. The same rules that apply to the student or inexperienced nurse in a novel situation apply also to the individual learning a new research technique. Here the emphasis must lie on 'appropriate' supervision – an otherwise experienced professional learning a new technique may not require the same kind of supervision as the greenhorn student. Nevertheless, a supervisory mechanism will be required. Supervisory mechanisms include piloting of the method, and peer review of the research design and of interim and final results, as well as more traditional means of educational supervision.

An important feature of supervision is that supervision is not identical to hierarchical reporting. So in a clinical team running a clinical trial, it may be that the principal investigator with overall responsibility for the trial, financially and administratively, is a new consultant physician. His or her research experience in this kind of clinical trial may be limited. The senior nurse on the team, acting as research nurse, may have considerable experience, however, even though from the point of trial management he or she reports to the principal investigator. (The Declaration of Helsinki requires any biomedical research project to be led by a physician, even if only nominally.) In this situation it is clear that the 'supervisory' role may in reality fall to the research nurse, rather than the designated principal investigator.

Each individual member of the clinical team is thus responsible for his or her own tasks, as well as participation in the generic task of quality oversight of the project. Hence in addition to each individual's competence (or 'supported competence' in the case of supervised work), there is 'team competence': can this group function effectively as a team to ensure that the ethical and quality obligations to carry out the research to a certain standard are met? This is a very brief summary of the implications of 'research governance' or 'good clinical practice' for research and clinical teams.

12.12   Recruitment and consent

The voluntary informed consent of the individual research participant is essential. In certain kinds of research consent may be impossible (for instance, research with babies or young children, or incapacitated subjects who are unable to give consent). In certain circumstances consent may not be sought because the research project is of great collective importance, consent would be impractical, and the risk of harm to the participants is minimal. The details of these exceptions are complex, and cannot be covered here; the reader is referred to the excellent guidelines prepared by the UK Medical Research Council on research with mentally incapacitated people and on the use of personal medical information in research. Consent is important because it respects the autonomy of individuals: their right to privacy, their right to determine what can be done to their bodies, and their right to choose whether or not to assist others in activities that may not benefit them directly. Justifications of departures from the consent standard may rest on legally shaky ground, but ethically two principles can be invoked. The first is that, in the case of individuals unable to consent by reason of lacking capacity to consent, medical and nursing innovations that will benefit them are required by the principle of beneficence. Research interventions that have a therapeutic component can directly benefit the individual, and enrolling an individual lacking capacity to consent would be justified by this. However, the principle of nonmaleficence requires that their special vulnerability to harm and exploitation be noted, and special care be taken to minimise the possibility of harm to them. Here, arguably, the principle of respect for autonomy is replaced by a principle of respect for the dignity of the vulnerable person.

A second justification for research without consent is that, where the harm and inconvenience caused to the individual is zero or negligible, all of us have, other things being equal, a duty to benefit others (especially if that involves no cost to us), and participation in socially useful research is one way to do that. This might be held to be supplemented in the United Kingdom by a sort of political claim that we are all members of the National Health Service, and all benefit from it, and all have an interest in its development and management. Hence, informally, we mandate it to carry out records-based research and audit, without the necessity to obtain consent, provided our privacy is protected. The former version is an argument from solidarity; the latter is an argument from social contract theory. But what is clear is that both arguments rest on a claim about the importance and utility of the research, a claim that the research is minimal risk and a claim that the rational individual would not object to their consent not being sought. All of these claims need proof in each situation, and the burden of proof lies with the researcher; these claims must be adjudicated by an independent research ethics committee. A more troubling worry about consent is the extent to which research on patients involves people who may be emotionally vulnerable, and who invest trust in health care professionals simply because they are professionals, or perhaps because they have come to like and rely on the particular individual professionals. They may not distinguish between the individual's roles as carer and as researcher, or they may think that they must somehow 'please' the member of staff in order to maintain good relationships or access to care. While this is explicitly ruled out by the Declaration of Helsinki, and patients must be told that their care will not be compromised if they refuse, this is sometimes difficult for patients to believe or accept.

A particular difficulty arises where a clinical trial is being managed by a research nurse who is requested by the principal investigator to recruit and enrol individuals in the trial. Strictly speaking, the consent must be obtained by the individual responsible for prescribing the study treatment – normally the physician principal investigator. This raises more general issues about the roles and responsibilities of the different members of the clinical team, which are beyond the scope of this chapter.

12.13   Research and care

Ethically, the issue of most profound concern about research involving patients is how research and care roles conflict. While the actions performed may be consistent with good medical and nursing care for the individual patient, there does seem to be a conflict in orientation. Research aims to benefit the community, and it must be pursued with scientific, methodical rigour. Care for the sick and vulnerable aims at benefiting the individual and is essentially personal and non-universalisable. The very idea of 'methodical care' seems to be an oxymoron, yet is implicit in the collection of clinical data and the carrying-out of research procedures at regular intervals, especially in the context of busy hospital settings, with the whole range of other clinical duties to be carried out by the researcher or his or her colleagues.

What is at stake here is an ethical relationship between the patient and the professional caring for them, which depends on respect for the dignity and autonomy of the patient, and maintenance of the integrity and professionalism of the carer. This can be a difficult balance to strike and is particularly acute when we reflect on the idea of the nurse as patient's advocate. To some extent this is possible where the nurse is not the principal investigator, but it is very difficult to maintain this stance where the nurse is both patient advocate and advocate of his or her own research. The risk here is that the nurse uncritically assumes that his or her goals are shared by the patient, hence that advocating the research is advocacy of the patient's interests and views. The ethical concept of most importance here is the concept of 'virtue': the researcher must maintain the virtues of the health care professional (care for the well-being of others, integrity and responsibility, for instance) at the same time as the virtues of the researcher (scrupulosity, honesty and curiosity, for instance).

This balance can be struck by many remarkable individuals, but it is more important that it is struck at the level of institutions – individuals working in teams with a shared institutional culture. The trend towards quality improvement and 'research governance' in part marks this attempt to achieve an institutional balance; there is a cultural shift in the health service to see research and treatment as complementary activities rather than activities in tension. A central question in research ethics today is whether this cultural shift is coherent, or whether it is a sort of institutional delusion.

12.14   Conclusion

Research will be an increasing part of the work of nurses in the coming years, and arguably this can only improve the care given by nurses. In this chapter I have described some of the ethical dilemmas that arise in research at a rather abstract and reflective level. As I point out at various places in this chapter, the growth in the role and importance of research outside of the narrow biomedical context that has historically shaped research ethics raises difficult philosophical and professional concerns, which guidelines alone will not solve. What is clear, however, is that attention to the core principles of good nursing – respect for the dignity and autonomy of patients, beneficence, non-maleficence, justice and integrity – will remain essential. The best research, and best practice in research, embodies and promotes these principles.

12.15   Acknowledgements

The author thanks Paul Wainwright and Heather Widdows for their helpful comments on drafts of this chapter.

12.16   Further reading

12.16.1   Handbooks

Baruch Brody, *The Ethics of Biomedical Research* (Oxford, Oxford University Press, 1998).
Trevor Smith, *Ethics of Medical Research: A Handbook of Good Practice* (Cambridge, Cambridge University Press, 1999).
Royal College of Nursing, *Ethics Related to Research in Nursing* (Harrow, Scutari Press, 1993).

12.16.2   Principles of ethics

Donna Dickenson, Richard Huxtable & Michael Parker, *The Cambridge Medical Ethics Workbook* (Cambridge, Cambridge University Press, 2010).
Leslie Gelling, Ethical principles in health care research, *Nursing Standard*, **13** (36) (1999), pp. 39–42.
Raanan Gillon, *Philosophical Medical Ethics* (Chichester, John Wiley, 1986).

12.16.3   Consent

Priscilla Alderson, Consent to research: The role of the nurse, *Nursing Standard*, **9** (36) (1995), pp. 28–31.
Len Doyal & Jeffrey S. Tobias (eds), *Informed Consent in Medical Research* (London, BMJ Books, 2000).
Sarah Edwards *et al.*, Ethical issues in the design and conduct of randomised controlled trials, *Health Technology Assessment*, **2** (15) (1998), pp. 1–128.

12.16.4   Recruitment

Richard Ashcroft *et al.*, Implications of sociocultural contexts for ethics of clinical trials, *Health Technology Assessment*, **1** (9) (1997), pp. 1–65.

Richard Ashcroft, Human research subjects, selection of, In Ruth Chadwick (ed.), *Concise Encyclopedia of Ethics of New Technologies* (San Diego, Plenum Press, 2000), pp. 255–66.

12.16.5   Research management

Richard Ashcroft, Ethical issues in outsourced clinical trials, In Roy Drucker & R. Graham Hughes (eds), *Outsourcing Health Care Development and Manufacturing* (Englewood, CO, Interpharm Press, 2000).

13 The Elderly

A Older People and Nursing Care

Jonathan Herring

Fellow in Law, Exeter College, University of Oxford, Oxford, and
Professor in Law, Director of Undergraduate Studies, Faculty of Law, University of
Oxford, Oxford

13.1 Introduction

In recent years the care of older people in the health care system has become a
major issue for the nursing profession. After a discussion of the nature of ageing,
this chapter will highlight some recent reports revealing the inadequate treatment of older people in hospitals and health settings. It will go on to examine
some of the key legal and ethical issues that arise in nursing. Some of these will
mirror issues raised in other chapters in the book (e.g. over-capacity) but it will
look at these issues particularly from the perspective of older people.

There is a general acceptance that in the past ageism was 'rampant' within the
NHS. The Department of Health accepts that 'older people and their carers have

Nursing Law and Ethics, Fourth Edition. Edited by John Tingle and Alan Cribb.
© 2014 by John Wiley & Sons, Ltd. Published 2014 by John Wiley & Sons, Ltd.

experienced age-based discrimination in access to and availability of services.'[1] But this should be in the past. The *NHS Constitution* states clearly:[2]

> The NHS provides a comprehensive service, available to all irrespective of gender, race, disability, age, sexual orientation, religion or belief. It has a duty to each and every individual that it serves and must respect their human rights. At the same time, it has a wider social duty to promote equality through the services it provides and to pay particular attention to groups or sections of society where improvements in health and life expectancy are not keeping pace with the rest of the population.

As we shall see later in this chapter this obligation, not to discriminate on the grounds of age, is now found in the Equality Act 2010.

In the outcry that has met some of the recent reports on the care of older people in health settings, nursing has faced the brunt of severe criticism. However, it should never be forgotten that older people face a bad deal at the hands of our society generally. They face ageism, social exclusion, poverty and disadvantage in many areas of life.[3] It is perhaps the public nature of the health care provision that makes ageism more visible than other contexts.

13.2   Ageing and health

In many people's mind old health and ill health are connected. However, a few moments' thought will show that to be a misplaced assumption. In part this is caused by an assumption that the way bodies change as they age amounts to ill health. The fact people seek help from doctors to 'treat' wrinkles perhaps indicates the assumption that natural ageing processes are illnesses. Even though old age is often connected with ill health, there is much debate over the extent to which socio-economic or environmental factors, rather than age itself, affects health among older people.

A forceful argument can be made that society has been keen to address the cosmetic issues surrounding old age, but not the more serious ones. As one commentator put it,

> We have botulinum toxin for the treatment of wrinkles, minoxidil for male pattern baldness, tooth whitening treatments; hormone replacement therapy for women (but not men, yet). But medicalisation of the two commonest social scourges of old age—poverty and loneliness—has not occurred.[4]

A major survey was recently published providing a snap shot of the health of older people in England in 2005.[5] It provides an important guide to health issues affecting older people. The key findings for those aged over 65 were summarised as follows:[6]

- More than half said their health was 'good' or 'very good'.
- More women than men – 65 per cent compared with 48 per cent – found it difficult to walk up a flight of 12 stairs without resting.
- 23 per cent men and 29 per cent of women had fallen in the last 12 months.

- CVD was the most common chronic disease reported by men (37 per cent).
- Arthritis was the most common chronic disease reported by women (47 per cent).
- Almost two-thirds were hypertensive.
- 22 per cent had visited their GP in the previous two weeks.
- 12 per cent of women and 9 per cent of men reported low levels of psycho-social well-being based on 12 items measuring general levels of happiness, depressions and anxiety, sleep disturbance and the ability to cope in the previous few weeks.

These figures demonstrate that we should reject any assumption that old age is normally accompanied by ill health. As many as 56 per cent of older people reported generally good or very good health, although, 71 per cent of over-65s reported long-standing illness. The popular misperception that older people cannot walk well is also challenged by the survey with only 39 per cent of men and 47 per cent of women reported any difficulty with walking a quarter of a mile.

13.3   Recent concerns

Recent discussions over the nursing of older people have been dominated by some shocking reports into the care of older people. This chapter will consider four of the main ones.

13.3.1   Care Quality Commission report

Between March and June 2011 the Care Quality Commission (CQC) undertook 100 unannounced inspections of acute NHS hospitals in England.[7] These focused on the standards of dignity and nutrition on wards caring for older people. Of the 100 hospitals, two were found to be putting people at unacceptable risk of harm. Less than half the hospitals (45) were fully compliant with the standards required for nutrition or dignity. Thirty-five met the standards in both, but needed to improve on one or both. Twenty did not meet one or both standards.

The picture painted in the report was grim: in particular, what the report noted about the standard of nursing care for older people. It is worth quoting from the introduction by Dame Jo Williams at length:

Time and time again, we found cases where patients were treated by staff in a way that stripped them of their dignity and respect. People were spoken over, and not spoken to; people were left without call bells, ignored for hours on end, or not given assistance to do the basics of life – to eat, drink, or go to the toilet.

Those who are responsible for the training and development of staff, particularly in nursing, need to look long and hard at why 'care' often seems to be broken down into tasks to be completed – focusing on the unit of work, rather than the person who needs to be looked after. Task-focused care is not person-centred care. It is not good enough and it is not what people want and expect. Kindness and compassion costs nothing.[8]

In fairness it is worth quoting what Dame Williams went on to say about resources:

> . . . resources have a part to play. Many people told us about the wonderful nurses in their hospital, and then said how hard pressed they were to deliver care. Having plenty of staff does not guarantee good care (we saw unacceptable care on well-staffed wards, and excellent care on understaffed ones) but not having enough is a sure path to poor care. The best nurses and doctors can find themselves delivering care that falls below essential standards because they are overstretched.
>
> Staff must have the right support if they are to deliver truly compassionate care that is clinically effective. In the current economic climate this is easy to say and far harder to deliver, but as the regulator our role is to cast an independent eye over care and reflect on what we see. There are levels of under-resourcing that make poor care more likely, and those who run our hospitals must play their part in ensuring that budgets are used wisely to support front line care staff.[9]

What is particularly chilling about this report is that there is little that is new here. We have known for a long time that too many older people are infantilised or ignored in hospital; that too often they fail to receive adequate hydration or nutrition; and that their dignity is not protected. In the report a long list of inappropriate conduct is listed, including:

- call bells being out of patient's reach
- curtains not being properly closed when personal care was being given
- staff speaking to patients in a rude or condescending manner
- patients not being given the help to eat
- patients being interrupted during meals and having to leave their food unfinished
- patients not being able to clean their hands before meal.

The report noted the following comments from patients and their relatives:

- 'The patient constantly called out for help and rattled the bedrail as staff passed by . . . We noted that 25 minutes passed before this patient received attention. When we spoke with the patient we observed that their fingernails were ragged and dirty.'
- 'We saw a staff member taking a female patient to the toilet. The patient's clothing was above their knees and exposed their underwear. The staff member assisted them to the toilet in full view of other patients on the ward, only closing the door when they left the toilet room.'
- 'When we spoke to one member of staff about how they managed to meet the needs of people on the ward, they said that they did not have enough time to care for patients. They said that when they are rushed they

cannot always meet people's needs and some things have to be delayed as a result.'[10]

13.3.2   Alzheimer's Society report

A report from the Alzheimer's Society[11] investigated the treatment of those suffering from dementia in hospital, noting that up to a quarter of hospital beds are occupied by people with dementia. The report found a very mixed picture with some excellent care, but also some neglectful care. The report found that:

- 47 per cent of carer respondents said that being in hospital had a significant negative effect on the general physical health of the person with dementia, which wasn't a direct result of the medical condition.
- 77 per cent of nurse managers and nursing staff said that antipsychotic drugs were used always or sometimes to treat people with dementia in the hospital environment.
- 77 per cent of carer respondents were dissatisfied with the overall quality of dementia care provided.

13.3.3   Health Service Ombudsman

In 2011 the Health Service Ombudsman reported in depth on ten investigations into the NHS care of older people.[12] The report concludes:

These accounts present a picture of NHS provision that is failing to respond to the needs of older people with care and compassion.[13]

The Report goes on:

These were individuals who put up with difficult circumstances and didn't like to make a fuss. Like all of us, they wanted to be cared for properly and, at the end of their lives, to die peacefully and with dignity. What they have in common is their experience of suffering unnecessary pain, indignity and distress while in the care of the NHS. Poor care or badly managed medication contributed to their deteriorating health, as they were transformed from alert and able individuals to people who were dehydrated, malnourished or unable to *communicate*.[14]

As the Ombudsman reports, such stories show the gulf between the fine rhetoric of the NHS Constitution and the reality for some older people. What this report highlights is that it is not so much a problem with complex cases or mistakes being made in emergencies, it is the day-in day-out basics of care. The Report found not only shocking treatment but that staff in dealing with complaints were 'dismissive' and showed 'a disregard for process and procedure and [an] apparent indifference . . . to deplorable standards of care'.[15]

One example from the report is sufficient to capture the kind of issues raised:

Older people are left in soiled or dirty clothes and are not washed or bathed. One woman told us that her aunt was taken on a long journey to a care home by ambulance. She arrived strapped to a stretcher and soaked with urine, dressed in unfamiliar clothing held up by paper clips, accompanied by bags of dirty laundry, much of which was not her own. Underlying such acts of carelessness and neglect is a casual indifference to the dignity and welfare of older patients.[16]

13.3.4 Centre for Policy on Aging

The Centre for Policy on Aging was commissioned to produce four reviews of the literature on age discrimination in the areas of primary and community health care;[17] social care; mental health services and secondary health care.[18] The reports note the difficulties in ascertaining when there is discrimination. In relation to primary care the report notes:

> There is evidence that older people are subject to covert, indirect discrimination. Stereotyping people on the basis of chronological age which can led to older people being excluded from treatments that are shown to be beneficial is a form of indirect discrimination . . . Evidence of covert discrimination is shown in limited preventative care for older people; reluctance to refer older people to specialist services; poor quality of care for conditions associated with ageing, which includes under treatment for conditions. Covert discrimination is demonstrated in shortfalls in receipt of basic recommended care by adults aged 50 or more with common health conditions.[19]

In relation to secondary care the report found very few instances of explicit policy-based age discrimination, but noted it was difficult to assess the extent to which there might be indirect discrimination as a result of subconscious ageist attitudes on behalf of staff. The report notes that older patients are less likely than middle-aged ones to describe their care as 'excellent' and that older people are most likely to report 'being talked over as if they weren't there'. The report also found some evidence that policies concerning mixed-sex wards and food provision operate particularly harshly on older people. Older patients less likely to be referred for surgical interventions for cancer, heart disease and stroke, although that could be explained on the basis of an assessment of chances of survival. The report's conclusion on cancer was that:

> Evidence of the under-investigation and under-treatment of older people in cancer care, cardiology and stroke is so widespread and strong that, even taking into account confounding factors such as frailty, co-morbidity and poly-pharmacy we must conclude that ageist attitudes are having an effect on overall investigation and treatment levels.[20]

13.3.4.1 Mental health

There are grave concerns over the provision of mental health services among older people. In its report *Securing Better Mental Health for Older Adults*[21] the Department of Health admitted that older adults had not benefitted from some of the developments in services which had assisted younger adults. Services were still failing to meet the mental health needs of older people. In the 2006 report *Living Well in Later Life* three inspectorates[22] found that the system of mental health had developed in an unfair way with an organisational division between care for adults 'of working age' and older people. Providers were 'struggling' to provide a full range of good-quality services to older people. One major research project found a widespread perception of those involved in older people's mental health services that:

> there were fewer services for older people and that they tended to be less well-staffed. Low levels of resources for identification and early intervention work was highlighted as having led to high levels of unmet need, particularly for older people with anxiety and depression.[23]

13.4 Professional guidance

The Nursing and Midwifery Council has produced Guidance for the Care of Older People.[24] The Guidance sets out what it regards as being at the heart of care for older people:

> The essence of nursing care for older people is about getting to know and value people as individuals through effective assessment, finding out how they want to be cared for from their perspective, and providing care which ensures that respect, dignity and fairness are maintained.[25]

As the guidance notes, in fact these principles can apply to any patient, of whatever age. Interestingly it seeks to encourage nurses to have a 'positive attitude' towards older people and 'embrace positive feelings of respect'. The fact that the Guidance needs to talk in these terms is perhaps an acknowledgement that some people may find themselves not naturally having the levels of empathy and care for older people that other patients will evoke.

The Guidance emphasises the importance of older people's human rights, including rights of dignity, beliefs, privacy and to make decisions about their care. They have the right to be free from exploitation and abuse. This requires:

> nurses who are efficient and able to deliver safe, effective, quality care by being:

- competent: having the right knowledge, skills and attitude to care for older people
- assertive: challenging poor practice, including attitude and behaviour and safeguarding older people
- reliable and dependable
- empathetic, compassionate and kind.[26]

Such nurses should be involved in delivering quality care which promotes dignity by nurturing and supporting the older person's self-respect and self-worth through:

- communicating with older people by not only talking with them, but listening to what they say
- assessment of need
- respect for privacy and dignity
- engaging in partnership working with older people, their families, carers and your colleagues.[27]

Throughout the Guidance the importance of empathy is stressed. It offers a useful definition of the concept:

> As a nurse you should demonstrate empathy, which means having a feeling for what someone is going through, perhaps by remembering or imagining yourself in a similar situation. In other words putting yourself in the person's place and trying to imagine how it would feel for you.[28]

As the Guidance emphasises this requires an understanding of the person's background and history.

13.5 Human rights

Human rights have come to take central stage in the law. Chapter 1 discusses the relevance of human rights generally for patients. In Age Concern's submission to the Joint Committee on Human Rights' *Inquiry into the Human Rights of Older Persons in Healthcare* the following were listed as examples where the rights of older people were ignored:

- Having hospital meals taken away before older patients can eat them (Articles 2 and 8).
- Being cared for in mixed-sex bays and wards (Article 8).
- Being repeatedly moved from one ward to another for non-clinical reasons (Articles 2 and 8).
- Deaths of residents within weeks of being moved from care homes (Article 2).
- Use of covert medication (Article 8).
- Carelessness about privacy in hospitals and care homes (Article 8)
- Refusal by a local authority to place couples in the same nursing home (Article 8).
- Being forced to go into residential care because of local authority's unwillingness to allocate resources for services in the person's home (Articles 8 and 14).
- Care home residents not being given their weekly personal expenses allowance by the home manager (Article 1, Protocol 1).
- 'Do not resuscitate' notices being used in hospitals without agreement of the individual concerned (Article 2).
- Unsatisfactory hospital care for older black and minority ethnic patients owing to a number of factors including insensitivity to cultural, religious and linguistic needs (Articles 8, 9 and 14).

- Homophobic prejudice against same sex couples in residential accommodation (Articles 8 and 14).[29]

This chapter will now consider the protection from age discrimination, which is a key aspect of the legal protection for older patients.

13.6   Non-discrimination

English law has been remarkably slow to respond to age discrimination. Its recognition has certainly lagged behind protection from sex or race discrimination. Indeed, it has only been in the last few years that legislation has been produced to address the issue.

The forms of ageism and age discrimination are varied. It is useful to distinguish ageism and age discrimination. Ageism refers to untrue assumptions and beliefs that are held about people based on their age. Age discrimination relates to behaviour in which a person is disadvantaged as a result of their age. Age discrimination often interacts with other sources of disadvantage such as race, class and sex discrimination. Ageism itself (having prejudicial beliefs based on age) is not unlawful, but acting on those beliefs to someone's disadvantage will be age discrimination and can now be unlawful.

The Equality Act 2010 now deals with the law on discrimination. Age is included as a 'protected characteristic',[30] that is a basis upon which a person may be unlawfully discriminated. The Act prohibits three kinds of age discrimination: direct discrimination, combined discrimination and indirect discrimination.

13.6.1   Direct discrimination

Section 13 of the Equality Act 2010 defines direct discrimination as follows:

(1) A person (A) discriminates against another (B) if, because of a protected characteristic, A treats B less favourably than A treats or would treat others.

(2) If the protected characteristic is age, A does not discriminate against B if A can show A's treatment of B to be a proportionate means of achieving a legitimate aim.

Direct discrimination requires proof that B was treated less favourably on account of his or her age. This would cover the most blatant forms of discrimination where, for example, a trust decided that patients over a certain age could not be given a particular treatment. It will be rare for such overt forms of discrimination to be found in formal policies of the NHS, although individual professionals might be guilty of treating a patient less favourably due to their age.

The concept of direct discrimination as expressed in section 13 requires proof that B was treated differently as compared with a person of a different age. One difficulty in applying this is finding an appropriate comparator. Imagine a 55-year old patient is denied treatment and claims age discrimination. She might point to a similar patient who was aged 30 and was provided the treatment.

However, the trust might point to a 50-year patient who was not. Is the comparison to be drawn with the 50-year old or the 30-year old? In the case of sex discrimination the comparator would be easy to find: a similarly qualified male worker. But in age there might be quite a number of different ages that could be used as comparators. Cases may become highly complex if each side introduces a range of possible comparators of different ages. There is evidence that this is what has happened in the USA. One solution is for the law to state that discrimination is made out if someone was treated less favourably on account of her age compared with any other age group. Then, it would be no defence for an NHS body to refer to other age groups who were treated as unfairly as the applicant was. After all, it should be no defence to a charge of discrimination that other people would have been treated in just as discriminatory a way as the applicant was.

13.6.2   Combined direct discrimination

Section 14 explains that combined discrimination can be claimed. This would be appropriate where the claim is that there has been discrimination against, for example, old women (rather than all old people):

(1)   A person (A) discriminates against another (B) if, because of a combination of two relevant protected characteristics, A treats B less favourably than A treats or would treat a person who does not share either of those characteristics.

(2)   The relevant protected characteristics are –
    (a)   age;
    (b)   disability;
    (c)   gender reassignment;
    (d)   race
    (e)   religion or belief;
    (f)   sex;
    (g)   sexual orientation.

(3)   For the purposes of establishing a contravention of this Act by virtue of subsection (1), B need not show that A's treatment of B is direct discrimination because of each of the characteristics in the combination (taken separately).

This deals with a case where it might be claimed that there is a policy that is not discriminating against all older people, but discriminates a protected group of them: such as old women or old gay people.

13.6.3   Indirect discrimination

Indirect discrimination is covered by section 19:

(1)   A person (A) discriminates against another (B) if A applies to B a provision, criterion or practice which is discriminatory in relation to a relevant protected characteristic of B's.

(2) For the purposes of subsection (1), a provision, criterion or practice is discriminatory in relation to a relevant protected characteristic of B's if –

    (a) A applies, or would apply, it to persons with whom B does not share the characteristic,

    (b) it puts, or would put, persons with whom B shares the characteristic at a particular disadvantage when compared with persons with whom B does not share it,

    (c) it puts, or would put, B at that disadvantage, and

    (d) A cannot show it to be a proportionate means of achieving a legitimate aim.

(3) The relevant protected characteristics are –

- age;
- disability;
- gender reassignment;
- marriage and civil partnership;
- race;
- religion or belief;
- sex;
- sexual orientation.

Indirect discrimination occurs where an apparently equal treatment in fact impacts more heavily on people of a particular age. Baroness Hale in *Rutherford (No.2)* v. *Secretary of State for Trade and Industry* explained the concept in this way:

> The essence of indirect discrimination is that an apparently neutral . . . provision, criterion or practice . . . in reality has a disproportionate adverse impact upon a particular group. It looks beyond the formal equality achieved by the prohibition of direct discrimination towards the more substantive equality of results. A smaller proportion of one group can comply with the requirement, condition or criterion or a larger proportion of them are adversely affected by the rule or practice. This is meant to be a simple objective enquiry. Once disproportionate adverse impact is demonstrated by the figures, the question is whether the rule or requirement can objectively be justified.[31]

An obvious example of indirect age discrimination would be a trust deciding not to fund treatment for a condition which is primarily found among older people. Although age is not mentioned, the rationing would have far greater an effect on older people and therefore, in effect, discriminates against them. A less obvious example would be a trust which provided food which older people in particular found it hard to eat. It may be found that such a policy would disproportionately affect older people in a negative way and hence amount to indirect discrimination.

Indirect discrimination is therefore less obvious than direct discrimination, and can raise some tricky questions. One problematic area concerns where the requirement only very slightly favours younger people, for example, 15.4 per cent of younger patients are affected, but 15.2 per cent of older patients are. It may be that the courts will take the fact that the impact on older patients is very slight as a matter that is relevant for the question of whether the discrimination is justified. Alternatively it may be that such a minor difference is simply insufficient to indicate discrimination.

A major difficulty with indirect age discrimination is that many commonly used health care practices are indirectly discriminatory. A doctor dealing with a very elderly patient with not long to live is unlikely to recommend the kinds of treatment that he or she would for a young patient with a similar medical condition. Health is not unusual in this regard. The same is true in employment law, where job criteria are indirectly discriminatory on the basis of age: experience, knowledge, emotional maturity or qualifications, for example, are all likely to favour older candidates. This means that although indirect age discrimination will be common, it will frequently be justified. The possibility of justification is, therefore, essential to the workability of the regulations in this area.

13.6.4 Justification

Sections 13 and 19, in the very definition of discrimination, states that discrimination will be justified where it is a 'proportionate means of achieving a legitimate aim'. This is all rather vague and there is plenty of scope for the courts to fashion a clearer approach as to when age discrimination will be justified.

In the employment context *Loxley* v. *BAE Systems* the Tribunal held:

> The principle of proportionality requires an objective balance to be struck between the discriminatory effect of the measure and the needs of the undertaking. The more serious the disparate adverse impact, the more cogent must be the justification for it. It is for the employment tribunal to weigh the reasonable needs of the undertaking against the discriminatory effect of the employer's measure and to make its own assessment of whether the former outweigh the latter. There is no 'range of reasonable response' test in this context.[32]

This suggests that the court will consider the severity of the impact of the discriminatory practice on the individual and the strength of the justification. The harsher the impact, the better the justification must be. However, for a court to strike this balance is complex. How can it determine whether, say, the denial of hip transplants for the over-80s is justified by the fact that the money saved can help keep prematurely new-born babies alive?

In *Palacios de la Villa* v. *Cortefiel Servicios* (2007)[33] the European Court of Justice rejected an argument that age discrimination should be regarded as easier to justify than sex or race discrimination. The court accepted that justification may be more common, but not that it would be easier. That is a revealing comment because it is generally accepted that very strong reasons are required to justify age or sex discrimination. It indicates that marginal benefits in terms of the legitimate aims will be insufficient.

It is notable that the Act only applies to those aged over 18. Under-18s will not be able to plead age discrimination. This is understandable as a matter of practicality: it will be hard enough dealing with all of the issues relating to adult age discrimination. But, as a matter of principle there is no reason unjustified discrimination on the ground of youth should be regarded as more acceptable than discrimination on the ground of old age.

13.6.5 Duties to promote equality

The Equality Act 2010 establishes a new legal duty on public bodies to have due regard to the need to eliminate discrimination, advance equality of opportunity and foster good relations in the exercise of its functions in relation to eight protected characteristics, including age.

13.6.6 What is wrong with age discrimination?

As the law develops, the courts will need to address in more depth the question of what it is the wrong of age discrimination. Discrimination law is seeking to outlaw the *improper* use of characteristics or groups membership as a factor in making public decisions. It ensures that the reasons used in making such decisions are acceptable ones and do not lead to disadvantage on the basis of the prohibited characteristics.

At the heart of discrimination is the notion of equality. At its most simple, to discriminate against a person is to treat then improperly as not equal to someone else. However, soon the disagreements appear. Equality can be conceived in at least three ways, as follows:

- Equality of treatment. This requires that the same set of rules apply to each person. As we have seen, this can lead to unequal results, but supporters of equality of treatment would argue that the answer to any differences that result in the use of equality of treatment, must be dealt with by other social changes. So if a university's admissions policies were leading to an under-representation of certain racial groups, for example, the answer would not be in changing the admissions requirements, but to improve standards of education for the affected group.
- Equality of outcome. Here the focus is on achieving an equality of result. So, using equality of outcome, the university just discussed would have lower entry requirements for disadvantaged groups to ensure a proportionate representation for each group. That would mean unfairness in one sense (different rules were applied to candidates) but the end result, supporters would say, would be fairer.
- Equality of opportunity. Here the focus is on providing equal opportunities. This does not require either equality of treatment or equality of outcome. Rather the focus is on giving everyone an equal chance to compete for particular benefits.

The arguments that may be used in favour of these different conceptions of equality are beyond the scope of this chapter,[34] but it will be apparent that strikingly different results will be produced depending on which approach is taken.

13.6.7   Applying age discrimination

It is difficult to find examples of overt ageism in the modern day provision of health services.[35] But there are plenty examples of covert age discrimination. Grimley Evans argues that too often in medical practice age is lazily used as the basis of prejudice about the needs and desires of older people. He regards this as unacceptable, arguing:

> Age is a number derived from a birth certificate and cannot be a cause of anything (apart from prejudice). Poorer outcomes from health care interventions, where these are not attributable to poorer treatment, are due to physiological impairments that may or may not be present in a particular individual even if the probability of their presence, where nothing else is known about the individual, rises with his or her age. If one knows enough about the physiological condition of the patient, age should drop off the end of the predictive equation for outcome.[36]

Medical decisions which are in fact based on ageist assumptions are usually presented on the basis of a clinical assessment. Abrams complains that:

> Instead of openly advising patients that economic and societal considerations are the constraint (to dialysis) they [patients] are led to believe a medical decision has been made, assumed (incorrectly) to be in the patient's best interests.[37]

When considering all these negatives, it should not be forgotten that there are ways in the NHS in which older people positively benefit from their age, with the over-60s being offered free prescriptions and eyesight tests.[38]

The Government has announced that it will not seek, as had originally been mooted, to exempt the NHS from the Equality Act, which came fully into force in April 2012.[39] The Care Services Minister, Paul Burstow, has stated:

> There can be no place for arbitrary age discrimination in the NHS. We know that older people are not always treated with the dignity they deserve because of ageist attitudes. Our population is ageing as more of us live longer. The challenge for the NHS is to look beyond a person's date of birth and meet the needs of older people as individuals. By not seeking any exception for the Equality Act, we are sending a clear message that there is no place for age discrimination in the NHS.[40]

However, the Government has made it clear that the new equality law means that:

> Commissioners and providers of NHS and social care services should continue to make sensible, clinically justifiable decisions based on age for relevant services such as eligibility for screening and vaccination programmes that are based on the best evidence available.[41]

Indeed the Government press release explicitly states that in its view clinical decisions based on age will be permitted in relation to the cervical cancer screening programme; NHS Health Checks; seasonal flu vaccination; IVF treatment; and NHS charges.[42] They do, however, list some factors which will be banned:

- making assumptions about whether an older patient should be referred for treatment based solely on their age, rather than on the individual need and fitness level
- not referring certain age groups for a particular treatment or intervention (such as those not of working age) that are considered mainly, but not exclusively for working age adults
- not considering the well-being or dignity of older people.

The Government aims to remove 'harmful' discrimination.[43] This implies an acceptance that some discrimination is non-harmful.

13.7   Capacity, incapacity and old age

It would be quite wrong to assume that with old age comes incapacity, or that incapacity only arises in old age. In fact, 78 per cent of those aged 85 and over have *no* cognitive impairment at all.[44] Nevertheless, for a significant minority of older people issues of mental capacity do arise. The issue is particularly relevant given the rising number of older people who suffer from dementia. It has been estimated that currently 700,000 people in the United Kingdom do, and it is estimated that by 2025 over a million will.[45] One third of those over the age of 95 suffer dementia.

The law governing incapacity has been reformed by the Mental Capacity Act of 2005, which now governs the area. This needs to be read alongside the *Code of Practice*,[46] which provides guidance on the application of the Act. The issues surrounding that Act are covered in Chapter 7 so I will only highlight here some of the key issues, as they may be relevant for older people.

(1)   There is a presumption that people are competent.[47] Therefore in borderline cases where it is unclear if a person has capacity or not, they should be treated as having it.

(2)   Lack of capacity can arise if, even though a person is able to make a decision, they are unable to communicate it.[48]
    A person may be able to consent to some issues but not others. So a person may be able to choose what kind of ice cream they like, but lack the mental abilities to decide whether or not to consent to heart surgery.[49] The general principle is helpfully and accurately encapsulated in the *Code of Practice*: 'An assessment of a person's capacity must be based on their ability to make a specific decision at the time it needs to be made, and not their ability to make decisions in general'.[50]

(3)   A person should not be found to lack capacity unless 'all practical steps to help him' or her reach capacity 'have been taken without success'.[51] This may include giving someone information in simple language or using visual aids.[52]

(4)   Capacity is not just about understanding the information but it is also about using it to make a decision. So a person who understands all the issues but cannot reach a decision (e.g. because they are too nervous) can be treated as incompetent. A person who refuses to believe a piece of information (e.g. they deny they are ill) can be found to lack the understanding necessary to have capacity.

(5)   According to section 1(4), 'A person is not to be treated as unable to make a decision merely because he makes an unwise decision'.[53] The Code of Practice States: 'Everybody has their own values, beliefs, preferences and attitudes. A person should not be assumed to lack the capacity to make a decision just because other people think their decision is unwise. This applies even if family members, friends or healthcare or social care staff are unhappy with a decision.'[54] This is an important point. It is all too easy to assume that a person who makes a decision you regard as foolish must lack capacity. Section 1(4) warns against making this assumption. Notice, however, the use of the word 'merely'. The fact a person is making a bizarre decision may be used along with other information to conclude that a person lacks capacity. This may be particularly where the decision is seen as out of character or puts the individual at a significant risk of harm.[55]

(6)   Section 2(3) warns against making assessment of lack of capacity based on prejudice. It states: 'A lack of capacity cannot be established merely by reference to: (a) a person's age or appearance, or (b) a condition of his, or an aspect of his behaviour, which might lead others to make unjustified assumptions about him.' Particularly relevant for our purposes is the reference to age. All too easily assumption of incapacity are made based on a person's age. This is prohibited by section 2(3).

(7)   Section 8 states that if a person has reasonable grounds for deciding the person lacks capacity, they will be protected from legal action even if in fact the person was not lacking capacity.

If a person is found to have capacity, then they have a complete right to refuse treatment, and this cannot be given to them without their consent. If a person lacks capacity, then decisions can be made on their behalf, based on what is in that person's best interests. Under the MCA, the 'best interests' principle is relevant to all substitute decisions involving 'acts in connection with care and treatment'.[56] This can involve a consideration of the views of family members and of the person's past wishes and feelings, but these all feed into an overall assessment of what is in the person's best interests. Where, for example, a person suffers dementia and has a different character, the weight attached to their past views may be less than the weight attached to their current preferences. Again the detail on this can be found in Chapter 7.

13.8   Elder abuse

The House of Commons Select Committee Report on the abuse of older people in 2004 declared that 'Abuse of older people is a hidden, and often ignored, problem in society.'[57] That report played an important role in galvanising responses to this problem. Increased public awareness of the problem of elder abuse and the political will to try to tackle it has meant that the Government is now taking positive steps to address it.

It is easy to image that elder abuse is just the result of the behaviour of wicked individuals. That ignores the wider societal responsibility for the problem and ignores the more insidious, if less dramatic forms of abuse. Abuse of older people reflects wider societal attitudes towards elder people. Further, the way that society arranges the care of older people enables, and to some sense causes, abusive behaviour. This is not to excuse or justify the abuse, but to argue that given the way care of older people is approached in our society, abuse is a predictable, maybe even inevitable, result. The 'wicked individual' image of elder abuse also overlooks the gendered nature of the abuse: that violent elder abuse is most commonly performed by men against women.

13.8.1   Definition of elder abuse

There is no standard definition of elder abuse.[58] The abuse of older people can take many forms. It can involve sexual abuse, financial abuse, misuse of medication, physical abuse, neglect and humiliating behaviour.[59] It can be carried out by relatives, carers, friends or strangers.

The World Health Organization has adopted the following definition: 'A single or repeated act or lack of appropriate action occurring within any relationship where there is an expectation of trust, which causes harm or distress to an older person'.[60]

There are certainly problems with this definition, but it is useful as a broad basis for discussion. In the UK Government's report *No Secrets* the following definition is used:

> Abuse is a violation of an individual's human and civil rights by any other person or persons. Abuse may consist of a single or repeated acts. It may be physical, verbal, or psychological, it may be an act of neglect or an omission to act, or it may occur when a vulnerable person is persuaded to enter into a financial or sexual transaction to which he or she has not consented, or cannot consent. Abuse can occur in any relationship and may result in significant harm to, or exploitation of, the person subjected to it.[61]

The report lists the following six forms of abuse:

- **physical abuse**, including hitting, slapping, pushing, kicking, misuse of medication, restraint, or inappropriate sanctions;
- **sexual abuse**, including rape and sexual assault or sexual acts to which the vulnerable adult has not consented, could not consent to or was pressured into consenting;
- **psychological abuse**, including emotional abuse, threats of harm or abandonment, deprivation of contact, humiliation, blaming, controlling, intimidation, coercion, harassment, verbal abuse, isolation or withdrawal from services or supportive networks;

- **financial or material abuse**, including theft, fraud, exploitation, pressure in connection with wills, property or inheritance or financial transactions, or the misuse or misappropriation of property, possessions or benefits
- **neglect and acts of omission**, including ignoring medical or physical care needs, failure to provide access to appropriate health, social care or educational services, the withholding of the necessities of life, such as medication, adequate nutrition and heating; and
- **discriminatory abuse**, including racist, sexist, that based on a person's disability, and other forms of harassment, slurs or similar treatment.

13.8.2   Statistics

We now have the benefit of a major recent study of elder abuse carried out for Comic Relief and the Department of Health.[62] This study found that 2.6 per cent of people aged 66 or over who were living in their own private household reported mistreatment[63] involving a family member, close friend or care worker in the past year. If the sample is an accurate reflection of the wider UK older population, it would mean 227,000 people aged over 66 suffering mistreatment in a given year. The figures rise to 4 per cent or 342,400 people, if incidents involving neighbours or acquaintances are included.[64] Three-quarters of those interviewed said that the effect of mistreatment was either serious or very serious. The researchers believed these figures to be on the conservative side, as they did not include care home residents in their survey, and some of those most vulnerable to abuse lacked the capacity to take part. Also, even among those interviewed, there may have been those who, for a variety of reasons, did not wish to disclose abuse.[65] Another UK survey found that a quarter of younger people knew an older person who was suffering neglect or mistreatment.[66]

13.8.3   Sexual abuse

The sexual abuse of older people is a disturbing issue. Sexual abuse in this context can be defined as the non-consensual sexual contact with an older person. This might include a violent sexual attack or the manipulation of a demented person into 'agreeing' to have sexual relations.[67] Little dispute surrounds the violent sexual assault, but less clear are cases where the individual suffers from some level of cognitive impairment. Consider, for example, a patient suffering from Alzheimer's who has virtually no short-term memory, but whose husband, her primary carer, continues to have sexual relations with her. There will be some for whom the issue is straightforward: sexual touching for which there is no active consent is impermissible. If the wife in this scenario is unable to give her consent due to her mental state, her husband may not engage in sexual contact with her. To others this is too strict an approach. Jennifer Hegerty Lingler[68] has argued that in a case like this the issue must be looked at in the context of the relationship between the parties. She argues that where there is no resistance and in the past there was no reluctance to engage in sexual relations, it may be permissible in the context of the relationship between the parties. Not to permit sexual relations causes her concern: 'The oppressive triad of ageism, sexism, and hyper-cognitivism puts women with dementia at risk of an inappropriate blanket condemnation of non-consensual sexual activity.'[69]

In *Re MM (an adult)*[70] Munby J held that the question of capacity to consent to sex depended on the woman 'having sufficient knowledge and understanding . . . of the sexual nature and character – of the act of sexual intercourse, and of the reasonably foreseeable consequences of sexual intercourse'. She must also have 'the capacity to choose whether or not to engage in it . . .'. This test he deliberately set fairly low to ensure that those suffering limited mental impairment were not prevented from enjoying sexual relations. In the case at hand he held, remarkably, that although the young woman lacked the capacity to decide where to live or with whom to have contact, she did have the capacity to consent to sexual relations. The test was developed further in *D Borough Council* v. *AB*,[71] where it was said capacity to consent to sex required an understanding and awareness of the mechanics of the act; that there were health risks involved; and that sex between a man and a woman might result in the woman becoming pregnant.

As courts have indicated the balance to be struck is between protecting a person from abuse and protecting their right to enjoy consensual sexual relations. To properly consider the issue would involve a detailed examination of the philosophical and legal literature on sexual contact and rape. That would take us well outside the scope of the book.

The Royal College of Nursing has produced a helpful guide to this issue: *Older People in Care Homes: Sex, Sexuality and Intimate Relationships*.[72] This provides some practical guidance in this area. They recommend that care home service providers should strive to:

- develop policies which support the rights of all the people who live, visit or work in care the homes;
- offer environments which facilitate individual rights and choices in sexuality expression and intimate relationships;
- offer support and appropriate education for staff in dealing with issues of sexuality, intimate relationships and sex.

13.8.4   Protection of vulnerable adults list

It is extraordinary that before 2000 there was virtually no regulation or control of those working with older people. Julia Neuberger writes:

> We have allowed our most vulnerable older people to be cared for by people to whom we show no respect. We have to do this properly, pay properly, train properly and support properly, the people who do the back-breaking work day after day, without the cost of care becoming prohibitive.[73]

There is now in place a system for the registration and regulation of professional social workers. Since 1 April 2003 such staff have to be accredited with an NVQ level 2 within three years of being registered.

One important limb of the current law protecting older people from abuse is the creation of the Protection of Vulnerable Adults list, which was introduced in July 2004 through the Care Standards Act 2000.[74] This requires employers to check whether an individual is on the list when employing workers or volunteers in regular contact with vulnerable adults. This is in addition to the need to do a Criminal Records Bureau Check.

Employers must refer to the list workers who have been guilty of misconduct that has harmed or put at risk of harm a vulnerable adult.[75] Once on the list, the individual cannot work with vulnerable adults, until their name is removed.

13.8.5 Criminal law

Of course, the standard criminal law applies just as much where the victim is an older person as anyone else. So an incident of elder abuse will often amount to one of the standard criminal offences such as assault or theft. I will here mention some of the criminal offences which are specifically related to older people.

13.8.6 Causing or allowing the death of a child or vulnerable adult

Section 5 of the Domestic Violence, Crime and Victims Act 2004 creates the offence of causing or allowing the death of a child or vulnerable adult. The offence can only be committed against a child or a vulnerable adult.[76] The offence can only be committed by a person who was living in the same household as the victim or had frequent contact with him or her. The offence can be committed in two ways. First, where the defendant did an act or omission which caused the death of the victim. Second, where the defendant 'failed to take such steps as he could reasonably have been expected to take to protect V from the risk' of significant physical harm by the unlawful act of a person living in the same household as V and having frequent contact with V.[77] There is no need for the prosecution to prove in which of these two ways the offence was committed, as long as the jury are convinced it was one or the other. The offence is particularly useful in cases where it is clear that one of two people killed the victim, but it is not clear which one did. The offence also, in effect, puts an obligation on a person living with a vulnerable adult to take steps to protect them from violence from an intimate.

13.8.7 Ill-treatment or neglect of a person lacking capacity

Section 44 of the Mental Capacity Act 2005 states:

(1) Subsection (2) applies if a person ('D') –
  (a) has the care of a person ('P') who lacks, or whom D reasonably believes to lack capacity,

>   (b)   is the donee of a lasting power of attorney, or an enduring power of
>   attorney (within the meaning of Schedule 4), created by P, or
>   (c)   is a deputy appointed by the court for P.
> (2)   D is guilty of an offence if he ill-treats or wilfully neglects P.

This offence is centred around the concept of ill-treatment or neglect.[78] It only applies where the victim lacks capacity. The key aspect of the offence is ill-treatment or wilful neglect. These are not well defined. First, there is the question of what mental element is required. In other words, does the offence require that the defendant intend to ill-treat or neglect the victim? One argument is that the use of the word 'wilful' is placed before 'neglect' and so presumably does not apply to ill-treatment. This might suggest that neglect must be intentional or reckless,[79] whereas ill-treatment only requires proof of negligence.

As to what counts as ill-treatment or neglect, it is notable that in *R* v. *Newington* the Court of Appeal interpreted the terms under the previous legislation as 'conduct by the appellant which could properly be described as ill-treatment irrespective of whether this ill-treatment damaged or threatened to damage the health of the victim.'[80] This indicates that even if there is not an identified 'harm', there may be ill-treatment. So leaving an older person naked in a public place would be ill-treatment, even if a specific harm may be hard to identify. There would be little doubt that inadequate feeding or heating could be covered, again even if no harm could be specified.

13.8.8   Mandatory reporting

It is clear that there is a strong incentive not to report suspected abuse. One survey found that 60 per cent of nurses feared reporting cases of elder abuse in case they had misinterpreted what they had seen.[81] A further 26 per cent said that fear of retaliation would prevent them reporting abuse.[82] Of course, many residents in care homes lack the capacity to make complaints themselves or are frightened of the repercussions if they do. The Government is undertaking con-sultation to see if complaints procedures can be improved.[83]

In part of the USA there are obligations to report cases of elder abuse.[84] In the United Kingdom there are provisions requiring the reporting by professionals of child abuse, but there is no equivalent for elder abuse. Given the human rights obligations on the state to ensure protection of people from serious cases of abuse, it is argued that imposing a mandatory reporting obligation would be desirable.

13.9   The social care and health care distinction

A central aspect of government policy concerning the health of older people is the distinction drawn between social care and health care. In short health care falls under the remit of the National Health Service, while social care falls under the auspices of the social services department of local authorities. The significance of this distinction is far greater than merely the jurisdiction of public bodies. NHS care is provided free of charge, but local authorities are able to charge for social or personal care.[85] The reinforcement of the distinction between health and social care in recent years has meant that services previous offered free under the NHS are now classified as personal care and need to be paid for. The kind of services in question include: washing someone; general personal hygiene; and foot care. As these services are primarily used by older people, this has led to claims that the state's failure to provide free personal care is a form of age discrimination.

Of course, this distinction can be criticised quite readily apart from reference to arguments of age. The point is powerfully made that those who are unable to provide their own personal care are in that position because they are suffering some kind of health problem. Their problems are therefore symptoms, at least, of their ill-health. Indeed, without the personal care they are likely to develop further health problems. So whether the inability to care is seen as an aspect of health promotion or dealing with the consequence of ill-health, the distinction is hard to justify. Indeed, it is hard to avoid the perception that the division has more to do with attempts to cut costs to the state, while holding on to the claim that health services are provided free at the point of delivery, than being one based on a sound policy.[86]

As mentioned, the local authority can require the client to pay as much of the cost of personal services as is reasonable.[87] The distinction thus created between health care services, which are free at the point of delivery, and community care, which is not, is one that is hotly debated. The Health and Social Care Act 2001, section 49 was enacted which provides that nursing care cannot be charged for by a local authority. This is defined as being care given by, or planned and supervised by, a registered nurse, unless it cannot be said to be required for a person. The section states:

(1) Nothing in the enactments relating to the provision of community care services shall authorise or require a local authority, in or in connection with the provision of any such services, to:
    (a) provide for any person, or
    (b) arrange for any person to be provided with, nursing care by a registered nurse.

(2) In this section 'nursing care by a registered nurse' means any services provided by a registered nurse and involving:
    (a) the provision of care, or
    (b) the planning, supervision or delegation of the provision of care, other than any services which, having regard to their nature and the circumstances in which they are provided, do not need to be provided by a registered nurse.

Local authorities' criteria for payment, based partly on this section, have been described as 'confusing and unsettled'.[88] The division between social and health care has led not only to difficulties in relation to payment but also difficulties in integrating the different services. As the Parliamentary Select Committee on Health stated in 1999:

If we were building a new service to provide long term care to vulnerable groups it would seem logical to have a single, integrated community care provider so that service users, their carers and families could move seamlessly between services they may require over time.[89]

In 2005 the same committee reported:

In nearly every inquiry undertaken in recent years, the absence of a unified health and social care structure has been identified as a serious stumbling block to the effective provision of care. The problems relate to structure, financial accountability and, fundamentally, to the distinction between health care, which is mainly free at the point of delivery, and social care, which is means-tested and charged to the individual. The evidence we have received in this inquiry once again indicates that the artificial distinction between health and social care lies at the heart of most of the difficulties that have arisen concerning eligibility for continuing care funding.[90]

One solution to the difficulties that the division has created is the use of a care manager from the health care staff who oversees all aspects of the older person's care.[91] The Government has recognised the problem that the distinction has caused in the provision of services and in their White Paper *Our Health, Our Care, Our Say* accepted that 'at the moment too much primary care is commissioned without integrating with the social care being commissioned by the local authority'.[92] The Government recognised the need to develop models and guidance to encourage joint commissioning and produced a shared framework. Notably, when Government organised a meeting of members of the public to discuss issues surrounding social care in 2007 integrating health and social care was voted as the priority issue.[93]

13.10 Notes and references

1. Department of Health, *National Service Framework for Older People* (London, Department of Health, 2001), p. 6.
2. National Health Service, *The NHS Constitution* (London, NHS, 2010), Principle 1.
3. J. Herring, *Older People in Law and Society* (Oxford, OUP, 2009).
4. S. Ebrahim, The medicalisation of old age. *British Medical Journal*, **324** (2002), p. 861.
5. R. Craig & J. Mindell, *Health Survey for England 2005* (London, Department of Health, 2007).
6. *Ibid.*, at 4.
7. Care Quality Commission, *Dignity and Nutrition for Older People* (London, Care Quality Commission, 2011).
8. Page 3.
9. Page 4–5.
10. Pages 11–12.
11. Alzheimer's Society, *Counting the Cost: Caring for People with Dementia on Hospital Wards* (London, Alzheimer's Society, 2009).
12. Health Service Ombudsman, *Care and Compassion?* (London, The Stationery Office, 2011).
13. At 7.

14. At 1.
15. At 8.
16. At 10.
17. Centre for Policy on Ageing, *Ageism and Age Discrimination in Primary and Community Health Care in the United Kingdom* (London, Centre for Policy on Ageing, 2009).
18. *Ibid*.
19. Page 65
20. Para. 11.2.
21. Department of Health, *Securing Better Mental Health for Older Adults* (London, Department of Health, 2005).
22. Department of Health, *Living Well in Later Life* (London, Department of Health, 2006).
23. J. Beecham, M. Knapp, J.-L. Fernández, P. Huxley, R. Mangalore, P. McCrone, T. Snell, W. Beth & R. Wittenberg, *Age Discrimination in Mental Health Services* (London, PSSRU, 2008).
24. Nursing & Midwifery Council, *Guidance for the Care of Older People* (London, Nursing and Midwifery Council, 2009).
25. At 3.
26. At 5.
27. At 5.
28. At 9.
29. Age Concern, *Submission to the Joint Committee on Human Rights' Inquiry into the Human Rights of Older Persons in Healthcare* (London, Age Concern, 2009), page 9.
30. Section 5.
31. Rutherford (No.2) v. Secretary of State for Trade and Industry [2006] UKHL 19, para, 71.
32. Loxley v. BAE Systems [2008] ICR 1348, para. 36.
33. Palacios de la Villa v. Cortefiel Servicios C-411/05 ECJ, October 16 2007.
34. S. Fredman, The age of equality, In S. Fredman & S. Spencer (eds), *Age as an Equality Issue* (Oxford, Hart, 2003).
35. Age Concern, *Submission to the Joint Committee on Human Rights' Inquiry into the Human Rights of Older Persons in Healthcare* (London, Age Concern, 2009).
36. J. Grimley Evans, Age discrimination: implications of the ageing process, In S. Fredman & S. Spencer (eds), *Age as an Equality Issue* (Oxford, Hart, 2003).
37. F. Abrams, Patient advocate or secret agent? *Journal of American Medical Association*, **256** (1986), p. 1784; D. Brahams, End-stage renal failure: the doctor's duty and the patient's right'. *The Lancet*, **1** (1984), p. 386.
38. J. Robinson, Age equality in health and social care, In S. Fredman & S. Spencer (eds), *Age as an Equality Issue* (Oxford, Hart, 2003).
39. Department of Health, *No more Age Discrimination in the NHS* (London, Department of Health, 2011).
40. *Ibid*.
41. *Ibid*.
42. The Equality Act 2010 contains a statutory exception so that where age-based charging mechanisms are set out in the law, they are exempted from the provisions in the Equality Act.
43. Government Equalities Office, *Equality Act 2010: Banning Age Discrimination in Services, Public Functions and Associations* (London, Government Equalities Office, 2011).
44. T. Poole, *Housing Options for Older People* (London, King's Fund, 2005), p. 2.
45. Alzheimer's Society, *Dementia UK* (London, Alzheimer's Society, 2007), p. 3.
46. Ministry of Justice, *Mental Capacity Act 2005, Code of Practice* (London, The Stationery Office, 2007). (hereafter, Code of Pratice).

47. Mental Capacity Act 2005, section1(2).
48. Mental Capacity Act 2005, section 3(1).
49. *Code of Practice*, Chapter 4.
50. *Code of Practice*, para. 4.4.
51. *Code of Practice*, para. 2.6.
52. Mental Capacity Act 2005, section 2(2).
53. Mental Capacity Act 2005, section 1(4).
54. *Code of Practice*, para. 2.10.
55. *Code of Practice*, para. 2.11.
56. Mental Capacity Act 2005, section 5.
57. House of Commons Health Committee, *Elder Abuse* (London, The Stationery Office, 2004), p. 1.
58. A. Brammer & S. Biggs, Defining elder abuse. *Journal of Social Welfare and Family Law*, **20** (1998), p. 385.
59. House of Commons Health Committee, *Elder Abuse* (London, The Stationery Office, 2004), p. 1.
60. World Health Organisation, *The Toronto Declaration on the Prevention of Elder Abuse* (Geneva, WHO, 2002).
61. Department of Health, *No Secrets* (London, Department of Health, 2000).
62. M. O'Keeffe, A. Hills, M. Doyle, C. McCreadie, S. Scholes, R. Constantine, A. Tinker, J. Manthorpe, S. Biggs & B. Erens, *UK Study of Abuse and Neglect of Older People Prevalence Survey Report* (London, Department of Health, 2008).
63. The report explains (at 3) ' "mistreatment" is used to describe both abuse and neglect. There are four types of abuse: psychological, physical and sexual abuse (sometimes referred to collectively as "interpersonal abuse") and financial abuse.'
64. M. O'Keeffe, A. Hills, M. Doyle, C. McCreadie, S. Scholes, R. Constantine, A. Tinker, J. Manthorpe, S. Biggs & B. Erens, *UK Study of Abuse and Neglect of Older People Prevalence Survey Report* (London, Department of Health, 2008), p. 4.
65. *Ibid.*, para. 7.4.
66. S. Hussein, J. Manthorpe & B. Penhale, Public perceptions of the neglect and mistreatment of older people: findings of a United Kingdom survey. *Ageing and Society*, **27** (2007), p. 919.
67. The Sexual Offences Act 2003 creates a variety of sexual offences which could be applicable including rape, sexual assault and a series of offences protecting those suffering from a mental disorder. They are discussed in, J. Herring, *Criminal Law: Text, Cases and Materials* (Oxford, OUP, 2010), Chapter 8.
68. J. Hegerty Linger, Ethical issues in distinguishing sexual activity from sexual maltreatment among women with dementia. *Journal of Elder Abuse and Neglect*, **15** (2003), p. 85.
69. However, there is no risk in this case that the woman will be subject to criminal proceedings.
70. [2007] EWHC 2003 (Fam), para. 87.
71. [2011] EWHC 101 (Fam).
72. Royal College of Nursing, *Older People in Care Homes: Sex, Sexuality and Intimate Relationships* (London, RCN, 2011).
73. J. Neuberger, *Not Dead Yet* (London, Harper Collins, 2008), p. 231.
74. Department of Health, *Protection of Vulnerable Adults Scheme in England and Wales for Care Homes and Domiciliary Care Agencies, A Practical Guide* (London, DoH, 2004).
75. *Ibid.*
76. 'A person aged 16 or over whose ability to protect himself from violence, abuse or neglect is significantly impaired through physical or mental disability or illness, through old age or otherwise.': section 5(6).

77. Section 5(1)(d).
78. Mental Health Act 1983, section 127. There is an offence to ill-treat or wilfully neglect a patient while they are receiving treatment for a mental disorder.
79. R v. Newington (1990) 91 Cr App R 247.
80. *R v. Newington* (1990) 91 Cr App R 247.
81. BBC News Online, Nurses fear elder abuse errors', 29 August 2007
82. K. Taylor & K. Dodd, Knowledge and attitudes of staff towards adult protection. *Journal of Adult Protection*, **3** (2005), p. 26.
83. Department of Health, *Making Experiences Count* (London, Department of Health, 2008).
84. M. Velick, Mandatory reporting statutes: a necessary yet underutilized response to elder abuse. *Elder Law Journal*, **3** (1995), p. 165.
85. NHS and Community Care Act 1990, section 47.
86. Ibid.
87. Health and Social Services and Social Security Adjudications Act 1983, section 17.
88. C. Newdick, *Who Should We Treat?* (Oxford, OUP, 2005), p. 118.
89. Parliamentary Select Committee on Health, *The Relationship between Health and Social Services* (London, Hansard, 1999).
90. Select Committee on Health, *Sixth Report* (London, Hansard, 2005), at para 24.
91. K. Weiner, J. Hughes, D. Challis & I. Pedersen, Integrating health and social care at the micro level: health care professionals as care managers for older people. *Social Policy and Administration*, **37** (2003), p. 498.
92. Department of Health, *Our Health, Our Care, Our Say* (London, Department of Health, 2006).
93. Department of Health, *Our Health, Our Care, Our Say – One Year On* (London, Department of Health, 2007).

B   Person-Centred Care, Personal Identity and the Interests of People with Dementia

Michael Dunn

Lecturer in Health and Social Care Ethics, The Ethox Centre, Department of Public Health, University of Oxford, Oxford

13.11   Introduction

Person-centred approaches have become a mantra for the delivery of high-quality health, nursing and personal care within UK policy and practice over recent years. Providing care in a way that is attuned to each individual person's wishes, values and needs is recognised as being the most appropriate way of meeting the ethical obligations to respect personal autonomy, to safeguard a person's dignity, and to enhance the well-being of the person. The legal developments that Herring outlines in Chapter 13A contribute to establishing the necessary foundations for these values to be translated into the care provided to all individuals. New statutory frameworks on human rights, equality, anti-discrimination and mental capacity should continue to assist in person-centred approaches becoming entrenched within hospital-based and community-based care settings for older adults.

People with dementia are one group of older adults who frequently receive health and nursing care interventions in hospital and community-based settings. Work on person-centred care in dementia identified four major elements that should guide care practices, as follows:[1]

1. valuing people with dementia and those who care for them
2. treating people as individuals
3. looking at the world from the perspective of the person with dementia
4. a positive social environment in which the person living with dementia can experience relative well-being.

One implication of this broad approach to conceptualising person-centred care has been the widespread agreement among nurses and other health care practitioners that personal autonomy considerations should trump paternalistic reasons to act in ways that will lead to a patient being better off or protected from harm. This ethical judgement means that all decisions made in the health care context should be responsive to the patient's own account of what is good for him/her, rather than being determined by an objective account of medical interests that are imposed in the process of making a decision. It is generally acknowledged, for example, that a person should be permitted to spend the last few days of life in their own homes, if they so desire, rather than being transported into hospital to receive treatment that could extend the length of their lives for a short period of time. However, as Herring discusses, numerous reports reveal how this ethical consensus has failed to lead to widespread improvements in the nursing care provided to older adults. There is clearly some way still to go before patient-centred, rather than task-centred care is infused throughout the health care service.

Notwithstanding the idea that patient-centred care is good care because it espouses clear ethical pathways for care provision (and that this is particularly the case for older adults and those with dementia), working in a patient-centred manner does not imply that philosophical or ethical issues concerning how care should be provided to a person will be eradicated from health and nursing care entirely.[2,3] In this commentary, the focus will be on two distinct challenges that are heightened precisely because of the four elements of person-centred care for people with dementia outlined above. The first challenge concerns the extent to which the onset of dementia impacts on personal identity, and what the implications of changes in personal identity mean for how decisions about the care provided to a person should be made. The second challenge concerns the difficulty in making judgements about a person's interests when there appears to be conflict between the person's previous life values and his/her present feelings.

13.12   Personal identity and dementia

There is a range of evidence that demonstrates that carers of people with dementia struggle to cope with the onset of the condition, and that these difficulties are explained by the cognitive impairments and personality changes that result from the onset of the condition.[4-6] While such changes have transformative impacts on caring relationships, they have also been taken to be evidence for a broader claim about the nature of the personal identity of people with dementia: whether a person with dementia is the same person s/he was before the onset of dementia, or whether the person with dementia is a person at all. Clearly, these debates about the nature of personal identity and personhood in the philosophical literature have profound implications for the possibility of providing person-centred care to people with dementia. How might we make sense of the arguments being made, and their relevance to the care provided to people with dementia? Hughes[7] draws attention to two competing approaches to understanding personal identity. The first approach determines a person's identity in terms of an account of psychological continuity and connectedness over time. The second approach determines a person's identity in terms of the situated, embodied and narrative nature of human existence.

The psychological continuity account of personal identity dominates the literature.[8,9] On this account, what it means to be a person amounts to nothing more than the continuity that exists over time between an individual's memories, intentions, thoughts, beliefs, affective states and dispositions.[7] Personal identity is reduced to the connectedness of an individual's mental states over time. In this sense, the different phases that could be said to define a person's life, differentiated on the basis of psychological changes that manifest themselves as shifts in the person's identity, sense of self, or personality, should in fact be considered as divisions between the lives of *different persons*.[10]

In contrast, the situated-embodied-agent account of personal identity contends that 'the person is best thought of as a human agent, a being of this embodied kind, who acts and interacts in a cultural and historical context in which he or she is embedded'.[7] Here, it is the external context of a person's life understood as lived in relation to other persons in the world that determines the personal identity of that person, rather than the internal continuity of an individual's psychological states over time. This situated account of personhood is often couched in the importance of a life narrative connecting the identity of a person with the rich detail of the existence that this person constructs for him/herself, and that is constructed about that person by other people, over time.[11–13]

Both of these accounts have significant implications for how the person with dementia should be thought about, and how the care practices provided to people with dementia are to be understood as legitimate. On the basis of the psychological continuity account, the changes associated with memory loss, cognitive impairment and personality changes that can accompany dementia imply that the person with dementia could be judged to be a different person from the person that existed before the onset of dementia. Moreover, in the more advanced stages of the condition, it is likely that there will be a complete loss of personal identity, in the sense that the individual only retains rudimentary perceptual or sensory capacities, unable to sustain memories or to exercise cognitive abilities. From the psychological continuity account of personhood, the individual with advanced dementia is no longer a person at all.

Equally, substitute decisions ought not to be made on the basis of the individual's previous values, wishes or beliefs. This is because, in essence, a decision made for one person (the person before the onset of dementia) would be being made on the basis of the wishes and values of a different person (the person after the onset of dementia). The provisions for advance refusals of treatment, and the relevant considerations to be taken into account in determining the best interests of a person with dementia who lacks capacity, under the Mental Capacity Act 2005 would also be rendered illegitimate on the basis of this account of personal identity. As Buchanan[14] puts it, advance directives would operate 'not as vehicles for self-determination, but as sinister devices to subjugate other persons'.

The situated-embodied-agent account of personal identity, on the other hand, implies that the onset of dementia does not impact on the person's personal identity. This is because the person would continue to exist in the same body, still standing in relation to other people giving meaning to the person's life in its broader social and familial context. In this sense, personal identity survives even the cognitive impairments that characterise advanced dementia, with dementia simply being one component of the rich narrative that characterises the trajectory of a person's life.

Accepting the dominant psychological continuity account means being forced to acknowledge that person-centred care for people with dementia is either unjustified, or that the component elements of person-centred care[1] are incongruent. In contrast, the situated-embodied-agent account of personal identity under-girds the elements of person-centred care for people with dementia, and is congruent with the legal and policy foundations that guide health and nursing care decision-making, particularly those outlined under the Mental Capacity Act 2005. Another reason for endorsing the situated-embodied-agent is because, as Hughes[7] argues, it is the account of personal identity that squares most closely with clinical experience, and the one that is likely to garner public acceptance due to its intuitive and common-sense appeal.

13.13   Balancing competing accounts of a person's interests

Even if it is accepted both that personal identity survives the onset of dementia, and that the person with dementia is the same person, the ethical challenge of how to weigh up a person's interests in order to make decisions for that person can arise. This is the case when people with dementia are judged to lack the capacity to make one or more decisions about their own care, and, therefore, that their autonomy cannot be respected in a straightforward way.

A clash between competing accounts of a person's interests can raise signifi-cant, practical dilemmas for nurses and other health and social care practitioners. A number of commentators have drawn attention to the following kind of example to illustrate the issue.[15–17] Mrs A is a 75-year-old woman who has devel-oped dementia and recently moved into a nursing home. Mrs A has been judged to lack the capacity to make decisions about her meal choices, but has been a vegetarian since the age of 14. For breakfast, many of the residents have an English breakfast consisting of bacon. Care staff in the home do not give Mrs A bacon because of her commitment to being a vegetarian. However, Mrs A is attracted by the smell of the bacon, takes a piece of bacon from another resident's plate, and eats it with obvious relish. A member of staff, seeing Mrs A acting in this way, takes the remainder of the piece of bacon from Mrs A's hand and moves the plate of bacon out of her reach. This causes Mrs A to get distressed and to shout out.

Was the staff member correct in acting as she did? No straightforward account of Mrs A's interests can provide the answer to this question. On the one hand, the values that have shaped Mrs A as a person across her entire life would suggest that the action taken was correct; every effort should be made to ensure that Mrs A does not eat meat, regardless of the fact that the onset of dementia has caused her to forget her moral or religious beliefs. On the other hand, Mrs A's current experiences are enhanced by allowing her to eat meat. She gains clear pleasure from doing so, and preventing her from eating meat might, in some situations, cause considerable distress to her.

Moreover, legal and professional guidance offers no assistance in reasoning through such scenarios. Making substitute decisions in a person's best interests under section 4 of the Mental Capacity Act 2005 requires decision-makers to take into account the person's past and present wishes and feelings, and the beliefs and values that would be likely to influence the person's decision if s/he were able to do so. No guidance is given on how to weigh present wishes and feelings against previous beliefs and values when these are in conflict. The values and beliefs that a person has endorsed prior to the onset of incapacity are only accorded primacy over current wishes and feelings if these values and beliefs were endorsed in an advanced decision to refuse treatment. In Chapter 13A, Herring suggests that 'where, for example, a person suffers dementia and has a different character, the weight attached to their past views may be less than the weight attached to their current preferences'. It should be noted, however, that other commentators have argued for the opposing position.

One reason for giving primacy to a person's previous values is derived from the ethical principle of respect for autonomy. If we accept that dementia threatens a person's autonomy because that person will, at some stage, lose the capacity to make one or more specific decisions about his/her care, endorsing the competent choices that the person has made about how they would like to be cared for in the future enables this principle to guide practice to the greatest extent. This is the ethical argument that underpins the validity of advance refusals of treatment under the Mental Capacity Act, and explains why substitute decision-makers must, when making judgements about a person's best interests, refer explicitly to any written statement made by that person when s/he had capacity.

A second reason for giving primacy to a person's previous values emerges out of a morally significant distinction between 'experiential' and 'critical' interests.[18] Experiential interests concern the quality of a person's experiences in terms of his/her state of mind. Experiential interests capture the interest that each person has in maximising the experience of pleasure (and other positive states of mind), and minimising the experience of pain (and other negative states of mind). Critical interests, on the other hand, refer to the interests that a person has in pursuing what that person believes is essential to what a good life would be for him/her. Critical interests are those things that articulate our aspirations in life, recognising, with Dworkin, that 'the place of each decision in a general program or picture of life the agent is creating and constructing, a conception of character and achievement that must be allowed its own distinctive integrity'.[19] This distinction – between individual decisions justified in light of the everyday experiences of a person, and a pathway of connected decisions justified by maintaining the person's integrity over time – leads Dworkin to advance a critical interests-based approach to the decisions made on behalf of people with dementia, particularly those decisions that relate to end-of-life care.

A number of observations follow from this distinction between experiential and critical interests. One observation is that applying the distinction between experiential and critical interests is not straightforward. Mrs A's commitment to vegetarianism might be due to religious beliefs, moral convictions, or due to a personal distaste for the texture of meat. These different kinds of reasons for committing herself to vegetarianism would impact on the status of Mrs A's critical interests, and might allow for her experiential interests to be given overriding weight in determining how care staff ought to act.[17]

A second issue is that prioritising a person's critical interests could also justify making decisions for a person by reference to another person's interests. Consider a situation in which Mrs B, in the early stages of dementia, outlines her preferences for artificial nutrition and hydration (ANH) towards the end of her life. She says that while she would wish to continue to receive ANH if it will keep her alive, the most important thing to her is that her husband is not distressed by any decisions made in the latter stages of her life. She makes it clear that the over-riding consideration for her is that nothing is done to her that would cause distress to the person she loves. On the grounds that Mrs B's relationship with her husband is judged critical to Mrs B's identity and character, prioritising the critical interest of not causing distress to her husband would justify withdrawing ANH from Mrs B when it would both extend her life, and equate with what she would have chosen otherwise.

13.14   Conclusions

This commentary has shown how the onset of dementia can give rise to specific challenges relevant to the practice of everyday care work. These challenges concern questions of personal identity, decision-making capacity, and the determination of a person's interests, and are both theoretical and practical in nature.

While health and nursing care policy and practice has endorsed the values of person-centred care and shared decision-making, asserting a person-centred approach does not act to sidestep the two issues raised, nor can person-centred approaches provide the necessary resources to address these two issues. This is precisely because questions about the nature of the person, and the interests of that person, lie at the heart of the judgements that need to be made. Moreover, the law and professional guidance only go some way to assist practitioners in answering these questions correctly. It is important that nurses and other health care practitioners are aware of the philosophical and ethical challenges posed by the practice of person-centred care for people with dementia, and are able to exercise their judgement in thinking through these issues in light of the considerations identified above.

13.15   References

1. D. Brooker, What is person-centred care in dementia? *Reviews in Clinical Gerontology*, **13** (2004), pp. 215–22.
2. L.M. McClimans, M. Dunn & A.-M. Slowther, Health policy, person-centred care and clinical ethics. *Journal of Evaluation in Clinical Practice*, **17** (2011), pp. 913–9.
3. C. Munthe, L. Sandman & D. Cutas, Person centred care and shared decision making: implications for ethics, public health and research. *Health Care Analysis*, **20** (2012), pp. 231–49.
4. R. Barnes, M. Raskind, M. Scott & C. Murphy, Problems of families caring for Alzheimer patients: use of a support group. *Journal of the American Geriatrics Society*, **29** (1981), pp. 80–5.
5. B. Chenoweth & B. Spencer, Dementia: the experience of family caregivers. *The Gerontologist*, **26** (1986), pp. 267–72.

6. M. Lezak, Living with the characterologically altered brain injured patient. *Journal of Clinical Psychiatry*, **39** (1978), pp. 592–9.

7. J. Hughes, Views of the person with dementia. *Journal of Medical Ethics*, **27** (2001), pp. 86–91.

8. D. Parfit, *Reasons and Persons* (Oxford, OUP, 1984).

9. R. Dresser, Advance directives, self-determination, and personal identity, In C. Hackler, R. Moseley & D.E. Vawter (eds), *Advance Directives in Medicine* (New York, Praeger, 1995).

10. R. Berghmans, Advance directives and dementia. *Annals of the New York Academy of Sciences*, **913** (2000), pp. 105–10.

11. A. MacIntyre, *After Virtue: A study in Moral Theory*, 2nd edn (London, Duckworth, 1985).

12. N. Rhoden, Litigating life and death. *Harvard Law Review*, **102** (1988), pp. 375–446.

13. C. Taylor, *Sources of the Self: The Making of the Modern Identity* (Cambridge, CUP, 1989).

14. A. Buchanan, Advance directives and the personal identity problem. *Philosophy and Public Affairs*, **17** (1988), pp. 277–302.

15. S. Holm, Autonomy, authenticity, or best interest: everyday decision-making and persons with dementia. *Medicine, Health Care, and Philosophy*, **4** (2001), pp. 153–9.

16. T. Hope, A. Slowther & J. Eccles, Best interests, dementia and the Mental Capacity Act (2005). *Journal of Medical Ethics*, **35** (2009), pp. 733–8.

17. T. Hope & J. McMillan, Advance decisions, chronic mental illness, and everyday care. *The Lancet*, **377** (2011), pp. 2076–7.

18. R. Dworkin, *Life's Dominion: An argument about abortion, euthanasia, and individual freedom* (London, Harper Collins, 1993).

19. R. Dworkin, Autonomy and the demented self. *Millbank Quarterly*, **64** (Suppl. 2) (1986), pp. 4–16.

Table of Cases

Note: page numbers with suffix 'n' refer to notes

The following abbreviations are used:

A – Atlantic Reporter (USA)
AC – Law Reports, Appeal Cases
ACC – Administrative Appeals Chamber
All ER – All England Reports
All ER (D) – All England Reports (Digest)
BMLR – Butterworths Medico-Legal Reports
CA – Quebec Official Reports, Court of Appeal
CCLR – Canadian Corporation Law Reporter
CCR – Crown Cases Reserved
Ch – Law Reports, Chancery Division
CLR – Commonwealth Law Reports (Australia)
CLY – Current Law Yearbook
CMLR – Common Market Law Reports
Cr App Rep – Court of Appeal Reports
CSOH – Scotland Court of Session, Outer House (neutral citation)
DLR – Dominion Law Reports (Canada)
ECHR– European Court of Human Rights Series A: Judgments and Decisions
ECJ – European Court of Justice
ECR – European Court Reports

Nursing Law and Ethics, Fourth Edition. Edited by John Tingle and Alan Cribb.
© 2014 by John Wiley & Sons, Ltd. Published 2014 by John Wiley & Sons, Ltd.

ECtHR – European Court of Human Rights
EHRR – European Human Rights Reports
EWCA – England and Wales Court of Appeal (neutral reference)
EWHC – England and Wales High Court (neutral reference)
Fam – Family Division Law Reports
FCR – Family Court Reports
FLR – Family Law Reports
HCA – High Court of Australia (neutral reference)
ICR – Industrial Cases Reports
IRLR– Industrial Relations Law Reports
KB – Law Reports, King's Bench Division
KIR – Knight's Industrial Reports
LR – Law Reports
Lloyds Rep Med – Lloyds List Medical Law Reports
LTL – Lawtel
Med LR – Medical Law Review
NSWLR – New South Wales Law Reports
OR – Ontario Reports
PIQR – Personal Injuries and Quantum Reports
PNLR– Professional Negligence and Liability Reports
QB – Law Reports, Queen's Bench Division
RPC – Reports of Patent, Design and Trademark Cases
UKEAT – United Kingdom Employment Appeal Tribunal (neutral reference)
UKHL – United Kingdom House of Lords (neutral reference)
UKUT – United Kingdom Upper Tribunal
WL – Westlaw Transcripts
WLR – Weekly Law Reports
WWR – Western Weekly Reports

Table of Statutes

Note: page numbers with suffix 'n' refer to notes

Index

Note: page numbers with suffix 'n' refer to notes

Nursing Law and Ethics, Fourth Edition. Edited by John Tingle and Alan Cribb.
© 2014 by John Wiley & Sons, Ltd. Published 2014 by John Wiley & Sons, Ltd.